A Clinical Guide to Anorexia Nervosa

A Clinical Guide to Anorexia Nervosa

Editor: Christopher Schneider

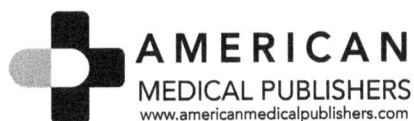

AMERICAN
MEDICAL PUBLISHERS
www.americanmedicalpublishers.com

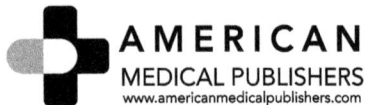

AMERICAN
MEDICAL PUBLISHERS
www.americanmedicalpublishers.com

Cataloging-in-Publication Data

A clinical guide to anorexia nervosa / edited by Christopher Schneider.
   p. cm.
Includes bibliographical references and index.
ISBN 978-1-63927-836-7
1. Anorexia nervosa. 2. Anorexia nervosa--Diagnosis. 3. Anorexia nervosa--Treatment.
4. Psychology, Pathological. 5. Psychiatry. I. Schneider, Christopher.
RC552.A5 C55 2023
616.852 62--dc23

© American Medical Publishers, 2023

American Medical Publishers,
41 Flatbush Avenue,
1st Floor, New York,
NY 11217, USA

ISBN 978-1-63927-836-7 (Hardback)

Contents

Preface

Every book is initially just a concept; it takes months of research and hard work to give it the final shape in which the readers receive it. In its early stages, this book also went through rigorous reviewing. The notable contributions made by experts from across the globe were first molded into patterned chapters and then arranged in a sensibly sequential manner to bring out the best results.

Anorexia nervosa refers to a mental health disorder where a person restricts food intake intentionally due to an intense fear of weight gain. The common symptoms of anorexia nervosa are constipation, hair loss, infertility, brittle nails, dry skin, abnormal heart rhythms, and low blood pressure. It can be caused due to multiple factors, such as genetics, trauma, environment, peer pressure and emotional health. There are several complications associated with this eating disorder including depression, anxiety disorders, borderline personality disorders, obsessive-compulsive disorder and substance use disorders. The diagnosis of anorexia nervosa is comprised of tests such as liver function tests, kidney function tests, urinalysis, bone density tests and complete blood count test. A combination of various methods, such as psychotherapy, medication, nutrition counseling, and hospitalization may be needed for the treatment of anorexia nervosa. This book includes some of the vital pieces of work being conducted across the world, on various topics related to anorexia nervosa. With state-of-the-art inputs by acclaimed experts of this field, it targets students and professionals.

It has been my immense pleasure to be a part of this project and to contribute my years of learning in such a meaningful form. I would like to take this opportunity to thank all the people who have been associated with the completion of this book at any step.

Editor

Lower Pattern Recognition Memory Scores in Anorexia Nervosa

Johanna Keeler[1]* [iD], Ellen Lambert[1], Miriam Olivola[1,2], Judith Owen[1], Jingjing Xia[1], Sandrine Thuret[3,4], Hubertus Himmerich[1], Valentina Cardi[1,5] and Janet Treasure[1]

Abstract

Background: There is extensive evidence for volumetric reductions in the hippocampus in patients with anorexia nervosa (AN), however the impact on function is unclear. Pattern separation and recognition are hippocampus-dependent forms of learning thought to underlie stimulus discrimination.

Methods: The present study used the Mnemonic Similarity Task to investigate pattern separation and recognition for the first time in patients with AN ($N = 46$) and healthy controls ($N = 56$). An Analysis of Covariance examined between-group differences, controlling for age, antidepressant use and method of task delivery (remote vs. in person).

Results: When controlling for covariates, pattern recognition memory scores were lower in the AN group with a medium effect size ($d = 0.51$). In contrast, there was a small effect whereby patients with AN had a greater pattern separation score than controls ($d = 0.34$), albeit this difference was not significant at the $p = 0.05$ threshold ($p = 0.133$). Furthermore, pattern separation and recognition memory abilities were not related to age, body mass index, eating disorder psychopathology or trait anxiety levels.

Conclusions: This preliminary study provides initial evidence for an imbalance in pattern separation and recognition abilities in AN, a hippocampus-dependent cognitive ability. Further studies should endeavour to investigate pattern separation and recognition performance further in AN, as well as investigate other hippocampus-dependent functions.

Keywords: Anorexia nervosa, Pattern separation, Recognition memory, Mnemonic similarity task, Hippocampus

Plain English summary

The hippocampus is an area of the brain that is vital for memory and learning, and it is not understood the extent to which its function is impaired in anorexia nervosa (AN). This paper used the Mnemonic Similarity Task to assess pattern separation, a hippocampus-dependent form of memory, in AN. This task involves showing participants a sequence of objects, who then categorise them as "indoor" or "outdoor" objects. Participants are later shown a

(Continued on next page)

* Correspondence: johanna.keeler@kcl.ac.uk
[1]Section of Eating Disorders, Institute of Psychiatry, Psychology and Neuroscience, King's College London, 103 Denmark Hill, London SE5 8AF, UK
Full list of author information is available at the end of the article

(Continued from previous page)

sequence of objects, although some of the images are replaced by a similar but slightly different image. The task involves recognising whether an image has previously been seen (pattern recognition) and also whether it is similar to, but distinct, from a previous image (i.e. pattern separation). In this study, individuals with AN showed reduced performance in pattern recognition, when statistically controlling for their age, how the task was delivered and their use of antidepressant medication. However, their performance in pattern separation was intact. This may indicate an imbalance in this hippocampus-dependent form of memory in AN.

Keywords: Anorexia nervosa, Pattern separation, Recognition memory, Mnemonic similarity task, Hippocampus

Introduction

Anorexia nervosa (AN) is a serious, complex psychiatric illness, with core characteristics including an avoidance of food, leading to severe dietary restriction and a significantly low body weight [1]. Many patients with AN have an enduring illness, with one study finding only a third recovered at a 9-year follow-up [2]. The protracted starvation impacts adversely on brain function and volume and the chronic state can be treatment resistant and often comorbid with depression (see the Cognitive Interpersonal Model [3];. Treatment resistance in other forms of severe psychiatric illnesses such as Major Depressive Disorder and schizophrenia has been linked to abnormal hippocampal function [4, 5]. In a scoping review, preliminary evidence was found for a reduction in the hippocampal structure in AN [6]. However, there were very few studies that examined hippocampal function in AN.

Adult hippocampal neurogenesis (AHN) is thought to be essential for specific forms of memory and learning processes [7]. AHN pertains to the birth of new neurons from stem cells in the granule layer of the dentate gyrus [8]. Reductions in AHN are associated with reductions in reversal learning and cognitive flexibility [9], both of which are impaired in AN [10, 11]. Reduced AHN in AN has been hypothesised due to aberrations in inflammatory molecules such as brain-derived neurotrophic factor and vascular-endothelial growth factor, which leads to secondary changes in affect and cognition, similar to proposed mechanisms within the depression literature [12–14]. Moreover, evidence from studies on rodents suggests that chronic mild stress [15] and starvation [16] reduces both AHN and hippocampus-dependent forms of learning. Both chronic stress (physiological and psychological) and chronic starvation are features of AN. Concurrently, animal models of AN have indicated preliminary evidence for abnormalities in hippocampal proliferation, which is the initial process towards AHN [17]. These findings raise the possibility that other neurogenesis-dependent functions of the hippocampus that have not yet been investigated, such as pattern separation and recognition, may be impacted in AN.

Pattern separation pertains to the process in which overlapping or similar representations are transformed into separate memory engrams, a crucial aspect of episodic memory. This allows the hippocampus to distinguish between highly similar but distinct representations at the time of encoding and storage. Pattern completion occurs at the time of retrieval, where the hippocampus reinstates the entire stored pattern in the case of a partial or degraded retrieval cue – rather than creating a new memory representation. Intact pattern separation at the time of encoding is vital to ensure distinct memory patterns are stored for their later retrieval. As such, interference after initial pattern separation can affect later recognition performance [18]. There is debate on whether pattern separation and completion are two ends of a unitary process, or whether they are distinct processes reliant on different neural networks [19, 20]. Indeed, individuals with hippocampal damage can be impaired in pattern separation but have preserved recognition performance [21]. The same pattern is often observed in age-related decline [22, 23]. As such, it is now generally thought that pattern separation and completion are distinct processes that are at odds with one another [24].

Age-related decreases in pattern separation have been associated with volumetric reductions in the dentate gyrus subfield of the hippocampus [25]. On the other hand, the cornu ammonis (CA) 3 subfield is thought to be a vital component of pattern recognition performance, which volumetrically is age-independent [25]. People with AN have been shown to have specific reductions in these subfields when controlling for total brain volume [26]. The processes of pattern separation and recognition have been linked to AHN, although there is a paucity of human evidence due to difficulties in directly measuring neurogenesis. However, this is possible in animal models. Cellular studies in rodents indicate that intact pattern separation is thought to link to "new" granule cell neurogenesis in the dentate gyrus, and pattern recognition is facilitated when these newly born cells are integrated into existing networks [27]. Specifically, "old" granule cells in the dentate gyrus may mediate the rapid retrieval of memory engrams from the CA3, thus facilitating pattern completion (i.e. pattern recognition). In many human fMRI studies, the CA3 and dentate gyrus are difficult to distinguish and thus signals are combined to reflect pattern separation, whereas cornu ammonis 1 (CA1) activity, which receives input from the CA3, is thought to reflect pattern completion [28].

Clinically, impaired pattern separation can lead to excessive overgeneralisation, whereby an individual perceives multiple stimuli as similar, even though they are dissimilar [29]. Pattern separation and completion impairments are particularly pronounced in mild cognitive impairment [30] and neurodegenerative diseases such as Alzheimer's disease [22]. Impairments in neurogenesis and hippocampal functioning are thought to be of relevance to a range of psychiatric and developmental disorders. For example, there is empirical evidence for pattern separation disturbances in schizophrenia [31], autism spectrum disorder [32] and depression and anxiety-related psychopathology [33–35]. The transdiagnostic features of psychosocial stress and sleep disturbances may contribute to these problems [36–39].

In animals, calorie restriction has been associated with changes in hippocampal functioning [40–42]. The negative effects of caloric restriction on hippocampal neurogenesis in rodents are particularly pronounced during adolescence [16]. An intermittent calorie-restricted diet used for the treatment of obesity in humans was associated with an increase in pattern separation performance, but a reduction in pattern recognition [43]. However, increases in pattern recognition performance have been found by promoting mastication through prescribing the daily chewing of gum [44]. Furthermore, exercise, especially in adolescents, also increases neurogenesis in animal models [45, 46]. Exercise in human studies has also been shown to increase pattern separation [47]. In summary, whilst caloric restriction and exercise may improve pattern separation, recognition abilities are impaired by restriction and promoted by high levels of mastication. Given that AN is characterised by dietary restriction (and thus lower mastication) and often compulsive exercise, it may be expected that pattern recognition abilities are impaired and pattern separation abilities are increased in this population.

Antidepressant usage has also been found to increase neurogenesis in both human and animal studies. The mechanism is thought to be by reducing hypothalamic-pituitary-adrenal (HPA) axis overactivation and cortisol release and increasing brain-derived neurotrophic factor (BDNF), which plays an important role in nerve growth and development [48]. Indeed, certain antidepressants have also been found to increase neurogenesis in both human and animal studies, and their ability to do so has been deemed relevant for the successful treatment of the psychiatric disorders they are used for [49]. Therefore, we considered the use of antidepressant an important

potential confounding factor influencing neurogenesis- and neuroplasticity-dependent hippocampal functions. There has been little examination of the behavioural effect of antidepressants on pattern separation and recognition abilities in the literature, although it has been suggested as a key avenue for future research (e.g. [50, 51]).

The present experimental study is to our knowledge the first investigation of pattern separation and recognition abilities in AN. From the literature we predicted that people with AN would show a reduction in pattern recognition with an increase in pattern separation. Moreover, we predicted that pattern separation and recognition memory performance would be confounded by variables such as antidepressant usage and age. Finally, we sought to examine the extent to which pattern separation and recognition abilities were related to clinical features such as trait anxiety, illness severity and weight.

Methods
Participants
The clinical group were recruited from the South London and Maudsley NHS trust and from recruitment websites, such as the eating disorder charity BEAT website (www.beateatingdisorders.org.uk). The healthy control group was recruited through the University internal recruitment circular email sent to staff and students. The clinical group included individuals aged between 18 and 60 with a formal or self-reported diagnosis of AN at varying stages of treatment and weight restoration. The healthy control (HC) group included individuals with no history of any mental health condition, including eating disorders, and were not taking psychiatric medication at the time of the study (ages between 18 and 61).

A total of 102 participants took part in this study (46 in the clinical group, 56 in the healthy control group). Previous studies using the mnemonic similarity task in novel populations have found clinically relevant effects with group sizes of 20–30 [30, 43, 52]. A compromise power analysis was conducted using G*Power software in order to assess the statistical power of this study, using effect sizes of varying sizes. Based on a small effect size of $d = 0.2$, a sample of 85 participants (the sample used in the pattern separation main analyses) entered into an ANCOVA model with three covariates yielded an estimated power of 0.58. With a moderate effect size of $d = 0.5$, the same model yielded an estimated power of 0.83.

Informed consent was obtained from all individuals before study participation and participants were reimbursed with a £5 voucher.

Procedure
Participants completed the pattern separation task before the self-report questionnaires. The Mnemonic Similarity Task was used (MST [30];). Participants completed

the task and questionnaires either on a study computer with the researcher present ($N = 55$; AN = 24, HC = 31) or on a personal computer with a stable internet connection ($N = 47$; AN = 22, HC = 25), via a remote version of the task delivered using Inquisit technology [53]. This was due to the COVID-19 pandemic interrupting the ability to conduct face-to-face research.

Measures

Self-report questionnaires: participants provided information in relation to their age, height, weight, current use of psychiatric medication and co-morbidities, ethnicity, clinical treatment status, living status (e.g. living with parents, in own accommodation), and level of educational attainment. We also asked participants questions based on their average sleep duration, specifically "on average how many hours of sleep do you think you get a night?". The Eating Disorder Examination Questionnaire (EDE-Q [54];) was included to assess current ED-related symptomology. The trait subscale of the State-Trait Anxiety Inventory (STAI-T [55];) was included to assess trait anxiety.

Pattern separation task: Participants were given standardised instructions for the task at the beginning of the session, which explained the stages of the task, identified the response keys and finally gave the opportunity for questions. Participants completing the task in person were read instructions from a script, whereas participants administered the task remotely read an identical script. For this latter group of participants, instructions in the second part of the task (recognition phase) were read aloud by an automated male voice. These participants were also not accompanied when completing the task, although they were encouraged to contact a researcher who was available at the time of testing, if they had any questions. Timings of the task are standardised by the Stark Laboratory, facilitating comparisons across datasets. During the initial encoding phase, participants viewed 128 object images on a computer screen. The images were colour photographs of everyday objects on a white background (see [30] for more details). Participants were instructed to classify the images as either "indoor" or "outdoor" objects (based on their opinion), by pressing specific buttons on their keyboard. Participants receiving the task remotely were given practice trials, in order to demonstrate the task procedure, albeit due to technological limitations this was not possible in person. Each image was presented for 2 s, and the inter-stimulus interval was 0.5 s. The encoding phase lasted for 5.3 min in total. After a delay of several minutes, a retrieval phase began. During the retrieval phase, participants viewed 192 object images; one third ($n = 64$) of which were completely new images (foils) one third of which were identical to the images presented in the encoding phase (targets or repeats), and a final third which were similar to the images presented during the encoding phase (lures). Foil, target and lure stimuli were presented randomly. Participants were instructed to classify these images as "new", "old" or "similar items", by pressing specific buttons on their keyboard. Each image was presented for 2 s, and the inter-stimulus interval was 0.5 s. The retrieval phase lasted for 8 min in total. All participants were presented with object stimuli from Sets C or D [30].

As in previous studies (e.g. [30]), the Lure Discrimination Index (LDI) is the main outcome measure. LDI was calculated as the difference between the rate of "similar" responses given to the lure items minus the rate of "similar" responses given to the foil items. A higher LDI reflects better behavioural pattern separation performance. The traditional recognition memory score for repeat items was calculated as the difference between the rate of "old" responses given to repeat items minus the rate of "old" responses given to the foil items. A higher recognition score reflects better general recognition abilities.

Data processing and analysis

Chi-squared tests and t-tests were used to compare demographic characteristics, EDE-Q scores and STAI-T scores between groups. Bonferroni corrections were applied to correct for multiple comparisons on subscales of the EDE-Q, with a significance level p of $(0.05/4) = 0.0125$.

Pattern separation and recognition memory scores were compared using an Analysis of Covariance (ANCOVA), in order to control for the effects of age, method of task delivery and antidepressant use. Age and antidepressant usage were selected as covariates due to the aforementioned findings that pattern separation abilities are known to decline over the lifespan and can theoretically be affected by the use of drugs such as selective serotonin reuptake inhibitors (SSRIs), which increase AHN [51]. Given the differences in procedure between the remote and in-person versions of the MST, method of task delivery was also included as a covariate. Relationships between variables (eating disorder psychopathology, trait anxiety, age, pattern separation and recognition memory scores) per group were assessed using Pearson product-moment correlation coefficients*.

For all analyses, effect sizes were established using Cohen's d and interpreted as small (0.2), medium (0.5) and large (0.8) [56]. A p-value of $<.05$ was interpreted to warrant further investigation. Analyses were conducted in SPSS version 25 (SPSS, Inc., USA, IBM SPSS Statistics for Windows, Version 25.0. Armonk, NY: IBM Corp.). A statistician at King's College London was consulted during the analysis process.

Process for dealing with missing data

Twelve participants did not contribute data to a selection of demographic and clinical variables, some of which were used as a covariate (e.g. antidepressant usage). These variables included: living status, level of education, relationship status, ethnicity, psychiatric comorbidities, medication usage, average sleep, STAI-T, EDE-Q Global Score and all subscales of the EDE-Q. The percentage of missing values varied between 11.7 and 18.4%, with a total of 298 out of 1247 records of these variables (19.3%) being incomplete. Supplementary Table 1 describes the missing data rates of each variable (see Additional file 1).

A Little's missing completely at random test of data patterns revealed that this missingness was not completely at random (MNAR). Furthermore, separate variance t-tests revealed that missing values were significantly correlated with values of one or more variables in the dataset, indicating missingness at random

(MAR). Thus, we performed multiple imputation, using the regression method in SPSS. Five imputed datasets were performed, which were pooled for analyses. All missing variables were also included in the imputation model as predictors, and age was added as an auxiliary variable.

Pooled data using multiple imputation is used in the analysis of demographic and clinical characteristics, as well as in the Pearson product-moment correlations. Due to software limitations, our main analyses could not be performed on the pooled imputed data. As such, we primarily report the ANCOVA models for complete-case analyses. For comparison, we also performed the analysis on each imputed model separately.

Results

Clinical and demographic characteristics

Table 1 describes the clinical and demographic characteristics of the participants in the control and clinical

Table 1 Clinical characteristics and memory scores of the participants by group

	Clinical Group (n = 46)	Healthy Controls (n = 56)	Between-groups difference			
	Mean (SEM)	Mean (SEM)	t	df	p	d
Age (Years)	30.43 (1.44)	26.63 (1.09)	−2.14	100	0.03*	−0.43
Body Mass Index (kg/m²)	15.00 (0.27)	22.07 (0.53)	11.33	100	< 0.001*	2.26
Trait Anxiety (total score)	65.11 (1.93)	39.40 (1.44)	−11.0	100	< 0.001*	−2.19
EDE-Q Global Score	3.97 (0.22)	0.92 (0.09)	−13.17	100	< 0.001*	−2.62
EDE-Q Restraint	3.64 (0.51)	0.57 (0.10)	−6.10	100	**< 0.001***	−1.21
EDE-Q Eating Concern	3.08 (0.26)	0.36 (0.06)	−10.85	100	**< 0.001***	−2.16
EDE-Q Shape Concern	4.65 (0.21)	1.58 (0.15)	−12.46	100	**< 0.001***	−2.48
EDE-Q Weight Concern	4.46 (0.22)	1.22 (0.13)	−12.90	100	**< 0.001***	−2.57
Pattern Separation (LDI)	0.33 (0.03)	0.29 (0.03)	−1.20	100	0.231	−0.24
Recognition Memory	0.74 (0.02)	0.75 (0.02)	0.75	94	0.451	0.09
	N (% of group)	N (% of group)	X² (p-value)			d
Highest level of education			9.18 (0.01)*			0.63
GCSE	**6 (13%)**	3 (5%)				
A-Levels	18 (39%)	10 (18%)				
Higher education	22 (48%)	43 (77%)				
Average sleep duration[†]			30.79 (< 0.001)*			1.32
>8 h	9 (20%)	2 (39%)				
6–7 h	9 (20%)	28 (50%)				
5–6 h	17 (37%)	6 (11%)				
0–5 h	11 (23%)	0 (0%)				
Medication use[†]			44.70 (<.001)*			1.77
Antidepressant	20 (44%)	0 (0%)				
Antipsychotic + Antidepressant	7 (15%)	0 (0%)				

Note. EDE-Q Eating Disorder Examination Questionnaire, *LDI* Lure Discrimination Index, *SEM* standard error of the mean, *p<0.05, [†]The pooled test statistic for this categorical variable was calculated using the median value [57]. For measures with multiple subscales, p-values which remained significant after applying Bonferroni Correction are displayed in bold groups after multiple imputation. Differences in demographic and clinical characteristics were identical when comparing the imputed dataset and the complete-case dataset.

There was one male participant and one participant who identified as non-binary. Participants in the clinical group were older than participants in the control group, were less ethnically diverse (91% AN vs 61% HC being white) and were more educated (see Table 1), but did not differ on any other demographic characteristics such as living status. As expected, participants in the clinical group had a significantly lower body mass index and reported significantly higher levels of eating disorder psychopathology. Participants in the clinical group had significantly different average sleep duration and medication usage.

Within the clinical group, 50% were receiving inpatient treatment, 26% were receiving outpatient treatment and 24% were not receiving any current treatment. Of this group, 24 participants had a confirmed diagnosis of AN (were recruited from within hospitals) and 22 had a self-reported diagnosis of AN. The majority (97%) of participants who reported their weight had a BMI lower than $18.5 \, \text{kg/m}^2$. Furthermore, 32% of participants in the clinical group reported having a comorbid anxiety disorder, 52% reported comorbid depression, 7% a comorbid diagnosis of emotionally unstable personality disorder and 2% "suspected" Autism Spectrum Disorder.

Mnemonic similarity task performance

There were small differences in LDI scores (pattern separation scores) between groups in the pooled t-test analyses, however effect sizes between groups for recognition memory were negligible (see Table 1 for effect sizes). Response proportions for each stimulus and response type are presented in Supplementary Table 2 (see Additional file 1).

Two individual one-way ANCOVAs were conducted using a complete-case analysis, to control for potential confounders of age, antidepressant use and the method of task delivery (i.e. in person vs. remote administration; see Table 2). In this analysis, medication usage was not recorded for 17 participants (HC = 2; AN = 17) thus these participants were excluded from analyses. Scores from seven participants (HC = 6; AN = 1) were identified as outliers in the recognition memory variable and thus were excluded from analyses in order to meet the assumptions of the statistical test. Levene's test and normality checks were carried out following this and assumptions were met for each dependent variable.

In this first ANCOVA there was no significant effect of diagnosis on pattern separation, however the clinical group had higher scores with a small effect size. A separate ANCOVA showed significant differences in recognition memory scores with lower scores in the clinical group. Furthermore, antidepressant usage emerged as a significant covariate in this model. Within the clinical group, participants who reported antidepressant usage had a higher pattern recognition score (M = 0.77, SD = 0.12) than those who were not taking antidepressant (M = 0.68, SD = 0.13) with a medium effect size (Cohen's d = 0.73).

Comparison with pooled multiple imputation analysis

As aforementioned, in other to verify the results of the complete-case ANCOVA, following the imputation of missing data, we performed identical ANCOVAs to above with each of the five imputed datasets. For both ANCOVA models, overall significance and individual covariate significant remained the same across all imputed datasets. This indicates the results are consistent when correcting for missing data.

Correlation analyses for pattern separation outcomes

Results of the Pearson product-moment correlation coefficients per group are presented in Supplementary

Table 2 Mnemonic Similarity Task between-groups ANCOVA controlling for age, antidepressant use and method of mnemonic similarity task delivery

	Clinical Group	Healthy Controls	Between-groups difference			
	Estimated Marginal Mean (SD), N	Estimated Marginal Mean (SD), N	F	df	p	d
Pattern Separation Scores (LDI)	0.36 (0.22), 31	0.28 (0.21), 54	2.22	1,80	0.133	0.34
Effect of Age			1.28	1,80	0.261	0.26
Effect of Antidepressant Use			1.05	1,80	0.309	0.23
Effect of Method of Delivery			1.05	1,80	0.308	0.23
Recognition Memory Scores	0.69 (0.14), 31	0.77 (0.14), 48	4.72	1,74	0.033*	0.51
Effect of Age			0.76	1,74	0.385	0.20
Effect of Antidepressant Use			5.17	1,74	0.026*	0.53
Effect of Method of Delivery			1.23	1,74	0.272	0.26

*Note. SD standard deviation, LDI Lure Discrimination Index, *p < 0.05*

Tables 3 and 4 (see Additional file 1). These analyses were based on pooled data from imputed datasets. Pattern Separation scores were positively associated with recognition memory scores ($p < 0.05$) in the clinical group but not in the control group. Pattern separation and recognition memory scores were not associated with age, body mass index, eating disorder symptoms or trait anxiety ($p > 0.05$) in both the clinical and control groups.

Discussion

The present study was the first investigation of pattern separation and recognition abilities in AN. Recognition memory was significantly lower in the AN group with a medium effect size when controlling for age, medication usage and task delivery. However when using the same covariates, there was a small increase in pattern separation scores albeit this statistically was not significantly different. There was no association of pattern separation or recognition scores with clinical features such as eating disorder psychopathology, BMI and trait anxiety levels.

Our main finding was the lower recognition memory scores specific to the AN group. This profile is similar to the previous findings in people with obesity, who followed a 4-week intermittent calorie restricted diet and showed a reduction in recognition memory [43]. Cellular studies using animal models have indicated that pattern separation is contingent on the birth of "new" adult born granule cells in the dentate gyrus, whereas pattern completion (i.e. recognition) is contingent on the survival and integration of these cells, which become "old" adult born granule cells [27]. Animal models have shown that factors such as dietary restriction reduces the survival of these newly born cells in the ventral dentate gyrus, due to the newly born cells being unstable [42]. This offers a possible explanation for our finding of reduced recognition memory in AN, since dietary restriction is characteristic of the disorder and is detrimental to both the survival of newly born cells in the dentate gyrus and pattern recognition performance. However, it is important to consider the difference of 0.08 (or 8%) in the context of clinical relevance. There are no published normative data for this task, although for a similar age group as in our study [20–39], previous research has indicated an average recognition memory score of approximately 0.80 (80%) in healthy individuals [58], which is generally stable across the lifespan. In populations with mild cognitive impairment (MCI [59];) and Alzheimer's Disease (AD [60];), recognition scores have been estimated at 0.57 (57%). The corrected recognition score for the AN sample used in this study was 0.69 (69%), which lies between estimates for healthy controls and for serious memory disorders such as MCI and AD. It has been suggested that recognition memory measured by the MST is sensitive to CA3 function in the

hippocampus, and thus our findings may be indicative of a subtle CA3 impairment [25]. However, a difference of 8% can be seen as marginal and with limited published data on recognition memory reductions measured by this task, it is difficult to speculate on how this translates to clinical relevance.

Moreover, this study also found that pattern separation and recognition performance was unrelated to clinical features of AN, such as eating disorder psychopathology and BMI. This is incongruent with the literature in depression, whereby depression scores were inversely related to performance on the MST [61]. However, the concept of "neuroprogression" has been recently introduced into the eating disorder literature [3, 62], which pertains to the pathological rewiring of the brain along the course of the illness (see [63] for a detailed overview of the term). This may contribute to impairments in cognitive processes as the illness progresses, partly due to the effects of persistent low weight and dietary restriction on the brain. Therefore, illness duration, as opposed to BMI, may be an important component of neuroprogression to examine in relation to pattern separation and recognition abilities in future research.

Interestingly, these results do not indicate that a tendency to overgeneralise learning exists in AN, as is thought to underlie other psychiatric disorders such as post-traumatic stress disorder [64], depression [65] and anxiety disorder [66]. This is especially pertinent given half of the clinical sample reported comorbid depression. The findings indicate that this sample can actually distinguish between stimuli during the encoding phase well (i.e. separate) but upon retrieval (i.e. completion) are less able to correctly retrieve the distinct representations they had stored. This may indicate an inability to store representations from a previous learning episode and apply this learning later on. Overall, our findings may suggest that an imbalance in this hippocampus-dependent system also exists in AN, albeit different to that observed in depression, which should be investigated further.

Crucially, when controlling for antidepressant usage, previously unseen deficits in pattern recognition performance emerged. Within the clinical group, those taking antidepressant medication also showed a greater pattern recognition performance than those not taking medication. Antidepressants are considered to produce their benefit through increasing hippocampal neurogenesis [9, 67]. Post-mortem studies have shown that individuals with major depressive disorder (MDD) undergoing chronic antidepressant treatment have a larger dentate gyrus than both untreated MDD and healthy controls [68]. They also have greater numbers of neural progenitor cells, which are cells capable of dividing and differentiating, and dividing cells, which become part of the granule layer of the dentate gyrus [68]. Furthermore, anterior hippocampus volume is increased in those with MDD who are receiving antidepressant treatment [69]. As such, it is possible that antidepressant treatment in the clinical sample normalised an imbalance in the hippocampus-dependent system, in this sample.

This study suffers from a number of methodological limitations that should be considered in the interpretation of our results and addressed in further investigation. Firstly, there are key variables known to impact pattern separation abilities that were not measured in this study. We did not have a measure of physical exercise, which has been found to promote pattern separation performance in humans [47]. Thus, the high levels of exercise often seen in AN might be a confounding factor, which should be measured in future studies. Other important factors that were not measured in this study include levels of mastication, which should be addressed in future research through measuring time chewing as well as their current dietary input. Measures of illness or amenorrhea duration, other psychopathologies (e.g. depression and stress) and indices of general cognitive ability (e.g. attention span, general intelligence) were not measured in this study. The AN group was more educated than the HC group in this study, and it is unclear from the literature whether education or IQ are influential on pattern separation and recognition abilities, although education has been found to have an influence on neuropsychological task performance (e.g. [70]). Therefore, these factors may be important confounds or moderators to consider when measuring these specific hippocampal abilities (e.g. [71]). As a result of missing data, a complete-case analysis was used in the primary analyses. However, following a multiple imputation of missing data, results across imputed datasets with a full dataset were consistent with results from the complete-case analyses. Finally, it is possible that the study was underpowered. Post-hoc compromise power analyses were conducted in order to assess the observed statistical power of this study. When assessing an ANCOVA model with three covariates, estimated power based on our observed effect sizes ranged from 0.70 ($d = 0.34$) to 0.82 ($d = 0.51$). Based on these estimations, there is a chance that the detection of effects was limited by our sample size, in the context of the pattern separation analyses. However, when considering these power estimates, it should be emphasised that estimates of power based on observed effects may be analytically misleading and may not reflect true power [72]. Nonetheless, the results from this study will be useful in development of future investigations and for future meta-analyses.

Conclusion

The present study provides preliminary evidence for the presence of lower pattern recognition memory yet intact pattern separation in individuals with AN. Clinically, individuals with AN often show memory lapses, problems with recalling specific details of episodic memories and difficulties in thinking about the future. Individuals with AN in this study were able to distinguish between details well but were also unable to correctly recall details of the stimuli. These findings may shed some light on their difficulties in thinking about the future and imagining recovery, since this requires the ability to flexibly recombine details from past memories [73]. The inability to imagine a future may act as a barrier to recovery and maintaining hope [74].

Further research would benefit from conducting a larger study in order to replicate these findings as well as distinguishing AN groups based on key variables that have strong effects on hippocampal neurogenesis and pattern separation performance (e.g. level of exercise and mastication) when examining pattern separation performance, in order to address potential confounds.

Abbreviations

AHN: Adult hippocampal neurogenesis; AN: Anorexia nervosa; ASD: Autism spectrum disorder; BDNF: Brain-derived neurotrophic factor; CA: Cornu ammonis; EDE-Q: Eating Disorder Examination Questionnaire; HC: Healthy control; HPA: Hypothalamic-pituitary-adrenal; LDI: Lure Discrimination Index; MAR: Missingness at random; MDD: Major depressive disorder; MNAR: Missingness not completely at random; MST: Mnemonic similarity task; SD: Standard deviation; SEM: Standard error of the mean; SSRIs: Selective serotonin reuptake inhibitors; STAI-T: State-Trait Anxiety Inventory – trait

Acknowledgements

V. Cardi, H. Himmerich, E. Lambert, & J. Treasure acknowledge funding from the National Institute for Health Research (NIHR) Biomedical Research Centre at South London and Maudsley NHS Foundation Trust and King's College London. J. Keeler & S. Thuret acknowledge funding from the Medical Research Council. The views expressed are those of the author(s) and not necessarily those of the NIHR or the Department of Health and Social Care.

Authors' contributions

JK, EL, MO, JO, JX, VC and JT have made substantial contributions to conception and design, acquisition of data, analysis or interpretation of data. JK, JT, EL and HH were involved in the drafting of the manuscript which was reviewed by all authors prior to publication. JK agreed to be accountable for all aspects of the work in ensuring that questions related to the accuracy or integrity of any part of the work are appropriately investigated and resolved. The authors read and approved the final manuscript.

Author details

[1]Section of Eating Disorders, Institute of Psychiatry, Psychology and Neuroscience, King's College London, 103 Denmark Hill, London SE5 8AF, UK. [2]Department of Mental Health and Addictions, Azienda Socio-Sanitaria Territoriale di Pavia, Pavia, Italy. [3]Department of Basic and Clinical Neuroscience, Institute of Psychiatry, Psychology and Neuroscience, King's College London, London, UK. [4]Department of Neurology, University Hospital Carl Gustav Carus, Technische Universität Dresden, Dresden, Germany. [5]Department of General Psychology, University of Padova, Padova, Italy.

References

1. American Psychiatric Association A. Diagnostic and statistical manual of mental disorders (DSM-5®): American Psychiatric Pub; 2013.
2. Eddy KT, Tabri N, Thomas JJ, Murray HB, Keshaviah A, Hastings E, et al. Recovery from anorexia nervosa and bulimia nervosa at 22-year follow-up. J Clin Psychiatry. 2017;78(2):184–9. https://doi.org/10.4088/JCP.15m10393.
3. Treasure J, Willmott D, Ambwani S, Cardi V, Clark Bryan D, Rowlands K, et al. Cognitive Interpersonal Model for Anorexia Nervosa Revisited: The Perpetuating Factors that Contribute to the Development of the Severe and Enduring Illness. J Clin Med. 2020;9(3).
4. Macqueen G, Frodl T. The hippocampus in major depression: evidence for the convergence of the bench and bedside in psychiatric research? Mol Psychiatry. 2011;16(3):252–64. https://doi.org/10.1038/mp.2010.80.
5. Huang J, Zhu Y, Fan F, Chen S, Hong Y, Cui Y, et al. Hippocampus and cognitive domain deficits in treatment-resistant schizophrenia: a comparison with matched treatment-responsive patients and healthy controls. Psychiatry Res Neuroimaging. 2020;297:111043. https://doi.org/10.1016/j.pscychresns.2020.111043.
6. Keeler J, Patsalos O, Thuret S, Ehrlich S, Tchanturia K, Himmerich H, et al. Hippocampal volume, function and related molecular activity in anorexia nervosa: a scoping review. Expert Rev Clin Pharmacol. 2020;13(12):1367–87. https://doi.org/10.1080/17512433.2020.1850256.
7. Ryan SM, Nolan YM. Neuroinflammation negatively affects adult hippocampal neurogenesis and cognition: can exercise compensate? Neurosci Biobehav Rev. 2016;61:121–31. https://doi.org/10.1016/j.neubiorev.2015.12.004.
8. Eriksson PS, Perfilieva E, Björk-Eriksson T, Alborn AM, Nordborg C, Peterson DA, et al. Neurogenesis in the adult human hippocampus. Nat Med. 1998;4(11):1313–7. https://doi.org/10.1038/3305.
9. Anacker C, Hen R. Adult hippocampal neurogenesis and cognitive flexibility - linking memory and mood. Nat Rev Neurosci. 2017;18(6):335–46. https://doi.org/10.1038/nrn.2017.45.
10. Brogan A, Hevey D, Pignatti R. Anorexia, bulimia, and obesity: shared decision making deficits on the Iowa gambling task (IGT). J Int Neuropsychol Soc. 2010;16(4):711–5. https://doi.org/10.1017/S1355617710000354.
11. Roberts ME, Tchanturia K, Stahl D, Southgate L, Treasure J. A systematic review and meta-analysis of set-shifting ability in eating disorders. Psychol Med. 2007;37(8):1075–84. https://doi.org/10.1017/S0033291707009877.
12. Dalton B, Bartholdy S, Robinson L, Solmi M, Ibrahim MA, Breen G, et al. A meta-analysis of cytokine concentrations in eating disorders. J Psych Res. 2018;103:252–64. https://doi.org/10.1016/j.jpsychires.2018.06.002.
13. Calabrese F, Rossetti AC, Racagni G, Gass P, Riva MA, Molteni R. Brain-derived neurotrophic factor: A bridge between inflammation and neuroplasticity. Front Cell Neurosci. 2014;8(430).
14. Audet MC, Anisman H. Interplay between pro-inflammatory cytokines and growth factors in depressive illnesses. Front Cell Neurosci. 2013;7(68).
15. Mineur YS, Belzung C, Crusio WE. Functional implications of decreases in neurogenesis following chronic mild stress in mice. Neurosci. 2007;150(2):251–9. https://doi.org/10.1016/j.neuroscience.2007.09.045.
16. Cardoso A, Marrana F, Andrade JP. Caloric restriction in young rats disturbs hippocampal neurogenesis and spatial learning. Neurobiol Learn Mem. 2016;133:214–24. https://doi.org/10.1016/j.nlm.2016.07.013.
17. Barbarich-Marsteller NC, Fornal CA, Takase LF, Bocarsly ME, Arner C, Walsh BT, et al. Activity-based anorexia is associated with reduced hippocampal cell proliferation in adolescent female rats. Behav Brain Res. 2013;236(1):251–7. https://doi.org/10.1016/j.bbr.2012.08.047.
18. Toner CK, Pirogovsky E, Kirwan CB, Gilbert PE. Visual object pattern separation deficits in nondemented older adults. Learn Mem. 2009;16(5):338–42. https://doi.org/10.1101/lm.1315109.
19. Guzowski JF, Knierim JJ, Moser EI. Ensemble dynamics of hippocampal regions CA3 and CA1. Neuron. 2004;44(4):581–4. https://doi.org/10.1016/j.neuron.2004.11.003.
20. Yassa MA, Stark CE. Pattern separation in the hippocampus. Trends Neurosci. 2011;34(10):515–25. https://doi.org/10.1016/j.tins.2011.06.006.
21. Kirwan CB, Hartshorn A, Stark SM, Goodrich-Hunsaker NJ, Hopkins RO, Stark CE. Pattern separation deficits following damage to the hippocampus. Neuropsychologia. 2012;50(10):2408–14. https://doi.org/10.1016/j.neuropsychologia.2012.06.011.
22. Ally BA, Hussey EP, Ko PC, Molitor RJ. Pattern separation and pattern completion in Alzheimer's disease: evidence of rapid forgetting in amnestic mild cognitive impairment. Hippocampus. 2013;23(12):1246–58. https://doi.org/10.1002/hipo.22162.
23. Doxey CR, Kirwan CB. Structural and functional correlates of behavioral pattern separation in the hippocampus and medial temporal lobe. Hippocampus. 2015;25(4):524–33. https://doi.org/10.1002/hipo.22389.
24. Hunsaker MR, Kesner RP. The operation of pattern separation and pattern completion processes associated with different attributes or domains of memory. Neurosci Biobehav Revi. 2013;37(1):36–58. https://doi.org/10.1016/j.neubiorev.2012.09.014.
25. Dillon SE, Tsivos D, Knight M, McCann B, Pennington C, Shiel AI, et al. The impact of ageing reveals distinct roles for human dentate gyrus and CA3 in pattern separation and object recognition memory. Sci Rep. 2017;7(1):14069. https://doi.org/10.1038/s41598-017-13853-8.
26. Myrvang AD, Vangberg TR, Stedal K, Ro O, Endestad T, Rosenvinge JH, et al. Hippocampal subfields in adolescent anorexia nervosa. Psychiatry Res Neuroimaging. 2018;282:24–30. https://doi.org/10.1016/j.pscychresns.2018.10.007.
27. Nakashiba T, Cushman JD, Pelkey KA, Renaudineau S, Buhl DL, McHugh TJ, et al. Young dentate granule cells mediate pattern separation, whereas old granule cells facilitate pattern completion. Cell. 2012;149(1):188–201. https://doi.org/10.1016/j.cell.2012.01.046.
28. Bakker A, Kirwan CB, Miller M, Stark CE. Pattern separation in the human hippocampal CA3 and dentate gyrus. Science. 2008;319(5870):1640–2. https://doi.org/10.1126/science.1152882.
29. Donaldson ZR, Hen R. From psychiatric disorders to animal models: a bidirectional and dimensional approach. Biol Psychiatry. 2015;77(1):15–21. https://doi.org/10.1016/j.biopsych.2014.02.004.
30. Stark SM, Yassa MA, Lacy JW, Stark CE. A task to assess behavioral pattern separation (BPS) in humans: data from healthy aging and mild cognitive impairment. Neuropsychologia. 2013;51(2):2442–9. https://doi.org/10.1016/j.neuropsychologia.2012.12.014.
31. Das T, Ivleva EI, Wagner AD, Stark CE, Tamminga CA. Loss of pattern separation performance in schizophrenia suggests dentate gyrus dysfunction. Schizophr Res. 2014;159(1):193–7. https://doi.org/10.1016/j.schres.2014.05.006.
32. South M, Stephenson KG, Nielson CA, Maisel M, Top DN, Kirwan CB. Overactive pattern separation memory associated with negative emotionality in adults diagnosed with autism Spectrum disorder. J Autism Dev Disord. 2015;45(11):3458–67. https://doi.org/10.1007/s10803-015-2547-x.
33. Lange I, Goossens L, Michielse S, Bakker J, Lissek S, Papalini S, et al. Behavioral pattern separation and its link to the neural mechanisms of fear generalization. Soc Cogn Affect Neurosci. 2017;12(11):1720–9. https://doi.org/10.1093/scan/nsx104.
34. Bernstein EE, McNally RJ. Exploring behavioral pattern separation and risk for emotional disorders. J Anxiety Disord. 2018;59:27–33. https://doi.org/10.1016/j.janxdis.2018.08.006.
35. Sahay A, Hen R. Adult hippocampal neurogenesis in depression. Nat Neurosci. 2007;10(9):1110–5. https://doi.org/10.1038/nn1969.
36. Nitschke JP, Giorgio LM, Zaborowska O, Sheldon S. Acute psychosocial stress during retrieval impairs pattern separation processes on an episodic memory task. Stress. 2020;23(4):437–43. https://doi.org/10.1080/10253890.2020.1724946.
37. Becker S, Macqueen G, Wojtowicz JM. Computational modeling and empirical studies of hippocampal neurogenesis-dependent memory: effects of interference, stress and depression. Brain Res. 2009;1299:45–54. https://doi.org/10.1016/j.brainres.2009.07.095.
38. Doxey CR, Hodges CB, Bodily TA, Muncy NM, Kirwan CB. The effects of sleep on the neural correlates of pattern separation. Hippocampus. 2018;28(2):108–20. https://doi.org/10.1002/hipo.22814.
39. Hairston IS, Little MT, Scanlon MD, Barakat MT, Palmer TD, Sapolsky RM, et al. Sleep restriction suppresses neurogenesis induced by hippocampus-

dependent learning. J Neurophysiol. 2005;94(6):4224–33. https://doi.org/1 0.1152/jn.00218.2005.

40. Rojic-Becker D, Portero-Tresserra M, Marti-Nicolovius M, Vale-Martinez A, Guillazo-Blanch G. Caloric restriction modulates the monoaminergic and glutamatergic systems in the hippocampus, and attenuates age-dependent spatial memory decline. Neurobiol Learn Mem. 2019;166:107107. https://doi. org/10.1016/j.nlm.2019.107107.

41. Dobashi S, Aiba C, Ando D, Kiuchi M, Yamakita M, Koyama K. Caloric restriction suppresses exercise-induced hippocampal BDNF expression in young male rats. J Phys Fit Sports Med. 2018;7(4):239–45. https://doi.org/10. 7600/jpfsm.7.239.

42. Staples MC, Fannon MJ, Mysore KK, Dutta RR, Ongjoco AT, Quach LW, et al. Dietary restriction reduces hippocampal neurogenesis and granule cell neuron density without affecting the density of mossy fibers. Brain Res. 2017;1663:59–65.

43. Kim C, Pinto AM, Bordoli C, Buckner LP, Kaplan PC, Del Arenal IM, et al. Energy Restriction Enhances Adult Hippocampal Neurogenesis-Associated Memory after Four Weeks in an Adult Human Population with Central Obesity; a Randomized Controlled Trial. Nutrients. 2020;12(3).

44. Kim C, Miquel S, Thuret S. A 3-month mastication intervention improves recognition memory. Nutr Healthy Aging. 2019;5(1):33–42. https://doi.org/1 0.3233/NHA-180047.

45. Kozareva DA, Cryan JF, Nolan YM. Born this way: hippocampal neurogenesis across the lifespan. Aging Cell. 2019;18(5):e13007. https://doi.org/10.1111/a cel.13007.

46. O'Leary JD, Hoban AE, Murphy A, O'Leary OF, Cryan JF, Nolan YM. Differential effects of adolescent and adult-initiated exercise on cognition and hippocampal neurogenesis. Hippocampus. 2019;29(4):352–65. https:// doi.org/10.1002/hipo.23032.

47. Suwabe K, Hyodo K, Byun K, Ochi G, Yassa MA, Soya H. Acute moderate exercise improves mnemonic discrimination in young adults. Hippocampus. 2017;27(3):229–34. https://doi.org/10.1002/hipo.22695.

48. Colucci-D'Amato L, Speranza L, Volpicelli F. Neurotrophic Factor BDNF, Physiological functions and therapeutic potential in depression, Neurodegeneration and brain cancer. Int J Mol Sci. 2020;21(20):7777. https:// doi.org/10.3390/ijms21207777.

49. Carli M, Aringhieri S, Kolachalam S, Longoni B, Grenno G, Rossi M, et al. Is adult hippocampal neurogenesis really relevant for the treatment of psychiatric disorders? Curr Neuropharmacol. 2020. https://doi.org/10.2174/1 570159X18666200818194948.

50. Ponzini GT, Steinman SA. Mnemonic discrimination and social anxiety: the role of state anxiety. Cogn Emot. 2020;34(8):1549–60. https://doi.org/10.1 080/02699931.2020.1779039.

51. Tanti A, Belzung C. Hippocampal neurogenesis: a biomarker for depression or antidepressant effects? Methodological considerations and perspectives for future research. Cell Tissue Res. 2013;354(1):203–19. https://doi.org/10.1 007/s00441-013-1612-z.

52. Poch C, Toledano R, García-Morales I, Prieto A, García-Barragán N, Aledo-Serrano Á, et al. Mnemonic discrimination in patients with unilateral mesial temporal lobe epilepsy relates to similarity and number of events stored in memory. Neurobiol Learn Mem. 2020;169:107117.

53. Inquisit. [Computer software]2018; Version 5. Available from: https:// millisecond.com. Accessed 10 Oct 2020.

54. Fairburn CG, Cooper Z, O'Connor M. The eating disorder examination. Int J Eat Disord. 1993;6:1–8.

55. Spielberger CD. State-trait anxiety inventory for adults; 1983.

56. Cohen J. Statistical Power Analysis for the Behavioural Sciences: Routledge; 1988.

57. Eekhout I, Van De Wiel MA, Heymans MW. Methods for significance testing of categorical covariates in logistic regression models after multiple imputation: power and applicability analysis. BMC Med Res Methodol. 2017; 17(1):129. https://doi.org/10.1186/s12874-017-0404-7.

58. Stark SM, Kirwan CB, Stark CE. Mnemonic similarity task: a tool for assessing hippocampal integrity. Trends Cog Sci. 2019;23(11):938–51. https://doi.org/1 0.1016/j.tics.2019.08.003.

59. Bennett IJ, Stark SM, Stark CE. Recognition memory dysfunction relates to hippocampal subfield volume: a study of cognitively Normal and mildly impaired older adults. J Gerontol Series B. 2019;74(7):1132–41. https://doi. org/10.1093/geronb/gbx181

60. Das T, Kim N, McDaniel C, Poston KL. Mnemonic similarity task to study episodic memory in Parkinson's disease. Clin Parkinsonism Relat Disord. 2020;3:100062. https://doi.org/10.1016/j.prdoa.2020.100062.

61. Shelton DJ, Kirwan CB. A possible negative influence of depression on the ability to overcome memory interference. Behav Brain Res. 2013;256:20–6. https://doi.org/10.1016/j.bbr.2013.08.016.

62. Treasure J, Stein D, Maguire S. Has the time come for a staging model to map the course of eating disorders from high risk to severe enduring illness? An examination of the evidence. Early Interv Psychiatry. 2015;9(3): 173–84. https://doi.org/10.1111/eip.12170.

63. Halaris A, Leonard BE. Unraveling the complex interplay of immunometabolic systems that contribute to the neuroprogression of psychiatric disorders. Neurol Psychiatry Brain Res. 2019;32:111–21. https:// doi.org/10.1016/j.npbr.2019.05.005.

64. Bernstein EE, Brühl A, Kley H, Heinrichs N, McNally RJ. Mnemonic discrimination in treatment-seeking adults with and without PTSD. Behav Res Ther. 2020;131:103650. https://doi.org/10.1016/j.brat.2020.103650.

65. Gandy K, Kim S, Sharp C, Dindo L, Maletic-Savatic M, Calarge C. Pattern separation: a potential marker of impaired hippocampal adult neurogenesis in major depressive disorder. Front Neurosci. 2017;11:571. https://doi.org/1 0.3389/fnins.2017.00571.

66. Kheirbek MA, Klemenhagen KC, Sahay A, Hen R. Neurogenesis and generalization: a new approach to stratify and treat anxiety disorders. Nat Neurosci. 2012;15(12):1613–20. https://doi.org/10.1038/nn.3262.

67. Levone BR, Cryan JF, O'Leary OF. Role of adult hippocampal neurogenesis in stress resilience. Neurobiol Stress. 2015;1:147–55. https://doi.org/10.1016/j. ynstr.2014.11.003.

68. Boldrini M, Underwood MD, Hen R, Rosoklija GB, Dwork AJ, Mann JJ, et al. Antidepressants increase neural progenitor cells in the human hippocampus. Neuropsychopharmacol. 2009;34(11):2376–89. https://doi. org/10.1038/npp.2009.75.

69. Boldrini M, Santiago AN, Hen R, Dwork AJ, Rosoklija GB, Tamir H, et al. Hippocampal granule neuron number and dentate gyrus volume in antidepressant-treated and untreated major depression. Neuropsychopharmacol. 2013;38(6):1068–77. https://doi.org/10.1038/npp.2 013.5.

70. Tripathi R, Kumar K, Bharath S, Marimuthu P, Varghese M. Age, education and gender effects on neuropsychological functions in healthy Indian older adults. Dementia Neuropsychol. 2014;8(2):148–54. https://doi.org/10.1590/S1 980-57642014DN82000010.

71. McGaugh JL, Introini-Collison IB, Cahill LF, Castellano C, Dalmaz C, Parent MB, et al. Neuromodulatory systems and memory storage: role of the amygdala. Behav Brain Res. 1993;58(1–2):81–90. https://doi.org/10.1016/01 66-4328(93)90092-5.

72. Zhang Y, Hedo R, Rivera A, Rull R, Richardson S, Tu XM. Post hoc power analysis: is it an informative and meaningful analysis? Gen Psychiatry. 2019; 32(4).

73. Schacter DL, Addis DR. The cognitive neuroscience of constructive memory: remembering the past and imagining the future. Philos Trans R Soc Lond Ser B Biol Sci. 2007;362(1481):773–86. https://doi.org/10.1098/rstb.2007.2087.

74. Fogarty S, Ramjan LM. Factors impacting treatment and recovery in anorexia nervosa: qualitative findings from an online questionnaire. J Eat Disord. 2016;4:1–9.

2

The Transition Process Between Child and Adolescent Mental Services and Adult Mental Health Services for Patients with Anorexia Nervosa: a Qualitative Study of the Parents' Experiences

Veronica Lockertsen[1,2]* ⓘ, Lill Ann Wellhaven Holm[3], Liv Nilsen[1], Øyvind Rø[2,4], Linn May Burger[5] and Jan Ivar Røssberg[1,2]

Abstract

Background: Patients with Anorexia Nervosa (AN) often experience the transition between Child and Adolescent Mental Health Services (CAMHS) and Adult Mental Health Services (AMHS) as challenging. This period tends to have a negative influence on the continuity of care for the adolescents and represents a demanding and difficult period for the parents. To our knowledge, no previous study has explored the parents' experience with the transition from CAMHS to AMHS. Therefore, this qualitative study examines how parents experience the transition process from CAMHS to AMHS.

Methods: In collaboration with a service user with carer experience, qualitative interviews were conducted with 10 parents who had experienced the transition from CAMHS to AMHS, some from outpatient care and others from both in- and outpatient mental care units in Norway. All had some experience with specialized eating disorder units. The interviews were analyzed with a Systematic Text Condensation (STC) approach. Service users' perspectives were involved in all steps of the research process.

Results: Six categories represent the parents' experiences of the transition: (1) the discharge when the child turns 18 years old is sudden; (2) the lack of continuity is often followed by deterioration and relapses in the patient; (3) the lack of involvement and information causes distress; (4) knowledge – an important factor for developing a trusting relationship between parents` and clinicians`; (5) parents have overwhelming multifaceted responsibilities; and (6) parents need professional support.

(Continued on next page)

* Correspondence: v.lockertsen@gmail.com
[1]Division of Mental Health and Addiction, Oslo University Hospital, P.O. Box 4959, Nydalen, Oslo, Norway
[2]Institute of Clinical Medicine, Faculty of Medicine, University of Oslo, 0318 Oslo, Norway
Full list of author information is available at the end of the article

(Continued from previous page)

Conclusion: Improving the transition by including parents and adolescents and preparing them for the transition period could ease parental caregiving distress and improve adolescents' compliance with treatment. Clinicians should increase their focus on the important role of parents in the transition process. The system should implement routines and guidelines to offer caregivers support and guidance during the transition process.

Keywords: Anorexia nervosa, Mental health transition, Adolescent, Carers, Parents' perspective, Caregivers' perspective, Qualitative research, Service user's perspective

Plain English summary

Adolescents with anorexia nervosa (AN) who receive care from Child and Adolescent Mental Health Services (CAMHS) often need further treatment from Adult Mental Health Services (AHMS). This study explores the transition between CAMHS and AHMS for parents of adolescents with AN in a naturalistic public mental health-care setting. Our study identified six themes concerning the transition between CAMHS and AMHS, based on parents' experiences of the process and what they considered influenced the transition. In general, parents and patients are both unprepared for the sudden discharge from CAMHS when the patient turns 18 years old. The transition is often characterized by a lack of continuity, leading to deterioration and relapses among patients. The lack of involvement and information parents experience in the transition causes distress, and parents have overwhelming multifaceted responsibilities in the transition period. Parents view knowledge to be the key to a successful transition, and they are stressed and need support in the transition.

Keywords: Anorexia nervosa, Mental health transition, Adolescent, Carers, Parents' perspective, Caregivers' perspective, Qualitative research, Service user's perspective

Introduction

Treatment guidelines recommend family interventions for adolescents with Anorexia Nervosa (AN) [1, 2]. Parents are often involved in the care while the adolescent AN patient is treated by Child and Adolescent Mental Health Services (CAMHS), but their role decreases when transitioning to Adult Mental Health Services (AMHS) [3]. The average onset for AN is the mid-teens, with an average duration of 6 years [4]. Thus, many patients are treated by both CAMHS and AMHS [5].

The development of AN is caused by a complex interplay of biological, psychological, social, developmental, and cultural factors. AN can manifest in a variety of ways, but often patients are ambivalent about treatment and do not regard themselves as ill [1, 6]. This ambivalence with treatment and fluctuating motivation for recovery creates additional challenges in the management of a successful transition.

Blum [7] defined an optimal transition as a purposeful, planned process that addresses the medical, psychosocial, and educational/vocational needs of adolescents. Many mental health-care systems fail to complete a seamless transition, mostly because of the lack of good cooperation between the services and different treatment philosophies [4, 8]. Four features of optimal transition have been identified: Information transfer, a period of parallel care, transition planning, and continuity of care [9]. Singh et. al studied transitions in an UK context involving six mental health trusts. They found that the majority of service users experience the transition as poorly planned, poorly executed, and poorly experienced [9, 10]. Studies show that only 4–13% of patients with a mental health disorder experience a satisfactory transition [11]. One of the most critical factors for a successful transition is preparation. Preparation implies acknowledging how important the therapeutic relationship in CAMHS can be in the adolescents' lives, and how leaving a secure relationship influences how the new relationship is established in AMHS [12–15].

Parents have an important caregiving role in treating patients suffering from AN, but their role changes when entering AMHS. In CAMHS, parents are used to having responsibility for the patients when it comes to both meal support and weight restoration. However, AMHS places the responsibility on the patient [3]. The different treatment approaches often create a barrier in the transition, as both patient and parents are often unprepared, and the changes are not made explicit. When parents experience themselves as being less involved in the treatment of AMHS, it can increase their feelings of loss and fear and lead to a sense of powerlessness [4, 8, 16]. Patients with AN often have disabilities that make them rely on their parents for emotional and financial support, even though they are emerging into adulthood [17]. Therefore, the transition should be guided by an individual transition plan that considers the need for the individual to practice self-sufficiency and family involvement [9, 18].

The emotional impact of caring for an individual with mental health problems is well established (Baronet, 1999). Parents of patients with AN appear to have poorer mental wellbeing than parents of other conditions [19]. Kyriacou, Treasure [20] found that more than 50% of parents with AN scored above the clinical threshold for anxiety, and 13% scored above the clinical threshold for depression. To decrease their own distress and increase involvement in the treatment of their adolescent, the parents expressed a need for information and support from the services [21, 22]. Without support, there is an increased risk of developing maladaptive coping strategies in their interactions with adolescents. To avoid conflict, parents can often develop family routines that in fact contribute to the adolescent maintaining their AN symptoms [23, 24].

Parents play an essential role in the transition period. However, to our knowledge, no previous studies have explored the parents' experiences of the transition from CAMHS to AMHS for patients with AN. Greater knowledge about how parents experience the transition process and the factors they experience as barriers to a more satisfactory transition for the patient might improve the transition process. This knowledge can also provide us with important information about what the parents need during the transition period to provide support for adolescents with AN. The main aim of this qualitative study was to examine how parents experience the transition process from CAMHS to AMHS.

Methods

Design

The present study is part of a service user-initiated qualitative research project focusing on the transition from CAMHS to AMHS for patients [14], professionals [24], and parents. The project is inspired by how the theme of challenging transitions to AMHS appeared repetitively in support groups for parents with children suffering from eating disorders. A parent with service use experience (LAWH) participated in the design of a semi-structured interview guide and moderated the interview in collaboration with the first author (VL). The research group also included a former service user (LMB) with patient experience, RN nurses (LN, VL), and psychiatrists (JIR and ØR).

Recruitment and participants

The study recruited 12 participants, three fathers and nine mothers, through snowball sampling methods. Eight of the participants were individual parents and four were couples; thus, the transitions of 10 adolescents were discussed. Three of the participants were invited to participate by their adolescents' therapists, who contacted participants they knew had experiences that could illuminate the research questions. The others made contact with the project manager after finding project information on an internet support site for eating disorders. None of the parents had relations to the patients included in a previous study [14]. The adolescents were aged 15, on average, when they first contacted the CAMHS. All parents had experience with the transition from CAMHS to AMHS. All but two of the adolescents had experience with in-patient treatment, and all had some experience with specialized eating disorder units. All parents had the main care of the adolescent while transitioning; one had received assistance from child welfare services until the transition. Three of the parents were separated and had the main responsibility for the adolescent during the transition. All transitions occurred the year their adolescents turned 18. The average time from transition to the qualitative interview was 4.5 years. Recruitment to the study took place between September 2018 and December 2019 in Norway. Written consent was obtained from all participants.

Data collection

In-depth, semi-structured interviews, guided by a thematic interview guide, were conducted by the first (VL) and the second (LAWH) authors. The interviews lasted between 60 and 90 min and were conducted in adapted settings chosen by the participants. The interviews were guided by our research question, which was to explore parents' experiences of parenting an adolescent with AN in the transition from CAMHS to AMHS. The participants were encouraged to describe their experience with the transition through specific examples. The questions focused on factors that influenced the transition process, regarding the treatment systems, the therapists, themselves, and their adolescents. Throughout the interview, we restated and summarized our understanding to validate our interpretations of their narratives. The first author audio-recorded and transcribed the interviews verbatim.

Qualitative data analysis

Data were analyzed using a systematic text condensation (STC) inspired by Giorgi [25, 26]. STC is an elaboration of Giorgi's principles, and the method focused on presenting the parents' expressed experiences, rather than a possible underlying interpretation of meaning. STC is a descriptive approach, presenting the participants' experience as expressed by themselves. However, STC shares the underlying theoretical foundations of social constructionism and has in this study been used more dynamically than the procedure may imply. By decontextualization and re-contextualization of the text, we analytically reduced the data and created a condensed text that represented the overall material [25]. Using STC, the moderators of interviews were considered co-producers of the data, and together with the participants, affected the interview process. STC comprises four main steps, where the end goal is to have a condensed text representing the validity and wholeness of the original context. Three of the authors listened and read the interviews several times, focusing on the parents' experiences with the transition between CAMHS and AMHS. Our research question developed dynamically as the research process influenced our understanding of the parents' experiences. After forming an overall impression of the material, texts that belonged together were grouped and encoded. By decontextualizing selections of meaning content from the created codes, we were able to reveal various aspects of the parents' experiences. This systematic way of renaming codes and processing the material was constantly conducted with the authenticity of the interviews in mind. Finally, our analysis revealed six themes that represented the answer to our research question. We used NVivo 11 to help organize and categorize the transcriptions (QSR International Pty Ltd.).

Results

Six categories describe the parents' experiences during the transition: (1) the discharge when the child turns 18 years old is sudden; (2) the lack of continuity is often followed by deterioration and relapses in the patient; (3) the lack of involvement and information causes distress for the parents; (4) parents have overwhelming multifaceted responsibilities in the transition; (5) knowledge is the key to a successful transition; and (6) parents are stressed and need support. The following paragraphs discuss each category in greater detail.

Sudden discharge from CAMHS at 18

The parents described the transition from CAMHS to AMHS as an abrupt end to treatment that is defined by age rather than a process. The parents were told that AMHS was responsible for the treatment when the patients turned 18 years old and that a transition phase with parallel care was impossible. The parents experienced stress, as they were unsure of how to proceed in the treatment system when their son/daughter was suddenly discharged from CAMHS. The parents felt powerless, with the sense that they had nothing to say, and they described the feeling of being left out of what was happening with their adolescent in AMHS.

The worst thing about the transition process is how she was discharged from outpatient care on her 18th birthday without any form of follow-up. She was all alone, and we, as parents, were not included or notified.

The parents expressed concern about the transition from CAMHS that was processed without consideration of the adolescents' capabilities or maturity.

I understand that the system must have limits, but she was treated like an adult from the first meeting between CAMHS and AMHS. When you are 18, you are not an adult. So, it should have been a transitional phase.

She met the CAMHS-therapist on Friday, turned 18 on Sunday—the following Monday she met with AMHS. She had been warned about how the transition was regulated by the calendar, but she was totally caught off guard.

One of the parents experienced that CAMHS wanted to continue treatment for a period, but the adolescent wanted to transfer to AMHS for a fresh start. To their surprise, CAMHS just let the adolescent go, without any contact information or help to transfer to AMHS.

She was all alone, and we, as parents, were not included or notified. There was a sharp separation between CAMHS and AMHS. CAMHS would not give us any assistance. They could at least have recommended someone or connected us with the outpatient clinic in AMHS.

Lack of continuity is often followed by deterioration and relapses

The parents frequently described the transition as going in circles between services, hospitalizations, and meetings with their primary care provider (PCP). For the parents, the transition period implied having to wait for adequate treatment, handle unstable adolescents, and face uncertainties about future treatment. This situation was described as a negative circle, putting the responsibility of the adolescent's health in the hands of the PCP and the parents and highlighting the important role continuity of treatment plays in the transition.

It is such a negative circle. Our PCP referred us to AMHS. It takes about 6 weeks to get an appointment at the outpatient clinic. Soon after the first meeting with our daughter, the therapist was going on vacation and she was left without a therapist. Soon after the vacation, the therapist went on paternity leave and our daughter was discharged without further consideration. Suddenly, once again, her PCP was her only therapist. This circle is not unique.

The parents described how their adolescents' health often deteriorated in waiting periods, with some patients being admitted to an acute psychiatric ward. Both the waiting time and the admission to the acute ward were difficult for the parents. The waiting time represented a period of feeling frightened and solely responsible for their adolescent. However, they found that the acute psychiatric ward was not attuned to their adolescent's needs and challenges, and they found it difficult leaving them in what they felt was an inhumane environment.

During the transition period, much of the parents' time was spent searching for adequate treatment facilities. The criteria for receiving treatment from AMHS were considered strict and focused mostly on the adolescent's BMI.

> How thin must one become to receive treatment? Actually, she lost weight just to meet their BMI criteria.

The parents described how their adolescent's ambivalence toward treatment created high levels of frustration during the transition period. The patients often dropped out of treatment, and the parents felt they were left responsible and followed up more closely as they were afraid of the consequences. How adolescents would become responsible for their own health without continuous professional support or preparation was of significant concern for the parents.

Although they considered it natural and important that their adolescents had something to say about treatment, they wanted the clinician to acknowledge the role patients' ambivalence plays in treating adolescents with AN and the impact it has on their self-sufficiency. They had experienced that their adolescent's disease made them make decisions they, in their parents' eyes, should not take.

> She refused potassium supplements because in her mind, she gained weight. That was more important than surviving. As she had turned 18, they gave her that choice and handed her a paper to sign, confirming she was familiar with the consequences of refusing treatment with a potentially fatal outcome.

Lack of involvement and information causes parental distress

The parents experienced a change in their role as caregivers when their adolescents started receiving treatment from AMHS. Despite still being responsible for the adolescent, after transferring to AMHS, there was a difference in their inclusion in the treatment and in the amount of information they received. The parents described how the lack of information made life at home difficult. They described a need for more guidance and knowledge about how to interact with their son/daughter.

> I understand that some things are confidential, but I literally got nothing and had to handle it on my own. With more information, I could have understood how serious it was, sooner.

Access to information was a topic already present in CAMHS, as the duty of confidentiality is set at age 16. Nevertheless, some describe a sudden change in their adolescents' attitudes to accessing AMHS. The parents experienced that the emphasis of AMHS on the individual's independence and self-sufficiency influenced the adolescents' attitudes. Parents that earlier had good cooperation with their adolescent and thereby access to information suddenly lost their overview of the situation.

> I felt, since it came so suddenly after transitioning, almost from 1 day to the next—it must have been the influence AMHS had. The idea of when you are 18, you are more responsible for your own life.

This sudden change in attitudes toward their involvement made the transition challenging for the parents. They often experienced that the amount of information they received and their cooperation with the adolescent were dependent on the adolescent's somewhat fluctuating state of disease. An easier flow of information to and from parents could benefit the transition. They questioned why their experience and knowledge were not requested by the health-care services, as in their view, it would make it easier for the clinician to understand the adolescent. Often, the adolescents found it straining to connect with a new clinician; thus, a more involved parents' role would be a positive bridging factor.

> I tried to speak with the doctors, but they looked at me like I was a nuisance. And as we did not receive any information, we kind of lost a way to understand her, so we felt very insecure and scared. They did not even let us know when she had escaped from the unit!

Knowledge – an important factor for developing a trusting relationship between parents and clinician's

The parents described how a successful transition often relied on trust in the clinician's competence with eating disorders. The adolescents tended to lose motivation for treatment and had difficulties in the therapeutic relationship when they sensed that the clinician knew less about eating disorders than they did themselves.

Developing trust was difficult, as N is really smart and has much knowledge about her own disease. She pulled him up on misinformation and then believed that he did not have the necessary competence.

During the transition, the parents experienced meetings with clinicians who seemingly lacked knowledge about what their caregiving role implied. Some parents described being met with a distrustful attitude, as they sensed that the professionals found it difficult to assess and trust their narrative. While some meetings in the transition increased their confidence and decreased their distress concerning their role as parents, others described how clinicians had increased their feelings of shame and lack of confidence in how they handled their situation. Consequently, their room for manoeuvre shrank during the transition period, and they felt lost.

There is no understanding of the parents' situation. Everywhere else I have been has confirmed that my reaction was normal to an abnormal situation. But it ruined me.

When met by experienced clinicians who embraced their situation and recognized their reactions, they felt calmer and had greater acceptance of their reactions. Health services ignoring the parents' knowledge and expertise in the transition was also of symbolic value to some parents. They used it as an example of what they perceived as professionals' tendency to focus on the somatic symptoms of the eating disorder, while overlooking the multidetermined aspects that their involvement could represent. They described how the adolescents were admitted and gained weight, but there was no psychological insight or motivation to maintain their weight. Nevertheless, they were discharged despite their parents' advice. This contributed negatively to a very unstable time, and from the parents' perspectives, many unnecessary transitions.

She [our child] said to us: When I am there, I just feel like a gigantic eating disorder. I am nothing else. She did not feel seen as a person, just a weight. And I understood her.

Overwhelming multifaceted responsibilities

The parents were overwhelmed by the many roles and their multifaceted responsibilities during the transition period. In addition to facilitating the transition for the adolescent and adapting to their needs, they had responsibilities toward other children, their work, and their own lives, yet they had difficulty meeting their other obligations. These ancillary pressures make the transition

period challenging. They describe the period as lonely and wearing. Their responsibilities for facilitating the treatment were time-consuming. They described their days as being mostly occupied with preparing food, offering meal support, following up after meals, and driving the adolescents to treatment appointments. As their adolescents often lacked the motivation or ability to administer their contact with different caring facilities, they obtained a coordination role for their adolescent. They emphasized how their adolescent still needed the same support from them as when they were underage. Meals were often followed with anxiety for the adolescent, parents, and other family members. The preparations and routines surrounding meals were adapted specifically around the patient and not for other family members. The parents expressed concern for their other children, as their adolescent with AN would often direct their strong emotions and aggression at them.

A mother's heart bleeds when I see how she treats her sister, but what can I do?

Since their lives were adapted to helping and looking after their adolescents, they relied on flexible jobs. Some described concerns about income, as they had increased expenses due to the need to purchase different foods and treatments. As their adolescents were often in-between treatment facilities, they felt as if they had to stay home and look after them, as they tended to be physically and mentally unstable. For the parents, this situation created stress as they were reliant on others being flexible on their behalf, which created insecure living conditions. They were left with no choice but to try to be with their adolescent and provide them with the security they needed. The transition period was thereby characterized by a lot of emotions, fear, and frustration. Some described difficulties sleeping and increased mental health problems. Nevertheless, as they had no choice, they had to endure.

I just did it. Had no choice really. That is the problem. And kids are your kids until they do not need you anymore. So, we have followed her very closely, but I think this is something all parents do.

Parents are in need of professional support

The parents described how they always had to be on guard, available, and prepared during the transition period, and they were therefore in need of support from the mental health care services. Some parents felt their adolescent had a hold on them and knew what to say to get their own way. Having experienced how life threatening their condition was and how unstable their adolescents became when setting their ground, they often submitted to their adolescents' wishes to keep the peace. They often lacked the support they needed to stand their ground and found it difficult to set boundaries.

> Because so much serious stuff has happened, I always must evaluate what is the consequence of me saying no to her. If I pay attention to myself, what could be the consequence for her? So, her consequence is always more important. There is a much greater risk for her.

They described how they stayed prepared and found it difficult to relax, as many of the parents had experienced their adolescents' self-harm and suicide attempts. This made sleeping at night difficult and affected the whole family.

> I often found her brother outside her door at night because she often ran away and went down to the railways.

They emphasized their need for support and to have somebody to talk to during the transition period. While some had an arrangement with their adolescent's clinic, others asked for help from voluntary support services or had good friends with similar experiences. The parents described that they could not focus on their own social lives, as they had to focus on their adolescents. Therefore, some felt alone and lonely. Others explained that they preferred to be alone, as they always had to be prepared for a phone call that would demand giving their attention to their adolescent.

Some found it difficult to be open with others, as they felt that their situation was an abnormal state, so they kept to themselves or used only family as support. They describe the support offered from the mental health care services as inconsistent. They missed having connections with other parents and access to more personal contact with their adolescents' clinicians to get more adapted advice and support. Once the transition period ended and things were more stable, they had different reactions. While some were able to regain their social life and reclaim their lives, others had more difficulty letting go and still felt the strain of the accumulated stress.

> In fact, for 2 years I have struggled a bit with fatigue. I kind of thought it might have something to do with the fact that I now can relax. You have walked on your toes for years, and suddenly there is no danger anymore. You feel so heavy in a way.

Discussion

To our knowledge, this study is the first to examine the transition process between CAMHS and AMHS,

focusing on the parents' perspective toward patients with AN. The present study revealed interacting factors important for the transition. The parents describe an abrupt discharge from AMHS based on age rather than maturity. They experienced a distance between the services that resulted in a gap in the care provided. This lack of continuity in treatment often caused negative treatment circles involving repetitive contacts with PCPs and AMHS, which led to a deterioration of the adolescent's health. Parents also described not being involved in the transition process. They felt left with the same responsibilities as in CAMHS but had less access to information. This loss of control triggered their need to be involved, not just informed. Trusting the therapists' knowledge was important. Combined with the responsibility they felt for their adolescent wellbeing, the parents had overwhelming multifaceted responsibilities they find difficult to balance. More parents need professional support to manage this challenging time to ease their distress.

Abrupt, discontinued transitions make parents feel responsible for coordinating the treatment

The current study shows that the parents find it important to consider the patients' readiness, rather than just age, to successfully transition from CAMHS to AMHS. Maturity and the ability to be self-sufficient are key patient-related factors that the parents perceive as underestimated in the treatment system. During the transition, the patients were unprepared for the difference in expectations toward them, which in some cases formed a care gap where the parents were left responsible. These findings are in line with our previous study that showed how patients felt unprepared for the expectations of self-sufficiency in the AMHS and how their parents' role changed during the transition phase [14]. The patients in our previous study found the transition process abrupt, and they had little influence on what they described as a critical period in their treatment. The loss of a safe environment and being expected to be more autonomous than what they were prepared for increased their anxiety and ambivalence. While supporting the adolescent, the parents in the current study spent much of their time during the transition process searching for adequate treatment. As they were often turned away by the AMHS, they had to assume responsibility for the patient in collaboration with their PCP. Other studies have found that, even though therapists in CAMHS expect the patient to need further treatment in AMHS, they are not directly referred to AMHS [11].

Dimitropoulos, Tran [27] showed that professionals acknowledged the parents' role in the transition and shared the concern of a more individual-oriented treatment that overlooked the need for more support by parents in the transition. Patients often had concerns over the parents' decreased role in their experience, as they were essential in their recovery process [27].

Additionally, the lack of continuity between CAMHS and AMHS left the parents and patients without support from CAMHS when establishing a safe connection with therapists in AMHS. Bucci, Roberts [28] underlined how planning transitions can buffer the loss of a secure base in CAMHS, as it would provide security and stability for both the patients and parents. Hill, Wilde [15] explained how preparing for the transition is difficult by acknowledging how treatment systems are fragmented and AMHS thresholds make accessing treatment more difficult. Nevertheless, it is important to try to overcome these practical barriers. The current study supports the arguments for securing the transition by considering the individual family's needs. An individual transition plan would help reduce stress and deterioration of illness, benefitting all those involved in the transition [29].

Knowledge and involvement – important for developing a trusting relationship between parents and clinician's

This study found that knowledge was an important part of the transition process and the basis of the parent's trust in the clinician. Regarding the clinician's knowledge about eating disorders, knowledge of the parents' role in the transition, and the clinicians' competence to include parents' knowledge during the transition period. Treasure, Whitaker [30] has argued that it is a misconception that adult services must exclude parents from the assessment and treatment of adult patients with AN to protect the patients' growing autonomy and confidentiality of the treatment. Clinicians treating patients with AN need competence to balance the patient's need for independence against the parents' involvement in treatment [30]. As our study reveals, it was sometimes difficult for clinicians to know when and how to involve the parents when treating patients with AN. As parents experience having the same responsibilities for the adolescent in the transition process as when they were treated in CAMHS, they feel left feeling alone with overwhelming responsibility. Adolescents transferring from CAMHS to AMHS often live with their families longer. In addition, their families tend to be involved to a larger degree in their diseased adolescents' lives compared with healthy peers [19]. Other studies and international guidelines have underlined the importance of involving parents in the transition [3, 31]. However, this study's results reveal that following up on these recommendations is challenging. Organizational factors, exemplified by a fragmented health-care system, and differences in treatment cultures, exemplified by a more individual approach in AMHS, can explain why the parents in our study experience are left uninvolved in treatment. Besides, according

to a previous study that explored professionals' experiences with the transition, clinicians have difficulties trusting their competence when treating patients with AN [32], which can influence how they trust their judgment concerning including parents. Hill, Wilde [15] identified that AMHS clinicians experience anxiety and lack confidence in their competence regarding developmental and adolescent issues; therefore, the transition period disclaims any training needs. This finding resonates with this study's findings, where parents experienced inconsistencies between clinicians in terms of their approaches to the parents and their consciousness of their adolescents' developmental stage. To ensure that the transition is effectuated with a high level of competence that includes the parent's expertise knowledge of the adolescent, we recommend updating the guidelines for eating disorders to prevent the random way transitions occur and support clinicians in a difficult treatment period.

Parents need professional support

Our study reveals how parents' distress during the transition period is related to a lack of support in a period in which they have an overwhelming degree of multifaceted responsibilities. The most obvious finding that emerges from the analysis is that parents put the adolescent's needs before much else due to their condition's severity. This finding is expected, as other studies have reported the heavy load and disruption to caregivers' lives due to the nature and demands of their adolescent's illness [20, 33]. It also pinpoints how differently parents experience their social support and how open and honest they can be with close friends and family. Kyriacou, Treasure [20] argued that both patients' and parents' needs must be identified and addressed in the transition. Earlier studies revealed how the development of overprotective parenting styles and expressing high emotion are common reactions for parents' caregiving for patients with AN. These reactions are associated with caregiver distress and burnout [30, 34]. Roots, Rowlands [35] found that parents experienced relief and unease when excluded from therapy, which resonates somewhat with this study's findings. The criterion is that parents need to feel safe and trust the patient's clinician. As in our study, Roots et al. (2009) found that parents and siblings need and value support from clinicians. We recommend that the clinicians facilitating the transition consider the important role parents have, being a secure epicenter for the adolescents in a turbulent period in their lives. Although studies have shown how social support can be a significant moderator of the stress following the caregiving role [36], we believe establishing family support within health care services could decrease the negative aspects of caregiving during the transition process.

Limitations

The study has generated findings from qualitative interviews concerning 10 transitions. The adolescents going through the transitions were all female, and the majority of the parents were also female. As the participants were recruited through therapists who perceived the transition to be an important theme and selected from volunteers, we may have recruited a biased sample most familiar with negative consequences with the transition process. Norwegian mental health system and cultural aspects may have provided this study with themes other than what other cultures would generate. However, our findings support those found in international literature and can be assumed to have relevance in other cultural settings.

Conclusion

Improving the transition by focusing on including parents and adolescents and preparing them for the transition period could ease parental distress and improve adolescents' compliance with treatment. Clinicians should increase their focus on the important role of parents in the transition process. There may be a need for more extensive service changes; the system should implement routines and guidelines to offer caregivers support and guidance during the transition process.

Abbreviations

CAMHS: Child and Adolescent Mental Health Services; AMHS: Adult Mental Health Services; AN: Anorexia Nervosa; PCP: Primary Care Doctor

Acknowledgements

Thank you to all participants who supported this research study.

,

Authors contributions

Design of the Mind the Gap study: LN, JIR, and LAWH. Data collection: VL and JIR. Drafting the article: VL, JIR, and LN. All authors contributed to data analysis, interpretation, and critical revision of the article as well as final approval of the version to be published.

Declarations

Ethics approval and consent to participate

The study was approved by the data protection authority at Oslo University Hospital (OUS; 2016/19732). The study was performed in accordance with the Declaration of Helsinki and evaluated by the Regional Committee for Medical and Health Research Ethics for the Southeast Region of Norway (2016/1259). The study is not viewed to be a medical or health-related research project regulated by the law of health research and is thereby not subject to presentation (cf. HFL. § 2).

Competing interests

The authors declare that they have no competing interests.

Author details

[1]Division of Mental Health and Addiction, Oslo University Hospital, P.O. Box 4959, Nydalen, Oslo, Norway. [2]Institute of Clinical Medicine, Faculty of Medicine, University of Oslo, 0318 Oslo, Norway. [3]Oslo, Norway. [4]Regional Department for Eating Disorders, Division of Mental Health and Addiction, Oslo University Hospital, Ullevål HF, Postboks 4950 Nydalen, 0424 Oslo, Norway. [5]Drammen, Norway.

References

1. Eating disorders: Recognition and treatment. Full guideline [Internet]. 2017 [cited 11.01.21]. Available from: https://www.nice.org.uk/guidance/ng69/evidence/full-guideline-pdf-161214767896.
2. Health TNDo. National treatmentguideline for eating disorders Oslo The Norwegian Directorate of Health. 2017 [cited 2020 23.11]. Available from: https://www.helsedirektoratet.no/retningslinjer/spiseforstyrrelser
3. Dimitropoulos G, Tran AF, Agarwal P, Sheffield B, Woodside B. Challenges in making the transition between pediatric and adult eating disorder programs: a qualitative study from the perspective of service providers. Eat Disord. 2013;21(1):1–15. https://doi.org/10.1080/10640266.2013.741964.
4. Treasure J, Schmidt U, Hugo P. Mind the gap: service transition and interface problems for patients with eating disorders. Br J Psychiatry. 2005; 187(5):398–400. https://doi.org/10.1192/bjp.187.5.398.
5. Herpertz-Dahlmann B. Adolescent eating disorders: definitions, symptomatology, epidemiology and comorbidity. Child Adolesc Psychiatr Clin N Am. 2009;18(1):31–47. https://doi.org/10.1016/j.chc.2008.07.005.
6. Fassino S, Piero A, Tomba E, Abbate-Daga G. Factors associated with dropout from treatment for eating disorders: a comprehensive literature review. BMC Psychiatry. 2009;9(1):67. https://doi.org/10.1186/1471-244X-9-67.
7. Blum R, Garell D, Hodgman C, et al. Transition from childcentered to adult health-care systems for adolescents with chronic conditions. J Adolesc Health. 1993;14(7):570–6. https://doi.org/10.1016/1054-139X(93)90143-D.
8. Winston AP, Paul M, Juanola-Borrat Y. The same but different? Treatment of anorexia nervosa in adolescents and adults. Eur Eat Disord Rev. 2012;20(2): 89–93. https://doi.org/10.1002/erv.1137.
9. Singh S, Paul M, Ford T, Kramer T, Weaver T, McLaren S, et al. Lost in transition: a multi-perspective study of process, outcome and experience of transition from child to adult mental health care (TRACK). Br J Psychiatry. 2010;197(4):305–12. https://doi.org/10.1192/bjp.bp.109.075135.
10. Singh SP, Paul M, Ford T, Kramer T, Weaver T, McLaren S, et al. Process, outcome and experience of transition from child to adult mental healthcare: multiperspective study. Br J Psychiatry. 2010;197(4):305–12. https://doi.org/10.1192/bjp.bp.109.075135.
11. Appleton R, Connell C, Fairclough E, Tuomainen H, Singh SP. Outcomes of young people who reach the transition boundary of child and adolescent mental health services: a systematic review. Eur Child Adolesc Psychiatry. 2019;28:1431–46.
12. Mulvale GM, Nguyen TD, Miatello AM, Embrett MG, Wakefield PA, Randall GE. Lost in transition or translation? Care philosophies and transitions between child and youth and adult mental health services: a systematic review. J Ment Health. 2016;28(4):379–88.
13. Paul M, Ford T, Kramer T, Islam Z, Harley K, Singh SP. Transfers and transitions between child and adult mental health services. Br J Psychiatry Suppl. 2013;54:s36–40. https://doi.org/10.1192/bjp.bp.112.119198.
14. Lockertsen V, Nilsen L, Holm LAW, Rø Ø, Burger LM, Røssberg JI. Experiences of patients with anorexia nervosa during the transition from child and adolescent mental health services to adult mental health services. J Eat Disord. 2020;8(1):1–11.
15. Hill A, Wilde S, Tickle A. Transition from child and adolescent mental health services (CAMHS) to adult mental health services (AMHS): a meta-synthesis of parental and professional perspectives. Child Adolesc Mental Health. 2019;24(4):295–306. https://doi.org/10.1111/camh.12339.
16. Lindgren E, Söderberg S, Skär L. Being a parent to a young adult with mental illness in transition to adulthood. Issues Ment Health Nurs. 2016; 37(2):98–105. https://doi.org/10.3109/01612840.2015.1092621.
17. Dimitropoulos G, Klopfer K, Lazar L, Schacter R. Caring for a sibling with anorexia nervosa: a qualitative study. Eur Eat Disord Rev. 2009;17(5):350–65. https://doi.org/10.1002/erv.937.

18. Hergenroeder AC, Wiemann CM, Cohen MB. Current issues in transitioning from pediatric to adult-based care for youth with chronic health care needs. J Pediatr. 2015;167(6):1196–201. https://doi.org/10.1016/j.jpeds.2015.08.005.

19. Linacre SJ. The wellbeing of carers of people with severe and enduring eating disorders (SEED). Leeds: University of Leeds; 2011.

20. Kyriacou O, Treasure J, Schmidt U. Understanding how parents cope with living with someone with anorexia nervosa: Modelling the factors that are associated with carer distress. Int J Eat Disord. 2008;41(3):233–42. https://doi.org/10.1002/eat.20488.

21. Anastasiadou D, Medina-Pradas C, Sepulveda A, Treasure J. A Systematic Review of Family Caregiving in Eating Disorders; 2014.

22. Fowler E. Supporting someone with an eating disorder: a systematic review of caregiver experiences of eating disorder treatment and a qualitative exploration of burnout management within eating disorder services; 2016.

23. Treasure J, Schmidt U. The cognitive-interpersonal maintenance model of anorexia nervosa revisited: a summary of the evidence for cognitive, socio-emotional and interpersonal predisposing and perpetuating factors. J Eat Disord. 2013;1(1):13. https://doi.org/10.1186/2050-2974-1-13.

24. Coomber K, King RM. Coping strategies and social support as predictors and mediators of eating disorder carer burden and psychological distress. Soc Psychiatry Psychiatr Epidemiol. 2012;47(5):789–96. https://doi.org/10.1007/s00127-011-0384-6.

25. Malterud K. Systematic text condensation: a strategy for qualitative analysis. Scand J Public Health. 2012;40(8):795–805. https://doi.org/10.1177/1403494812465030.

26. Giorgi A. Sketch of a psychological phenomenological method. In A. Giorgi (Ed.), Phenomenology and psychological research: essays. Pittsburgh: Duquesne University Press; 1985.

27. Dimitropoulos G, Tran AF, Agarwal P, Sheffield B, Woodside B. Navigating the transition from pediatric to adult eating disorder programs: perspectives of service providers. Int J Eat Disord. 2012;45(6):759–67. https://doi.org/10.1002/eat.22017.

28. Bucci S, Roberts NH, Danquah AN, Berry K. Using attachment theory to inform the design and delivery of mental health services: a systematic review of the literature. Psychol Psychother Theory Res Pract. 2015;88(1):1–20. https://doi.org/10.1111/papt.12029.

29. Farre A, Wood V, McDonagh JE, Parr JR, Reape D, Rapley T. Health professionals' and managers' definitions of developmentally appropriate healthcare for young people: conceptual dimensions and embedded controversies. Arch Dis Child. 2016;101(7):628–33. https://doi.org/10.1136/archdischild-2015-309473.

30. Treasure J, Whitaker W, Whitney J, Schmidt U. Working with families of adults with anorexia nervosa. J Fam Ther. 2005;27(2):158–70. https://doi.org/10.1111/j.1467-6427.2005.00308.x.

31. NICE. Transition from children's to adults' services for young people using health or social care services. In: Excellence TNIfHaC, editor. UK: NICE; 2016.

32. Lockertsen V, Nilsen L, Holm LAW, Rø Ø, Burger LM, Røssberg JI. Mental health professionals' experiences transitioning patients with anorexia nervosa from child/adolescent to adult mental health services: a qualitative study. BMC Health Serv Res. 2020;20(1):1–9.

33. Maurin JT, Boyd CB. Burden of mental illness on the family: a critical review. Arch Psychiatr Nurs. 1990;4(2):99–107. https://doi.org/10.1016/0883-9417(90)90016-E.

34. Whitney J, Currin L, Murray J, Treasure J. Family work in anorexia nervosa: a qualitative study of carers' experiences of two methods of family intervention. Eur Eat Disord Rev. 2012;20(2):132–41. https://doi.org/10.1002/erv.1077.

35. Roots P, Rowlands L, Gowers SG. User satisfaction with services in a randomised controlled trial of adolescent anorexia nervosa. Eur Eat Disord Rev. 2009;17(5):331–7. https://doi.org/10.1002/erv.944.

36. MacMaster SA. Differences in the well-being of family caregivers of adults with mental illness and a co-occurring substance abuse disorder: Case Western Reserve University; 2001.

3

Oxidative Status in Plasma, Urine and Saliva of Girls with Anorexia Nervosa and Healthy Controls

Alexandra Gaál Kovalčíková[1]*⬤, Ľubica Tichá[1], Katarína Šebeková[2], Peter Celec[2,3,4], Alžbeta Čagalová[1], Fatma Sogutlu[5] and Ľudmila Podracká[1]

Abstract

Background: Anorexia nervosa (AN) is a serious psychosomatic disorder with unclear pathomechanisms. Metabolic dysregulation is associated with disruption of redox homeostasis that might play a pivotal role in the development of AN. The aim of our study was to assess oxidative status and carbonyl stress in plasma, urine and saliva of patients with AN and healthy controls.

Methods: Plasma, spot urine, and saliva were collected from 111 girls with AN (aged from 10 to 18 years) and from 29 age-matched controls. Markers of oxidative stress and antioxidant status were measured using spectrophotometric and fluorometric methods.

Results: Plasma advanced oxidation protein products (AOPP) and advanced glycation end products (AGEs) were significantly higher in patients with AN than in healthy controls (by 96, and 82%, respectively). Accordingly, urinary concentrations of AOPP and fructosamines and salivary concentrations of AGEs were higher in girls with AN compared with controls (by 250, and 41% in urine; by 92% in saliva, respectively). Concentrations of thiobarbituric acid reactive substances (TBARS) in saliva were 3-times higher in the patients with AN than in the controls. Overall antioxidants were lower in plasma of girls with AN compared to the controls, as shown by total antioxidant capacity and ratio of reduced and oxidized glutathione (by 43, and 31%, respectively).

Conclusions: This is the first study assessing wide range of markers of oxidative status in plasma, urine and saliva of the patients with AN. We showed that both, higher levels of markers of oxidative stress and lower antioxidants play a role in redox disruption. Restoration of redox homeostasis might be of the clinical relevance

Keywords: Eating disorder, Malnutrition, Oxidative status, Antioxidants, Biomarkers

* Correspondence: alexandra.kovalcikova114@gmail.com
[1]Department of Paediatrics, The National Institute of Children's Diseases and Faculty of Medicine, Comenius University, Limbová 1, 83340 Bratislava, Slovakia
Full list of author information is available at the end of the article

Plain English summary

Anorexia nervosa is a serious psychosomatic disorder with increasing incidence worldwide. Numerous general medical complications affecting most major organ systems are caused by progressive malnutrition and rapid weight loss. However, precise pathomechanism involved in the pathogenesis of anorexia nervosa remains to be elucidated. A potential role of oxidative stress caused by metabolic disruption in the etiology of anorexia nervosa was already described in plasma or blood components. This study aimed to investigate whether redox imbalance could be detected even in alternative body fluids of patients with anorexia nervosa - urine and saliva. Samples from female patients ($n = 111$) with anorexia nervosa and healthy controls ($n = 29$) were collected and analysed in this study. Our results indicated that changes in redox homeostasis could be detected not only in plasma, but also in urine and saliva of patients with anorexia nervosa. This was shown by higher markers of oxidative stress - advanced oxidation protein products, fructosamines and advanced glycation end-products. Oxidative damage of biomolecules might have direct cytotoxic effect associated with increased expression of proinflammatory cytokines, growth factors etc. Thus, many medical complications of anorexia nervosa might be directly connected to the accumulation of oxidatively damaged biomolecules.

Introduction

Anorexia nervosa (AN) is a serious mental disorder characterized by an intense fear of weight gain and by a disturbed body image, which motivates severe dietary restriction or other weight loss behaviours (e.g. purging, excessive physical activity). Its prevalence among adolescents is increasing worldwide over the last few decades [1]. Metabolic dysregulation and homeostasis disruption that are directly attributable to extreme weight loss and malnutrition play an important role in dermatological, osteological [2], neuroendocrine [3], gastrointestinal [4], cardiovascular, and immune system disorders [5] leading to premature death [2], but precise pathomechanisms are not fully understood.

Oxidative stress is an imbalance between the production of free radicals (e.g., reactive oxygen species – ROS; reactive nitrogen species – RNS; Fig. 1) and the antioxidants caused either by the overproduction of the free radicals, the insufficiency of an antioxidant defence mechanism, or by a combination of both [6]. Oxidative stress may damage the biomolecules, impair the cell structures, and deteriorate the organ functions (Fig. 1) [7]. It activates various transcription factors that are involved in several pathological processes, including inflammation and immunity [8].

Since redox reactions are intracellular processes and a half-life of ROS is short, in clinical practice, oxidative status is usually quantified indirectly, via determination of concentrations of damaged substrates, often using non-specific methods. Malondialdehyde (MDA) is the end-product of lipid peroxidation. Thiobarbituric acid reactive substance (TBARS) assay is a standard non-specific method for the measurement of the levels of MDA and other aldehydes that might react with thiobarbituric acid [9]. Advanced oxidation protein products (AOPP) are formed by myeloperoxidase, during neutrophil activation [10]. The most common markers of carbonyl stress - fructosamines and advanced glycation end-products (AGEs) are formed during early and late stage, respectively, of non-enzymatic glycation of amino groups of proteins by the carbonyl compound of sugars or reactive aldehydes [11, 12]. A ratio of reduced (GSH) to oxidized glutathione (GSSG) serves as a marker of antioxidant status. GSH is considered to be one of the most essential scavengers of the free radicals [13]. Ferric reducing antioxidant power (FRAP) and total antioxidant capacity (TAC) evaluate overall endogenous and exogenous antioxidant capacity, without need for measuring of the individual antioxidants [14, 15].

Oxidative stress is associated with various mental disorders that might be interrelated to AN, including depression or anxiety [16]. Compared to the healthy controls, the patients with depression presented lower activities of the antioxidant enzymes, such as superoxide dismutase and catalase or lower concentrations of glutathione [17, 18]; and higher levels of MDA or AOPP [19, 20]. Moreover, the antidepressants and the psychotherapy increased the concentrations of the antioxidants and led to the decrease of MDA [19].

So far, only a few studies evaluated the oxidative status in patients with AN [21–23]. It has been shown that the effective treatment resulting in weight gain is associated with an improvement of oxidative status in patients with AN [23, 24]. Nevertheless, these studies mostly focused on plasma or blood components [21–23]. Saliva and urine represent a promising alternative to the blood sampling, as their collection is non-invasive, painless and does not require trained personnel [25].

Thus, the aim of our study was to compare the markers of oxidative status and carbonyl stress in different body fluids, including plasma, urine and saliva in the patients with AN and in the healthy controls. We hypothesised that reduced food intake and metabolic disruption lead to an increased production of oxidative -

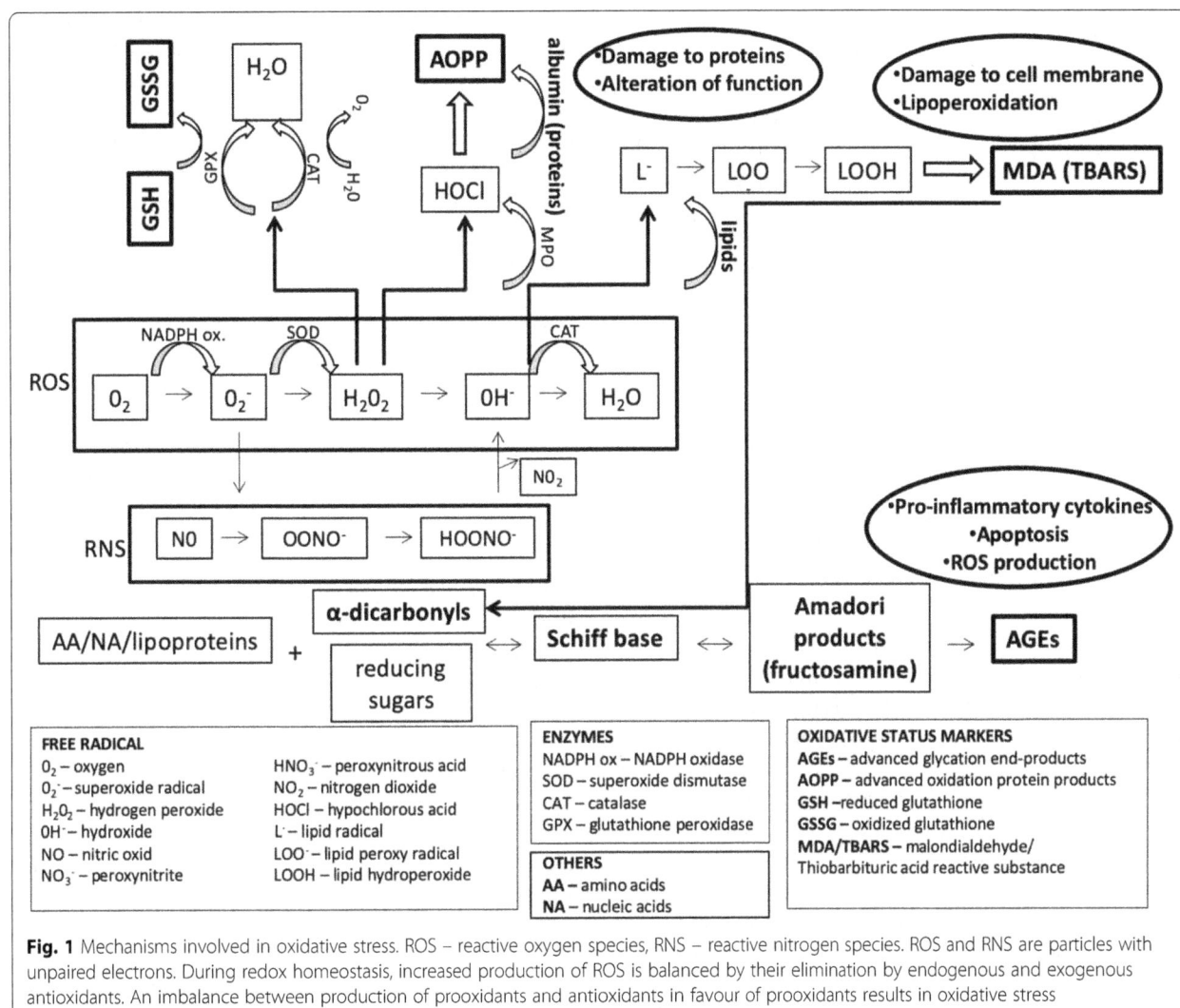

Fig. 1 Mechanisms involved in oxidative stress. ROS – reactive oxygen species, RNS – reactive nitrogen species. ROS and RNS are particles with unpaired electrons. During redox homeostasis, increased production of ROS is balanced by their elimination by endogenous and exogenous antioxidants. An imbalance between production of prooxidants and antioxidants in favour of prooxidants results in oxidative stress

and carbonyl-stress markers and a decrease in the levels of antioxidants that would be manifested not only on the plasma level, but also in the alternative body fluids – urine and saliva.

Methods

Participants

In this study, 111 consecutive female patients aged from 10 to 18 (median age: 14.9, interquartile range - IQR: 13.4–16.1) years, hospitalized at the Paediatric endocrinology clinic or the Psychiatric clinic of the National Institute of Children's Diseases (NICD) from February 2016 to February 2020 with a diagnosis of restrictive subtype of AN were enrolled. Diagnosis of AN was based on the new Diagnostic and Statistical Manual of Mental Disorders 5th Edition (DSM-5) [26]. E.g., the patient had to meet the following criteria: persistent restriction of energy intake that leads to a low body weight, intense fear of gaining weight, distorted

perception of body weight and shape, undue influence of weight on self-evaluation or lack of the recognition of severity of the illness [26]. Manifestation of other psychiatric comorbidities (e.g., binge eating/purging subtype of AN, depression, anxiety) as diagnosed by the psychiatrists, and the presence of peripheral oedema (indicating volume overload) were the exclusion criteria. All anthropometric measurements and collections of samples in patients with AN were performed at the time of recruitment i. e. before initiation of refeeding, and pharmacological treatment.

Twenty-nine healthy age-matched girls (median age: 14.0; IQR: 11.0–16.3), recruited from regular check-ups in the practice of a general paediatrician at the same institution served as healthy controls. Inclusion criteria were BMI between 90th and 10th percentile for sex and age, no past or current mental disorder, and no involvement in weight reduction regimen [26].

Other exclusion criteria for all participants were pregnancy, lactation, hormonal contraception, and acute or chronic inflammation (C-reactive protein - CRP>10 mg/l).

Anthropometric and blood pressure measurements

Anthropometric measurements were performed by the trained nurses according to the standard protocols of the NICD clinics. Briefly, the height was measured in standing position using stable stadiometer; body weight was measured by digital scales. BMI was calculated. Standard deviation (SD) of height, weight, and BMI was expressed using the current reference data of Slovak children and adolescents [27]. Three blood pressure measurements were taken on a dominant arm after 5 min resting in sitting position, using an automated device (Omron HBP-1100, Kyoto, Japan). The mean of the last two measurements was recorded. Blood pressure SD was calculated according to the guidelines for percentiles of blood pressure in normal-weight children and adolescents [28].

Samples collection and handling

Biological material was collected in the morning hours, between 6.00 and 8.00 am. Blood was collected after overnight fasting, from median cubital vein, into K$_3$EDTA, lithium-heparin, and SST™ II Advance tubes (BD Vacutainer Plastic Tube, Becton Dickinson, Czech Republic). At the Department of Clinical Biochemistry of NICD, blood was centrifuged; plasma was subjected to immediate blood chemistry analyses and aliquots were stored at $-80\,°C$ for measurements of markers of oxidative status and carbonyl stress. Spot urine was collected into 50 ml sterile Falcon tubes (Sarstedt, Numbrecht, Germany). To prevent saliva contamination, all participants were asked not to drink, eat or teeth brush optimally 60 min before sampling. Unstimulated saliva was collected according to the standard protocol [25], by spitting for 10 min into 15 ml sterile Falcon tubes (Sarstedt, Numbrecht, Germany). Urine and saliva were centrifuged at 1600 g for 10 min to remove cell debris. Supernatants were frozen until analyses.

Laboratory measurements

Plasma glucose, albumin, total cholesterol, high-density lipoprotein cholesterol (HDL-C), triacylglycerols (TAG), bilirubin, aspartate aminotransferase (AST), alanine aminotransferase (ALT), creatinine, urea, uric acid, and high sensitive CRP were analysed using standard laboratory methods (Cobas c501, Roche Diagnostics, Mannheim, Germany). Measurement of cystatin C was performed using Biolis 24i Premium analyser (Tokyo Boeki Machinery, Tokyo, Japan). Blood count analyses were conducted using the Sysmex XN-1000™ Hematology Analyser (Sysmex Group's, Kobe, Japan).

All methods used for determination of markers of oxidative status and carbonyl stress are described in detail in the Additional file 1. Briefly, TBARS [9], AGE-associated fluorescence [11], and GSH and GSSH [13] were determined fluorometrically; spectrophotometric methods were used to quantify fructosamines [12], AOPP [10], FRAP [14], and TAC [15].

Creatinine in urine was measured using Jaffé method [29], while urinary proteins were quantified using the pyrogallol-red method [30]. Plasma proteins were determined using a commercial kit (SERVA Electrophoresis GmbH, Heidelberg, Germany). Measurements of oxidative status markers and carbonyl stress were performed on a Synergy HT Multi-Mode Microplate Reader (BioTekInstruments, Inc., Winooski, VT, USA); and all chemicals were purchased from Sigma Aldrich (Steinheim, Germany).

Assessment of kidney functions

Glomerular filtration rate (eGFR) was estimated using the cystatin C based Schwartz formula [31]. Urine protein to creatinine ratio (PCR) was calculated.

Statistical analysis

Total number of participants required for the study was estimated according to G Power analysis using G*Power 3.1.9.4 software (Universität Kiel, Germany) from our preliminary results on TAC, to 72 individuals (noncentrality parameter $\delta = 3.31$; critical $t = 1.67$; df = 70; actual power = 0.95). Similar results were obtained when data on AOPP (noncentrality parameter $\delta = 3.34$; critical $t = 1.66$; df = 94; actual power = 0.95; total samples size = 94) or fructosamines (noncentrality parameter $\delta = 3.36$; critical $t = 1.67$; df = 62; actual power = 0.95; total samples size = 64) were evaluated. GraphPad Prism software v. 6.01 was used for statistical analysis (GraphPad Software, San Diego, California, USA). The normality of the data distribution was tested using the D'Agostino-Pearson omnibus test. Outliers were detected using the Grubbs´ test. Patients and controls were compared employing two-sided Student's t-test. To compare not normally distributed data, Mann-Whitney U test was used. Spearman correlation analysis and regression analysis was performed. Data are expressed as a mean ± SD or as a median and IQR. For auxological data, which are directly dependent on division into patients and controls, $p < 0.05$ was considered statistically significant. Due to multiple comparison in the assessment of oxidative and carbonyl stress markers, two groups were tested against a Bonferroni-adjusted (Bonf.) alpha level of 0.0071 (0.05/7), 0.001 (0.01/7), and 0.0001 (0.001/7) for plasma or saliva, and 0.0083 (0.05/6), 0.002 (0.01/6) and 0.0002 (0.001/6) for urine.

Results

In our cohort, the median of AN duration was 10.9 months (IQR: 6.1–18.1). Fifteen girls (13.5%) were presented with primary amenorrhea; while 65 (58.6%) suffered from secondary amenorrhea, with a median of duration of 9.0 months (IQR: 4.6–15.3).

Anthropometric and blood chemistry data

Auxological data of patients and controls are presented in Table 1. Two groups did not differ by age, height, and height SD ($p>0.05$). Body weight, body weight SD, BMI, and BMI SD significantly differed between patients with AN and controls ($p<0.001$). Concentrations of endogenous antioxidants including albumin, bilirubin, and uric acid were lower in the patients compared with the controls (albumin; bilirubin: $p<0.001$; uric acid: $p<0.01$);

however, none of the patients with AN presented hypouricaemia, hypobilirubinaemia or hypoalbuminemia. Concentrations of markers of liver function AST and ALT in girls with AN were within reference range. Concentrations of urea and TAG ($p<0.05$) were significantly higher, while glycaemia was lower ($p<0.01$) in the girls with AN compared with the controls albeit within the reference range. Concentrations of urinary PCR were higher in the AN group compared with the controls ($p<0.001$). Neither cholesterol, CRP, nor eGFR differed significantly ($p>0.05$) between the groups (Table 1).

Markers of oxidative stress

In patients with AN, plasma and urinary TBARS concentrations were similar to those in the control group (plasma: $p_{Bonf.}>0.0071$; urine: $p_{Bonf.}>0.0083$, Table 2). In

Table 1 Clinical and biochemical characteristics of patients with anorexia nervosa and healthy controls

	Anorexia nervosa	Healthy controls	p
Age (years)	14.9 (13.4–16.1)	14.0 (11.0–16.3)	NS
BMI (kg/m^2)	15.1 (13.7–16.8)	19.8 (18.9–21.2)	<0.001
BMI SD	−1.8 (−2.4−−1.1)	0.03 (−0.4–0.8)	<0.001
Height (cm)	164.5 (159.5–169.7)	162.0 (148.0–169.5)	NS
Height SD	0.2 ± 1.1	0.5 ± 1.0	NS
Body weight (kg)	41.5 ± 8.3	52.1 ± 10.1	<0.001
Body weight SD	−1.0 (−1.6−−0.1)	0.4 (−0.1–0.9)	<0.001
Systolic blood pressure (mm Hg)	112 ± 11	ND	
Systolic blood pressure SD	0.05 ± 0.96	ND	
Diastolic blood pressure (mm Hg)	71 ± 8	ND	
Diastolic blood pressure SD	0.47 ± 0.74	ND	
Glucose (mmol/l)	4.3 (4.0–4.6)	4.7 (4.2–4.9)	<0.01
Cholesterol (mmol/l)	4.56 ± 0.96	4.39 ± 0.71	NS
HDL-cholesterol (mmol/l)	1.72 ± 0.41	1.14 ± 0.22	<0.001
Triacylglycerols (mmol/l)	0.76 (0.61–1.12)	0.72 (0.53–0.84)	<0.05
Albumin (g/l)	46.7 (44.1–48.9)	49.9 (47.5–51.8)	<0.001
Total proteins (g/l)	69.9 (66.0–73.5)	70.5 (67.6–73.2)	NS
Uric acid (μmol/l)	218 (195–258)	264 (216–309)	<0.01
Bilirubin (μmol/l)	3.8 (2.7–4.8)	9.3 (6.0–13.7)	<0.001
AST (μkat/l)	0.39 (0.32–0.47)	ND	
ALT (μkat/l)	0.34 (0.25–0.52)	ND	
Urea (mmol/l)	4.6 (3.4–5.6)	3.7 (3.0–4.7)	<0.05
Creatinine (μmol/l)	66 ± 13	72 ± 15	<0.05
Cystatin C (mg/l)	0.70 (0.62–0.83)	0.79 (0.69–0.83)	NS
eGFR (ml/min/1.73m^2)	99 (84–110)	89 (84–100)	NS
C-reactive protein (mg/l)	0.1 (0.1–0.4)	0.2 (0.1–0.5)	NS
Leukocytes (10^9/l)	5.4 (4.4–6.2)	ND	
Urinary PCR (mg/mmol)	35.5 (22.2–48.8)	15.7 (12.7–24.0)	<0.001

AST aspartate aminotransferase, *ALT* alanine aminotransferase, *BMI* body mass index, *eGFR* estimated glomerular filtration rate, *HDL* high density lipoprotein, *ND* not determined, *NS* non-significant, *PCR* protein to creatinine ratio, *SD* standard deviation; Results are expressed as mean ± SD (normally distributed data) or as median (interquartile range), (skewed data) whole group of participants, Spearman analyses revealed positive correlations between plasma and urinary concentrations of TBARS (r = 0.50, $p_{Bonf.}$<0.0001). Salivary concentrations of TBARS were 3-fold higher in the AN group compared with the controls ($p_{Bonf.}$<0.0001, Table 2).

The group with AN displayed significantly higher concentrations of AOPP in plasma (by 96%, $p_{Bonf.}$<0.0001, Fig. 2a), as well as in urine (by 250%, $p_{Bonf.}$<0.0002, Fig. 2b) – compared with the controls. In the whole group of participants, Spearman analysis revealed a positive correlation between plasma and urinary AOPP (r = 0.48, $p_{Bonf.}$<0.0001). Salivary concentrations of AOPP in the girls with AN were similar to the controls ($p_{Bonf.}$ > 0.0071, Fig. 2c).

Markers of carbonyl stress
In comparison to the healthy controls, the group with AN displayed significantly higher concentrations of AGE-Fl in plasma (by 82%, $p_{Bonf.}$<0.0001, Fig. 2d); as well as in saliva (by 92%, $p_{Bonf.}$<0.0071, Fig. 2e).

Concentrations of fructosamines in plasma, and saliva did not differed between girls with AN and controls ($p_{Bonf.}$ > 0.0071, Table 2), while urinary levels of fructosamines in girls with AN were higher by 41% - compared with controls ($p_{Bonf.}$<0.0083, Table 2).

Markers of antioxidant status
Two groups did not differ in plasma, and salivary concentrations of FRAP ($p_{Bonf.}$>0.0071, Table 2). In comparison to controls, urinary concentrations of FRAP were 3-fold higher in girls with AN ($p_{Bonf.}$<0.0002, Table 2).

Patients with AN had plasma TAC concentrations lower by 43% ($p_{Bonf.}$<0.0001, Fig. 3a), while urinary TAC concentrations were 3-fold higher - compared with controls ($p_{Bonf.}$<0.0002, Fig. 3b). Salivary TAC concentrations in patients with AN were similar to controls ($p_{Bonf.}$>0.0071, Fig. 3c).

In patients with AN, GSH/GSSG ratio in plasma was lower by 31% ($p_{Bonf.}$<0.0001, Fig. 3d), while in saliva it was higher by 132% ($p_{Bonf.}$<0.001, Fig. 3f) – compared to controls. In the whole group of participants, an inverse correlation between plasma and salivary GSH/GSSG was revealed using Spearman analysis (r = − 0.30, $p_{Bonf.}$<0.0071), as well as using regression analysis (beta = − 0.206, p<0.05). We did not find relation between plasma and salivary GSH (beta = 0.114, p>0.05), while negative relation between plasma GSSG and salivary GSSG was revealed (beta = − 0.304, p<0.001). Urinary of GSH/GSSG ratio did not differ between AN and control group ($p_{Bonf.}$ > 0.0083, Fig. 3e).

The effect of the duration of AN
Regression analyses revealed positive relation between duration of the disease and plasma markers of oxidative stress – TBARS, AOPP (TBARS: beta = 0.294, p<0.01; AGEs: beta = 0.264, p<0.01) and carbonyl stress – AGEs

(beta = 308, p<0.001). Moreover, a marker of antioxidant status TAC inversely correlated with disease duration (beta = − 0.250, p<0.001). While, positive relation was found between disease duration and urinary AOPP and TAC (AOPP: beta = 0.231, p<0.05; TAC: beta = 0.253, p<0.05, respectively), negative correlation was revealed with urinary fructosamines (beta = − 0.234, p<0.05; Additional file 2).

The effect of BMI SD and menstrual status
In the whole group of participants, we found inverse correlations between BMI SD, and plasma AOPP (beta = − 0.143; p<0.05). Moreover, positive relation between BMI SD, and plasma TAC was revealed (beta = 0.213; p<0.05). Further, BMI SD correlated negatively with salivary TBARS and AGEs (TBARS: beta = − 0.200, p<0.05; AGEs: beta = − 0.234, p<0.01) and urinary AOPP, respectively (beta = − 0.227, p<0.05). Regarding the effect of menstrual status on oxidative status, inverse relation between the duration of secondary amenorrhea and FRAP was found (beta = − 0.369, p<0.01). Moreover, a trend to a positive correlation was revealed between LH and TAC (beta = 0.254, p = 0.06).

Discussion
To the best of our knowledge, this is the first study assessing a wide range of markers of oxidative status and carbonyl stress in plasma, urine and saliva of the patients with AN. In addition to confirming former data that AN is associated with the markers of increased oxidative stress [22–24, 32], our data also suggest the presence of enhanced carbonyl stress. We confirmed our hypothesis that anorexia-associated redox imbalance and enhanced carbonyl stress are reflected by changes in their markers even in the alternative body fluids. However, the alterations in the markers assessed in non-invasively collected body fluids, i.e., urine and saliva, do not completely mirror those observed in plasma – considered as indicators of systemic changes.

Previous meta-analyses of Solmi et al. [23, 24] indicated a potential association between AN and systemic oxidative stress, as reflected by higher serum levels of oxidative stress marker apolipoprotein B and lower levels of antioxidants including superoxide dismutase, glutathione and albumin in patients with AN compared with the controls. Moreover, weight gain was associated with an improvement in oxidative status [23, 24].

Another studies demonstrated an impairment of oxidative status in blood elements [22, 32]. Erythrocyte tocopherol levels and superoxide dismutase activities were significantly lower in patients with AN compared to the controls [32]. Moreover, impairment of mitochondrial function associating with decreased mitochondrial O_2 consumption, low GSH levels, and increased ROS

Table 2 Concentrations of markers of oxidative and carbonyl stress in patients with anorexia nervosa and healthy controls

Markers	Plasma			Urine			Saliva		
	AN	CTRL	P$_{Bonf}$	AN	CTRL	P$_{Bonf}$	AN	CTRL	P$_{Bonf}$
TBARS	5.74 (3.47–10.82) µmol/l	3.88 (3.15–6.48)	NS	1.60 (0.38–6.73) µmol/mmol creatinine	1.16 (0.28–1.45)	NS	0.48 (0.22–0.90) µmol/l	0.11 (0.08–0.13)	<0.0001
AOPP	0.84 (0.54–1.26) µmol/g proteins	0.33 (0.23–0.84)	<0.0001	48.4 (25.7–81.3) µmol/mmol creatinine	12.0 (9.8–16.6)	<0.0002	8.20 (2.8–23.4) µmol/l	24.5 (6.1–34.9)	NS
AGEs	0.030 (0.020–0.040) g/g proteins	0.023 (0.018–0.024)	<0.0001	ND g/mmol creatinine	ND		0.47 (0.28–0.82) g/l	0.31 (0.16–0.43)	<0.0071
FRUCTOS	1.85 (1.39–2.20) mmol/l	1.36 (1.24–1.97)	NS	0.72 (0.52–1.03) mmol/mmol creatinine	0.48 (0.37–0.54)	<0.0083	0.21 (0.14–0.39) mmol/l	0.09 (0.04–0.30)	NS
FRAP	592 ± 129 µmol/l	600 ± 153	NS	1555 (613–5309) µmol/mmol creatinine	552 (395–819)	<0.0002	131 (66–267) µmol/l	143 (105–161)	NS
TAC	393 (235–674) µmol/l	879 (502–1164)	<0.0001	1652 (699–4533) µmol/mmol creatinine	573 (481–958)	<0.0002	567 (260–776) µmol/l	393 (234–541)	NS
GSH/GSSG	5.46 (4.51–9.16) ratio	8.99 (6.03–12.51)	<0.0001	0.81 (0.70–1.14) ratio	1.32 (0.78–1.54)	NS	0.66 (0.38–1.42) ratio	0.37 (0.30–0.43)	<0.001

AGEs advanced glycation end products, AN anorexia nervosa, AOPP advanced oxidation protein products, FRAP ferric reducing antioxidant power, FRUCTOS fructosamines, GSH/GSSG a ratio of reduced and oxidized glutathione, NS non-significant, TAC total antioxidant capacity, TBARS thiobarbituric acid reactive substance; Results are expressed as mean ± SD (normally distributed data) or as median (interquartile range), (skewed data)

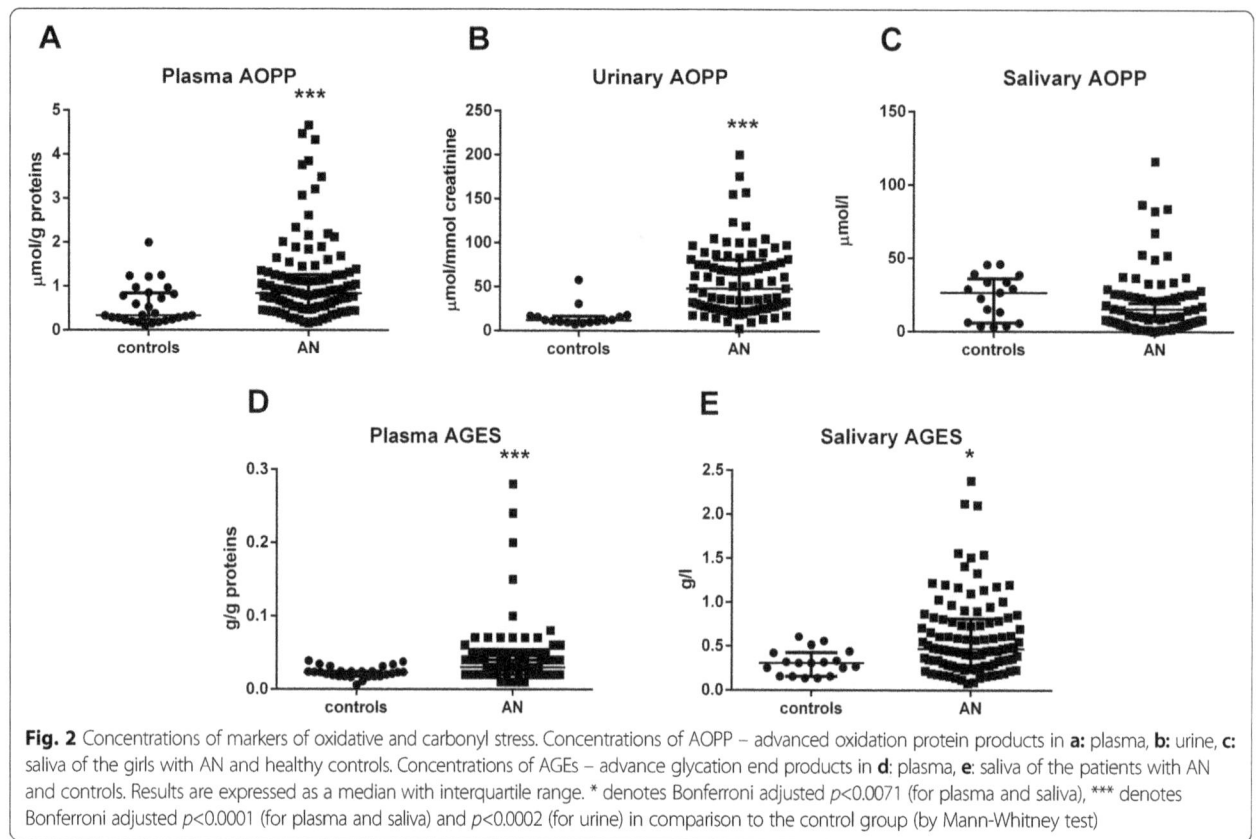

Fig. 2 Concentrations of markers of oxidative and carbonyl stress. Concentrations of AOPP – advanced oxidation protein products in **a**: plasma, **b**: urine, **c**: saliva of the girls with AN and healthy controls. Concentrations of AGEs – advance glycation end products in **d**: plasma, **e**: saliva of the patients with AN and controls. Results are expressed as a median with interquartile range. * denotes Bonferroni adjusted $p<0.0071$ (for plasma and saliva), *** denotes Bonferroni adjusted $p<0.0001$ (for plasma and saliva) and $p<0.0002$ (for urine) in comparison to the control group (by Mann-Whitney test)

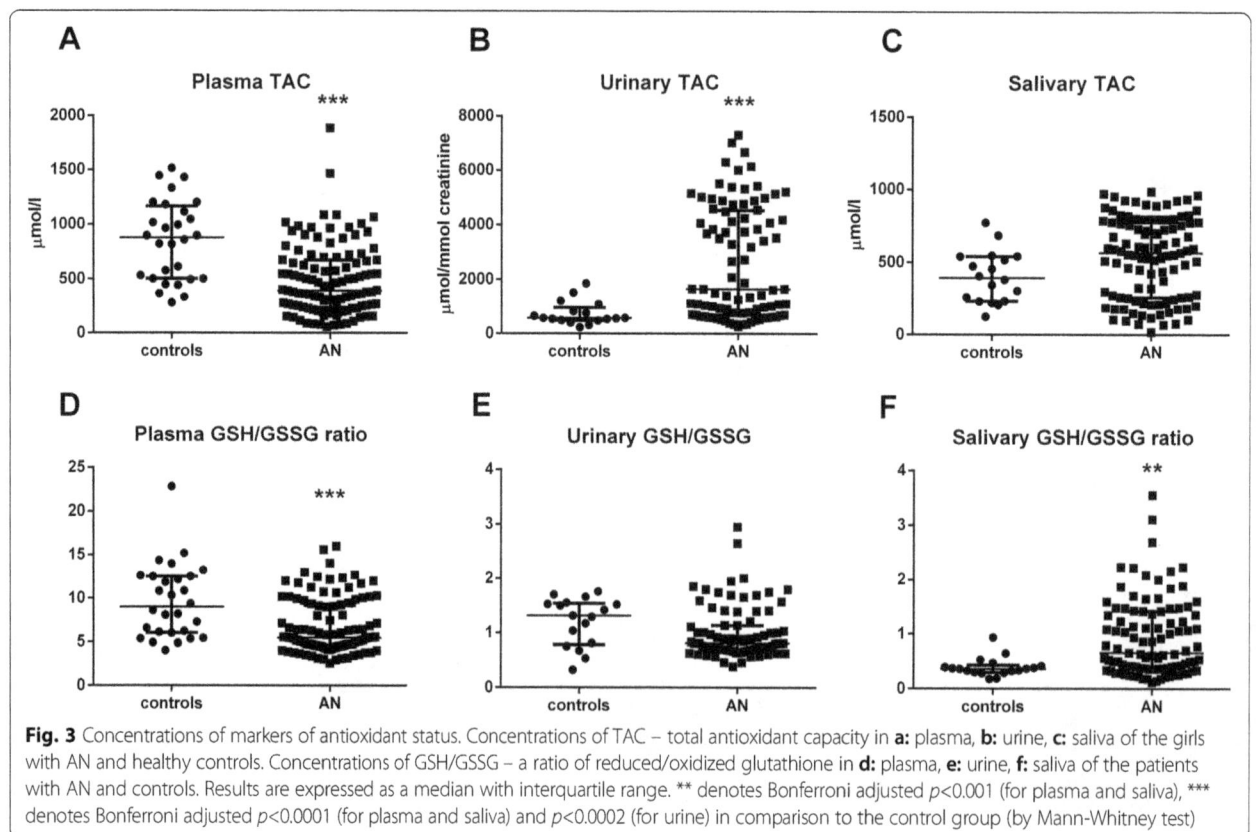

Fig. 3 Concentrations of markers of antioxidant status. Concentrations of TAC – total antioxidant capacity in **a**: plasma, **b**: urine, **c**: saliva of the girls with AN and healthy controls. Concentrations of GSH/GSSG – a ratio of reduced/oxidized glutathione in **d**: plasma, **e**: urine, **f**: saliva of the patients with AN and controls. Results are expressed as a median with interquartile range. ** denotes Bonferroni adjusted $p<0.001$ (for plasma and saliva), *** denotes Bonferroni adjusted $p<0.0001$ (for plasma and saliva) and $p<0.0002$ (for urine) in comparison to the control group (by Mann-Whitney test)

production was revealed in leukocytes of the patients with AN [22].

ROS produced by mitochondria act as signalling molecules that are involved in different intracellular processes including autophagy. Autophagy is a catabolic process that is essential for the removal of cytoplasmic material or damaged organelles playing an important role in cellular homeostasis. During starvation or enhanced oxidative stress, autophagy is up-regulated to produce nutrients and to protect cells from apoptosis, respectively. An impairment of autophagy contributes to oxidative damage to lipids, proteins and nucleic acids especially due to slower mitochondria turnover. This bidirectional relation between oxidative stress and autophagy might be involved in various pathologies including AN [33].

Increased concentrations of plasma lipids in the patients with AN are associated with several mechanisms including alternation in hormonal regulation, and enhanced lipid reabsorption [34]. We assumed that the rise in plasma lipid levels in the patients with AN results in their higher susceptibility to oxidative damage and thus, systemic levels of TBARS would be elevated in patients with AN. Despite higher plasma lipid concentrations in girls with AN, plasma and urinary TBARS concentrations were not changed. On the other hand, higher salivary TBARS levels in the patients with AN could be connected to higher incidence of dental caries in patients with AN [35] that are implicated in higher salivary levels of TBARS [36]. Further, we observed inverse correlations of salivary TBARS and AGE-Fl with BMI. Previous study showed higher salivary MDA and AGEs in overweight and obese children compared with the normal weight children, and their positive correlation with BMI, respectively [37]. It seems that both obesity and underweight might affect salivary markers of oxidative stress.

Plasma AOPP are generated on proteins via hypochlorous acid produced by myeloperoxidase released from activated phagocytes [38], and may act as inflammatory mediators [39]. Thus, higher plasma AOPP levels in girls with AN compared with controls may indicate the activity of neutrophils or monocytes and inflammation. This is in line with previous study of Dalton et al. [40], showing that some inflammatory markers, including interleukin-6, interleukin-15 or tumor necrosis factor-beta are altered in patients with AN. However, the majority of quantified inflammatory markers including CRP, did not differ between patients with AN and healthy subjects [40]. Oxidative stress and changes in autophagy stimulate the release of proinflammatory cytokines [33]. In our study, CRP as a non-specific marker of inflammation did not differ between patients and controls. Increased plasma AOPP, however, suggest that the immune system is or at least was active. Given the lack

of infection the inflammatory response can be judged as inadequate although more inflammatory markers are needed to better characterize the immune status [41] that might contribute to multiorgan dysfunction associated with AN. Since urinary oxidative status could reflect changes of local as well as systemic oxidative status [42], the rise of plasma concentrations of AOPP in girls with AN probably caused elevation of their urinary levels.

Fructosamines – reversible early glycation products reflect plasma glucose levels over approximately the last two weeks. However, in the presence of hydrogen peroxides, fructosamines might be formed on albumin even under normoglycaemic conditions, and may in turn contribute to protein damage via the generation of ROS [43]. In our study, we did not reveal any changes in plasma and salivary fructosamines. Similarly, to AOPP, the rise of urinary fructosamines could be attributed to higher protein content in urine of the girls with AN.

On the other hand, concentrations of AGEs – irreversible glycation products - were elevated in plasma and saliva of the girls with AN. Cytotoxic effects AGEs, mediated through ROS and inflammatory cytokines production, are implicated in various diseases [44]. Exogenous sources of AGEs, such as smoking or a high dietary intake of AGEs-rich foods [45], increased production under persistent hyperglycaemia [46], or decreased renal elimination [44] as sources contributing to the rise in plasma AGEs in AN might be excluded. Alternative pathways of AGEs formation in vivo include reactions of proteins with α-dicarbonyls, produced, among others, via lipid peroxidation [47]. However, we did not observe increased TBARS concentrations in patients with AN. On the other hand, previously shown local accumulation of peroxidated lipid products in liver of patient with AN [48] might indirectly support this mechanism. Paradoxically, plasma AGEs are lower in obese compared to lean subjects [49], probably since lipophilic AGEs are preferentially trapped into fat tissue [50]. Whether in the case of anorexia-associated low body fat content its trapping capacity is exceeded with a consequent increase in plasma AGEs concentrations remains to be elucidated in further studies. Nevertheless, an increase of plasma AGEs probably creates concentration gradients for diffusion of low molecular weight AGEs into saliva [25].

Total antioxidant capacity of plasma is a non-specific method assessing the overall endogenous and exogenous antioxidants [14, 15]. Glutathione is an important endogenous antioxidant protecting cells from oxidative damage [13]. Plasma concentrations of uric acid, bilirubin, and albumin - substances that serve as endogenous scavengers of ROS - were lower in the patients with AN than in the controls. Albeit their concentrations were within the age- and sex-specific reference ranges, their lower levels in girls with AN could contribute to diminished concentrations of markers of antioxidant status - TAC and GSH/GSSG ratio. Although we cannot fully explain higher urinary TAC in patients with AN, it might be caused by increased urinary excretion of these substances [51, 52]. On the contrary, salivary GSH/GSSG ratio in the patients with AN was elevated, which is a consequence of lower GSSG in these patients. Since, GSSG is generated during reduction of peroxides via glutathione peroxidise, lower GSSG could be associated with decreased glutathione peroxidise activity or its increased turnover that is in line with previous study [53]. It suggests that salivary antioxidants could mirror local status rather than systemic changes. Differences in the salivary antioxidants could be associated with alternations of periodontal status related to the changes in oral microbiome [54] that often occurs in patients with AN [35].

The advantage of this study is a reasonably large cohort of young girls with AN, and analysis of several markers of oxidative status in different body fluids. We provide the first data on carbonyl stress markers in AN. The main limitation of the study is its cross-sectional nature, allowing only for comments on associations. Although the power analysis calculated for unequal sizes of groups was sufficient, the size of control group is quite small.

Our present study is the first study assessing wide range markers of oxidative and carbonyl stress in different body fluids, which represents a basis for further research. It has a cross-sectional design, which does not allow to analyze the effect of weight gain on changes of oxidative stress markers. Therefore, our next study should have a longitudinal design with regular check-ups during the follow up. Moreover, the link between oxidative status, autophagy and an inflammation in AN should be elucidated.

Conclusions

Our study demonstrated that anorexia-associated redox imbalance is accompanied by accumulation of oxidatively damaged proteins, which might exert a direct cytotoxic effect. Products of protein oxidation and glycation - AOPP, AGEs or fructosamines activate stress-sensitive pathways associated with increased expression of proinflammatory cytokines, growth factors, procoagulants, and adhesion molecules leading to micro- and macrovascular complications [55]. These pathways are also implicated in various chronic pathologies, such as inflammation, neurodegenerative, cardiovascular, nutritional diseases, atherosclerosis, etc. Thus, several complications of AN including dermatological signs, osteoporosis, myocardial atrophy, arrhythmias, nephropathy, gastrointestinal and neurological complications [2, 56] might be a direct consequence of accumulation of modified biomolecules over prolonged periods under diminished oxidative defence status. As disruption of redox homeostasis in young girls with AN appears to be an early finding, it could have a predictive value for development of disorders associated with AN. However, confirmation of this assumption requires longitudinal studies.

Abbreviations

AGEs: Advanced glycation end-products; AGE-FI: Advanced glycation end-products associated fluorescence; ALT: Alanine aminotransferase; AN: Anorexia nervosa; AOPP: Advanced oxidation protein products; AST: Aspartate aminotransferase; BMI: Body mass index; DSM-5: Diagnostic and Statistical Manual of Mental Disorders 5th Edition; eGFR: Estimated glomerular filtration rate; FRAP: Ferric reducing antioxidant power; GSH/GSSG: A ratio of reduced and oxidized glutathione; HDL-C: High density lipoprotein cholesterol; IQR: Interquartile range; MDA: Malondialdehyde; NICD: The National Institute of Children's Diseases; PCR: A ratio of protein and creatinine; RNS: Reactive nitrogen species; ROS: Reactive oxygen species; SD: Standard deviation; TAC: Total antioxidant capacity; TAG: Triacylglycerols; TBARS: Thiobarbituric acid reactive substances

Acknowledgements

This study was supported by the Grant of Ministry of Health of the Slovak republic 2018/36-LFUK-10 and by the Grant Agency of Ministry of Education, Science, Research and Sport of the Slovak Republic VEGA 1/0613/17. We are grateful to the Dr. Táňa Nováková from the practice of general paediatrician (National Institute of Children's diseases), who recruited healthy girls. We would like to thank the children and parents who participated in the study.

Authors' contributions

All authors significantly contributed to the design and implementation of the research, to the analysis of the results and to the writing of the manuscript. A.G.K, Ľ.P. and K.Š. conceived and designed research, Ľ.T. and A.Č. examined the patients, A.G.K, Ľ.T. and A.Č. collected the samples, A.G.K. and F.S. measured the samples and analyzed the data, A.G.K., K.Š. and L.P. interpreted results, A.G.K. drafted the manuscript, K.Š., P.C. and Ľ.P. edited the manuscript, all authors read and approved the final version.

Competing interests

The authors declare that they have no competing interest.

Author details

[1]Department of Paediatrics, The National Institute of Children's Diseases and Faculty of Medicine, Comenius University, Limbová 1, 83340 Bratislava, Slovakia. [2]Institute of Molecular Biomedicine, Faculty of Medicine, Comenius University, Bratislava, Slovakia. [3]Institute of Pathophysiology, Faculty of Medicine, Comenius University, Bratislava, Slovakia. [4]Department of Molecular Biology, Faculty of Natural Sciences, Comenius University, Bratislava, Slovakia. [5]Department of Medical Biology, Faculty of Medicine, Ege University, Bornova, Izmir, Turkey.

References

1. Herpertz-Dahlmann B. Adolescent eating disorders: update on definitions, symptomatology, epidemiology, and comorbidity. Child Adolesc Psychiatr Clin N Am. 2015;24(1):177–96. https://doi.org/10.1016/j.chc.2014.08.003.

2. Gibson D, Workman C, Mehler PS. Medical complications of anorexia nervosa and bulimia nervosa. Psychiatr Clin North Am. 2019;42(2):263–74. https://doi.org/10.1016/j.psc.2019.01.009.

3. Naisberg Y, Modai I, Weizman A. Metabolic bioenergy homeostatic disruption: a cause of anorexia nervosa. Med Hypotheses. 2001;56(4):454–61. https://doi.org/10.1054/mehy.2000.1199.

4. Nagata JM, Park KT, Colditz K, Golden NH. Associations of elevated liver enzymes among hospitalized adolescents with anorexia nervosa. J Pediatr. 2015; 166: 439–443.e1. doi: https://doi.org/10.1016/j.jpeds.2014.10.048.

5. Dalton B, Bartholdy S, Robinson L, Solmi M, Ibrahim MAA, Breen G, et al. A meta-analysis of cytokine concentrations in eating disorders. J Psychiatr Res. 2018;103:252–64. https://doi.org/10.1016/j.jpsychires.2018.06.002.

6. Berg D, Youdim MBH, Riederer P. Redox imbalance. Cell Tissue Res. 2004; 318(1):201–13. https://doi.org/10.1007/s00441-004-0976-5.

7. Valko M, Leibfritz D, Moncol J, Cronin MTD, Mazur M, Telser J. Free radicals and antioxidants in normal physiological functions and human disease. Int J Biochem Cell Biol. 2007;39(1):44–84. https://doi.org/10.1016/j.biocel.2006.07.001.

8. Morgan MJ, Liu Z. Crosstalk of reactive oxygen species and NF-κB signaling. Cell Res. 2011;21(1):103–15. https://doi.org/10.1038/cr.2010.178.

9. Behuliak M, Pálffy R, Gardlík R, Hodosy J, Halčák L, Celec P. Variability of thiobarbituric acid reacting substances in saliva. Dis Markers. 2009;26(2):49–53. https://doi.org/10.3233/DMA-2009-0606.

10. Witko-Sarsat V, Friedlander M, Capeillère-Blandin C, Nguyen-Khoa T, Nguyen AT, Zingraff J, et al. Advanced oxidation protein products as a novel marker of oxidative stress in uremia. Kidney Int. 1996;49(5):1304–13. https://doi.org/10.1038/ki.1996.186.

11. Münch G, Keis R, Weßels A, Riederer P, Bahner U, Heidland A, et al. Determination of advanced glycation end products in serum by fluorescence spectroscopy and competitive ELISA. Eur J Clin Chem Clin Biochem. 1997;35(9):669–77. https://doi.org/10.1515/cclm.1997.35.9.669.

12. Chung H, Lees H, Gutman S. Effect of nitroblue tetrazolium concentration on the fructosamine assay for quantifying glycated protein. Clin Chem. 1988;34(10):2106–11. https://doi.org/10.1093/clinchem/34.10.2106.

13. Zitka O, Skalickova S, Gumulec J, Masarik M, Adam V, Hubalek J, et al. Redox status expressed as GSH:GSSG ratio as a marker for oxidative stress in paediatric tumour patients. Oncol Lett. 2012;4(6):1247–53. https://doi.org/10.3892/ol.2012.931.

14. Benzie IF, Strain JJ. The ferric reducing ability of plasma (FRAP) as a measure of "antioxidant power": the FRAP assay. Anal Biochem. 1996;239(1):70–6. https://doi.org/10.1006/abio.1996.0292.

15. Erel O. A novel automated direct measurement method for total antioxidant capacity using a new generation, more stable ABTS radical cation. Clin Biochem. 2004;37(4):277–85. https://doi.org/10.1016/j.clinbiochem.2003.11.015.

16. Kim Y, Vadodaria KC, Lenkei Z, Kato T, Gage FH, Marchetto MC, et al. Mitochondria, metabolism, and redox mechanisms in psychiatric disorders. Antioxid Redox Signal. 2019;31(4):275–17. https://doi.org/10.1089/ars.2018.7606.

17. Kumar B, Kuhad A, Chopra K. Neuropsychopharmacological effect of sesamol in unpredictable chronic mild stress model of depression: behavioral and biochemical evidences. Psychopharmacology. 2011;214(4): 819–28. https://doi.org/10.1007/s00213-010-2094-2.

18. Diniz BS, Mendes-Silva AP, Silva LB, Bertola L, Vieira MC, Ferreira JD, et al. Oxidative stress markers imbalance in late-life depression. J Psychiatr Res. 2018;102:29–33. https://doi.org/10.1016/j.jpsychires.2018.02.023.

19. Kaufmann FN, Gazal M, Mondin TC, Cardoso TA, Quevedo LÁ, Souza LDM, et al. Cognitive psychotherapy treatment decreases peripheral oxidative stress parameters associated with major depression disorder. Biol Psychol. 2015;110:175–81. https://doi.org/10.1016/j.biopsycho.2015.08.001.

20. Maes M, Bonifacio KL, Morelli NR, Vargas HO, Moreira EG, St. Stoyanov D, et al. Generalized anxiety disorder (GAD) and comorbid major depression with GAD are characterized by enhanced nitro-oxidative stress, increased lipid peroxidation, and lowered lipid-associated antioxidant defenses. Neurotox Res. 2018;34(3):489–510. https://doi.org/10.1007/s12640-018-9906-2.

21. Rodrigues Pereira N, Bandeira Moss M, Assumpção CR, Cardoso CB, Mann GE, Brunini TMC, et al. Oxidative stress, l-arginine–nitric oxide and arginase pathways in platelets from adolescents with anorexia nervosa. Blood Cells Mol Dis. 2010;44(3):164–8. https://doi.org/10.1016/j.bcmd.2009.12.003.

22. Victor VM, Rovira-Llopis S, Saiz-Alarcon V, Sangüesa MC, Rojo-Bofill L, Bañuls C, et al. Altered mitochondrial function and oxidative stress in leukocytes of anorexia nervosa patients. PLoS One. 2014;9(9):e106463. https://doi.org/10.1371/journal.pone.0106463.

23. Solmi M, Veronese N, Luchini C, Manzato E, Sergi G, Favaro A, et al. Oxidative stress and antioxidant levels in patients with anorexia nervosa after oral re-alimentation: a systematic review and exploratory meta-analysis. Eur Eat Disord Rev. 2016;24(2):101–5. https://doi.org/10.1002/erv.2420.

24. Solmi M, Veronese N, Manzato E, Sergi G, Favaro A, Santonastaso P, et al. Oxidative stress and antioxidant levels in patients with anorexia nervosa: a systematic review and exploratory meta-analysis. Int J Eat Disord. 2015;48(7): 826–41. https://doi.org/10.1002/eat.22443.

25. Celec P, Tóthová Ľ, Šebeková K, Podracká Ľ, Boor P. Salivary markers of kidney function — potentials and limitations. Clin Chim Acta. 2016;453:28–37. https://doi.org/10.1016/j.cca.2015.11.028.

26. Schorr M, Thomas JJ, Eddy KT, Dichtel LE, Lawson EA, Meenaghan E, et al. Bone density, body composition, and psychopathology of anorexia nervosa spectrum disorders in DSM-IV vs DSM-5. Int J Eat Disord. 2017;50(4):343–51. https://doi.org/10.1002/eat.22603.

27. Regecová V, Hamade J, Janechová H, Ševčíková Ľ. Comparison of Slovak reference values for anthropometric parameters in children and adolescents with international growth standards: implications for the assessment of overweight and obesity. Croat Med J. 2018;59(6):313–26. https://doi.org/10.3325/cmj.2018.59.313.

28. National High Blood Pressure Education Program Working Group on High Blood Pressure in Children and Adolescents. The fourth report on the diagnosis, evaluation, and treatment of high blood pressure in children and adolescents. Pediatrics. 2004;114:555–76 https://doi.org/10.1542/peds.114.2.S2.555.

29. Badiou S, Dupuy AM, Descomps B, Cristolead JP. Comparison between the enzymatic vitros assay for creatinine determination and three other methods adapted on the olympus analyzer. J Clin Lab Anal. 2003;17(6):235–40. https://doi.org/10.1002/jcla.10103.

30. Watanabe N, Kamei S, Ohkubo A, Yamanaka M, Ohsawa S, Makino K, et al. Urinary protein as measured with a pyrogallol red-molybdate complex, manually and in a Hitachi 726 automated analyzer. Clin Chem. 1986;32(8): 1551–4. https://doi.org/10.1093/clinchem/32.8.1551.

31. Schwartz GJ, Schneider MF, Maier PS, Moxey-Mims M, Dharnidharka VR, Warady BA, et al. Improved equations estimating GFR in children with chronic kidney disease using an immunonephelometric determination of cystatin C. Kidney Int. 2012;82(4):445–53. https://doi.org/10.1038/ki.2012.169.

32. Moyano D, Sierra C, Brandi N, Artuch R, Mira A, García-Tornel S, et al. Antioxidant status in anorexia nervosa. Int J Eat Disord. 1999;25(1):99–103. https://doi.org/10.1002/(sici)1098-108x(199901)25:1<99::aid-eat12>3.0.co;2-n.

33. Mizushima N, Levine B. Autophagy in human diseases. Longo DL, editor. N Engl J Med. 2020;383(16):1564–76. https://doi.org/10.1056/NEJMra2022774.

34. Hussain AA, Hübel C, Hindborg M, Lindkvist E, Kastrup AM, Yilmaz Z, et al. Increased lipid and lipoprotein concentrations in anorexia nervosa: a systematic review and meta-analysis. Int J Eat Disord. 2019;52:611–29. https://doi.org/10.1002/eat.23051.

35. Sato Y, Fukudo S. Gastrointestinal symptoms and disorders in patients with eating disorders. Clin J Gastroenterol. 2015;8(5):255–63. https://doi.org/10.1007/s12328-015-0611-x.

36. Tóthová L, Kamodyová N, Červenka T, Celec P. Salivary markers of oxidative stress in oral diseases. Front Cell Infect Microbiol. 2015;5:73. https://doi.org/10.3389/fcimb.2015.00073.

37. Zalewska A, Kossakowska A, Taranta-Janusz K, Zięba S, Fejfer K, Salamonowicz M, et al. Dysfunction of salivary glands, disturbances in salivary antioxidants and increased oxidative damage in saliva of overweight and obese adolescents. J Clin Med. 2020;9(2):548. https://doi.org/10.3390/jcm9020548.

38. Capeillère-Blandin C, Gausson V, Descamps-Latscha B, Witko-Sarsat V. Biochemical and spectrophotometric significance of advanced oxidized protein products. Biochim Biophys Acta. 1689;2004(2):91–02. https://doi.org/10.1016/j.bbadis.2004.02.008

39. Liu SX, Hou FF, Guo ZJ, Nagai R, Zhang WR, Liu ZQ, et al. Advanced oxidation protein products accelerate atherosclerosis through promoting oxidative stress and inflammation. Arterioscler Thromb Vasc Biol. 2006;26(5): 1156–62. https://doi.org/10.1161/01.ATV.0000214960.85469.68.

40. Dalton B, Campbell I, Chung R, Breen G, Schmidt U, Himmerich H. Inflammatory markers in anorexia nervosa: an exploratory study. Nutrients. 2018;10(11):1573. https://doi.org/10.3390/nu10111573.

41. Fajgenbaum DC, June CH. Cytokine storm. N Engl J Med. 2020;383(23): 2255–73. https://doi.org/10.1056/NEJMra2026131.

42. Gyurászová M, Kovalčíková A, Janšáková K, Šebeková K, Celec P, Tóthová Ľ. Markers of oxidative stress and antioxidant status in the plasma, urine and saliva of healthy mice. Physiol Res. 2018;67(6):921–34. https://doi.org/10.3354 9/physiolres.933866.

43. Vlassopoulos A, Lean MEJ, Combet E. Oxidative stress, protein glycation and nutrition – interactions relevant to health and disease throughout the lifecycle. Proc Nutr Soc. 2014;73(3):430–8. https://doi.org/10.1017/S002 9665114000603.

44. Heidland A, Sebekova K, Schinzel R. Advanced glycation end products and the progressive course of renal disease. Am J Kidney Dis. 2001;38(4):S100–6. https://doi.org/10.1053/ajkd.2001.27414.

45. Šebeková K, Brouder ŠK. Glycated proteins in nutrition: friend or foe? Exp Gerontol. 2019;117:76–90. https://doi.org/10.1016/j.exger.2018.11.012.

46. Goh SY, Cooper ME. The role of advanced glycation end products in progression and complications of diabetes. J Clin Endocrinol Metab. 2008; 93(4):1143–52. https://doi.org/10.1210/jc.2007-1817.

47. Thornalley PJ, Langborg A, Minhas HS. Formation of glyoxal, methylglyoxal and 3-deoxyglucosone in the glycation of proteins by glucose. Biochem J. 1999;344(1):109–16. https://doi.org/10.1042/0264-6021:3440109.

48. Tajiri K, Shimizu Y, Tsuneyama K, Sugiyama T. A case report of oxidative stress in a patient with anorexia nervosa. Int J Eat Disord. 2006;39:616–8. https://doi.org/10.1002/eat.20326.

49. Šebeková K, Somoza V, Jarčušková M, Heidland A, Podracká L. Plasma advanced glycation end products are decreased in obese children compared with lean controls. Int J Pediatr Obes. 2009;4:112–8. https://doi. org/10.1080/17477160802248039.

50. Gaens KH, Da Stehouwer C, Schalkwijk CG. Advanced glycation endproducts and its receptor for advanced glycation endproducts in obesity. Curr Opin Lipidol. 2013;24(1):4–11. https://doi.org/10.1097/MOL.0b013e32835aea13.

51. Sitar ME, Aydin S, Çakatay U. Human serum albumin and its relation with oxidative stress. Clin Lab. 2013;59(9-10):945–52.

52. Stheneur C, Bergeron S, Lapeyraque AL. Renal complications in anorexia nervosa. Eat Weight. 2014;19(4):455–60. https://doi.org/10.1007/s40519-014-0138-z.

53. Karincaoglu Y, Batcioglu K, Erdem T, Esrefoglu M, Genc M. The levels of plasma and salivary antioxidants in the patient with recurrent aphthous stomatitis. J Oral Pathol Med. 2005;34(1):7–12. https://doi.org/10.1111/j.1600-0714.2004.00253.x.

54. Celecová V, Kamodyová N, Tóthová Ľ, Kúdela M, Celec P. Salivary markers of oxidative stress are related to age and oral health in adult non-smokers. J Oral Pathol Med. 2013;42(3):263–6. https://doi.org/10.1111/jop.12008.

55. Bigagli E, Lodovici M. Circulating oxidative stress biomarkers in clinical studies on type 2 diabetes and its complications. Oxidative Med Cell Longev. 2019:5953685–17. https://doi.org/10.1155/2019/5953685.

56. Cost J, Krantz MJ, Mehler PS. Medical complications of anorexia nervosa. Cleve Clin J Med. 2020;87(6):361–6. https://doi.org/10.3949/ccjm.87a.19084.

4

Adapting a Neuroscience-informed Intervention to Alter Reward Mechanisms of Anorexia Nervosa: a Novel Direction for Future Research

Ann F. Haynos[1*], Lisa M. Anderson[1], Autumn J. Askew[1], Michelle G. Craske[2] and Carol B. Peterson[1]

Abstract

Accumulating psychobiological data implicate reward disturbances in the persistence of anorexia nervosa (AN). Evidence suggests that individuals with AN demonstrate decision-making deficits similar to those with mood and anxiety disorders that cause them to under-respond to many conventionally rewarding experiences (e.g., eating, interacting socially). In contrast, unlike individuals with other psychiatric disorders, individuals with AN simultaneously over-respond to rewards associated with eating-disorder behaviors (e.g., restrictive eating, exercising). This pattern of reward processing likely perpetuates eating-disorder symptoms, as the rewards derived from eating-disorder behaviors provide temporary relief from the anhedonia associated with limited responsivity to other rewards. Positive Affect Treatment (PAT) is a cognitive-behavioral intervention designed to target reward deficits that contribute to anhedonia in mood and anxiety disorders, including problems with reward anticipation, experiencing, and learning. PAT has been found to promote reward responsivity and clinical improvement in mood and anxiety disorders. This manuscript will: (1) present empirical evidence supporting the promise of PAT as an intervention for AN; (2) highlight nuances in the maintaining processes of AN that necessitate adaptations of PAT for this population; and (3) suggest future directions in research on PAT and other reward-based treatments that aim to enhance clinical outcomes for AN.

Keywords: Anorexia nervosa, Positive affect, Reward, Treatment, Intervention, Neuroscience

Plain English summary

Past research has shown that people with anorexia nervosa (AN) have trouble experiencing positive emotions in response to many common life events (e.g., socializing, winning money). This tendency to under-respond to positive events is similar to that found in people with mood and anxiety disorders. However, people with AN also appear to feel more positive emotions when they think about or engage in eating-disorder behaviors (e.g., cutting

(Continued on next page)

* Correspondence: afhaynos@umn.edu
[1]Department of Psychiatry and Behavioral Sciences, University of Minnesota, 2450 Riverside Ave., Minneapolis, MN 55454, USA
Full list of author information is available at the end of the article

(Continued from previous page)
back on their eating, exercising, thinking about being very thin). For this reason, people with AN may continually turn to eating-disorder behaviors, rather than other actions, to feel good about themselves and their lives. In this paper, we describe a new treatment, Positive Affect Treatment (PAT), that we believe has the potential to help individuals with AN gain more happiness and fulfillment from their lives outside of their eating disorder. Our expectation is that such a change may result in individuals with AN no longer needing their eating disorder to feel good.

Introduction

Anorexia nervosa (AN) is a psychiatric disorder associated with serious physiological and psychological morbidity, increased risk of mortality, and, for some, enduring illness courses [1–3]. One empirically-supported treatment has emerged with the strongest efficacy for treating adolescent AN [4]. However, despite recent growth in efficacious treatments for adult AN, no existing intervention has emerged clearly superior over others [5]. As such, there have been calls for increased efforts to develop innovative interventions for this population that may more precisely target the maintenance mechanisms of this disorder [6]. Indeed, one potential barrier to effective treatment for AN is that many treatments to date have been limited in their incorporation of the field's growing knowledge on the maintaining mechanisms of AN [6, 7].

Several theories have suggested that aberrations in the experience of positive affect may perpetuate the symptoms of AN [8, 9]. These reward-based theories have been bolstered by an expansion of neuroimaging research that demonstrates abnormalities in the ways in which the brain processes reward in AN [10]. Despite a preponderance of evidence suggesting that problems with processing reward and positive affect play a critical role in the symptomatology of AN, no treatments for this population have been designed that designate increasing positive affect as a primary intervention target.

Here we briefly review evidence that reward processes present viable targets for AN treatment. We then outline and describe one potential approach for targeting reward abnormalities in AN: Positive Affect Treatment (PAT), a novel psychotherapy intervention that has been used to alter positive affect and reward processes in anxiety and mood disorders [11]. We suggest a proposed adaptation of this treatment for AN that we are currently testing (PAT-AN), and highlight potential avenues for future research. In addition to describing a promising treatment for AN, this manuscript highlights the need to consider positive affect as a critical target in interventions for AN.

Evidence for reward disturbances in AN

Many have comprehensively reviewed the reward literature in AN [8–10, 12–14]. Below we provide a selective overview of the literature in AN relevant to specific reward targets that have been determined to influence other mental health concerns [15], and to serve as appropriate

treatment targets in psychiatric populations [11]. Reward system dysregulation has been implicated in a number of psychiatric disorders [16]. Prominent neurobiologically-informed reward theories suggest that reward processing can be decomposed into three stages that occur before, during, and after reward receipt: reward anticipation (or "wanting"), experiencing (or "liking"), and learning [15, 17]. Reward anticipation refers to positive expectancy, desire, or effort for a future pleasant experience. Reward experiencing is the ability to derive pleasure from rewards once they are obtained. Reward learning reflects the ability to internalize the information provided by rewards and to use it to guide future approach behavior. A deficit in any one of these stages of the reward process could result in low positive affect or an inability to direct behavior towards valued life goals. Existing research indicates that individuals with psychiatric disorders vary on the degree to which reward anticipation, experience, or learning are impacted [18]. For instance, each of these reward stages appears to be impaired in depressive disorders [15, 18], but reward anticipation deficits appear to feature most prominently in schizophrenia [18].

Thus, we will review the evidence on the functioning of reward anticipation, experiencing, and learning in AN. Additionally, we will review the literature on disorder-specific reward processes (heightened reward anticipation, experiencing, and learning related to weight-loss cues) that differentiate AN from other disorders.

Reward anticipation

On self-report temperament measures, individuals with AN score lower on sensation-seeking measures, which capture drive to seek novel hedonic rewards, compared to healthy comparison (HC) and other eating-disorder groups [19]. Further, compared to HCs, individuals with AN demonstrate lower implicit and explicit anticipation of reward from palatable foods [20, 21] and interpersonal experiences, such as prosocial touch [22]. Individuals with AN, especially restricting subtype, also exhibit greater preference for delayed over immediate monetary gains compared to HCs and individuals with bulimia nervosa or binge eating disorder [23]. This pattern of delay discounting findings has been commonly attributed to decreased desire for immediate rewards, or increased engagement of cognitive control over immediate rewards [10].

Activity in particular brain regions, especially the ventral tegmental area, amygdala, and ventral striatum, has been associated with reward anticipation [15, 17]. There evidence of aberrant neural responding during anticipation of monetary rewards in AN. Some studies have found that individuals with AN over-engage brain regions promoting cognitive control and punishment, such as the dorsolateral prefrontal cortex and insula, during reward anticipation [24, 25]. This over-engagement of control- and punishment-related brain regions could indicate that the expectation of a positive event evokes fear or desire to exert top-down control over emotions. This hypothesis corresponds with data identifying that individuals with AN avoid positive, in addition to negative, emotional experiences [26]. Indeed, reducing prefrontal cortex activity (and, thereby, cognitive control) during reward anticipation has been associated with greater weight gain during treatment [24]. Individuals with AN also display less activation of brain regions traditionally linked to reward anticipation, such as the striatum, when delaying monetary receipt [27]; thus, expectation of immediate gratification may be less appealing in this group.

Reward experiencing

Research using implicit and explicit measures has shown that typically rewarding experiences, such as viewing or consuming palatable foods [20, 21, 28, 29] watching humorous videos [30, 31], or perceiving prosocial emotions or touch [22, 32, 33] are less subjectively pleasant, and in some cases more aversive, for individuals with AN compared to HCs. Reward experiencing has been shown to engage similar brain structures as reward anticipation, most notably the ventral tegmental area and striatum interacting with the orbitofrontal cortex [15, 17]. Individuals with AN exhibit less activation in reward-related brain regions (e.g., ventral tegmental area, dorsal striatum) in response to palatable food cues compared to those with bulimia nervosa [21, 34]. Paralleling the literature on reward anticipation, individuals with AN also show greater activation of cognitive control circuitry (e.g., medial or dorsolateral prefrontal cortex) during the receipt of food [35–37], social [38], and monetary [25] rewards compared to HC participants. Further, while hunger enhances reward experiencing among HC participants, reflecting a biological tendency to seek rewards (such as food) in a deprived state, reward-related brain activation is unaffected by hunger in AN [39]. Further, amphetamine-stimulated dopamine release in the ventral striatum, which is experienced by most as euphoric, is experienced instead as anxiogenic among individuals with AN [40]. The anxiogenic quality of dopamine release may explain why individuals with

AN find immediate, high-intensity, and uncontrollable rewarding stimuli less enjoyable [10].

Reward learning

Individuals with AN have been found to perform poorly on decision-making games that require them to learn to obtain rewards based on feedback [41]. Individuals with AN tend to demonstrate inflexible decision-making on these and other decision tasks; once rewarded, their responses persist without incorporating new and changing reward information [42]. The bias towards previously-rewarded stimuli parallels the presentation of AN, in which weight-loss behaviors persist well beyond the point at which they no longer garner reward [7].

Reward learning is most typically associated with activation among varied regions of the prefrontal cortex that process signals received from subcortical reward structures [15, 17]. There is evidence that individuals with AN demonstrate less differentiation between rewards and losses in the ventral striatum during reward learning tasks, suggesting a possible disruption of signal from this region interrupting consolidation of learning in the prefrontal cortex [43]. Similar findings pertain to prediction error (the discrepancy between expected and actual outcomes), which can be viewed as a learning signal, in AN. Greater prediction error (surprise at an unexpectedly good or bad outcome) typically leads to greater adjustment to future expectations. However, individuals with AN show abnormal prediction error responses to unexpected losses and gains of general stimuli (money) and disorder-specific stimuli (food) characterized by greater responsivity in punishment-related regions (e.g., insula) [24, 44]. Thus, findings relating to predictor error may reflect a tendency to prioritize punishment information over reward information in making future decisions.

Reward from weight loss cues and behaviors

In contrast to the above research on processing of disorder-irrelevant rewards, there is evidence for *elevated* reward anticipation, experiencing, and learning specifically in the context of weight loss in AN. This cue-specific reward responsivity differentiates AN from other psychiatric disorders (e.g., mood and anxiety disorders), which show deficit reward processing across contexts [15]. In AN, drive and activity for reward is enhanced in anticipation of weight-loss behaviors, such as restrictive eating and exercise [45, 46]. Additionally, individuals with AN show enhanced implicit and explicit reward experiencing in response to weight-loss cues, such as low-calories foods [20, 47, 48], exercise stimuli [49], and underweight bodies [50, 51]. Similarly, ecological momentary data collected from individuals with AN in real-time have found that positive affect is elevated during restrictive eating and exercise episodes [52, 53]. Self-conscious positive affect (e.g., pride) appears to be an especially important class of reinforcers maintaining eating-disorder behavior in AN. Studies have found that self-assurance increases in anticipation of exercise and following restrictive eating episodes in AN samples [53, 54] and that enhancing pride is cited as one of the primary motivators for restrictive eating among individuals with eating disorders, including AN [55].

There is also initial evidence for neural underpinnings of enhanced disorder-relevant reward in AN. Compared to HCs, individuals with AN demonstrate increased activity in the ventral striatum in response to pictures of underweight bodies [50, 56]. Further, activation and connectivity in cognitive control regions is decreased in response to low-calorie food and exercise images in AN [47, 57], suggesting that reward responding to these disorder-specific stimuli, in contrast to other rewards, is less constrained by cognitive control.

Summary and theoretical model

Theories developed through the investigation of reward-based behavior and brain activity suggest that reward anticipation, experiencing, and learning in AN are often diminished in response to certain situations (i.e., those involving food, social interaction, and monetary rewards). Further, there are data highlighting neurobiological disturbances in the functioning of reward-related neural circuitry in AN. There is also evidence of a complex interplay between cognitive control mechanisms and reward in AN, which may reflect cognitive barriers

impeding the ability to expect or experience reward. Paradoxically, rewards related to AN symptoms (i.e., weight loss) are highly appealing to this population.

As highlighted in Fig. 1, transactions between low levels of positive affect derived from typically rewarding experiences (unrelated to the eating disorder) and elevated positive affect from weight-loss cues may maintain eating-disorder symptoms over time. Limited access to reward from most positive experiences (due to low trait reward responsivity or cognitive control applied too frequently or inflexibly) can generate an aversive anhedonic state. In this case, if reward responding is heightened to weight loss and related cues, the resulting momentary positive affect enhancement could serve as a powerful instrumental reinforcer, thus strengthening eating-disorder symptoms. The more an individual engages in eating-disorder behavior and receives a subsequent reward, the more likely an individual will be behaviorally and biologically compelled to seek out disorder-related, as opposed to disorder-unrelated, rewards. Thus, over time, disrupted reward processing may increase the desire to engage in eating-disorder behavior, and eating-disorder behavior may enhance reward system abnormalities. Further, as starvation is prolonged and individuals become underweight, reward responding becomes biologically dampened to all stimuli [58], potentially enhancing the need to rely on the most compelling or practiced reward-eliciting experiences (e.g., weight-loss behaviors) to feel good. This cycle presents several critical targets that have not yet been addressed in AN treatment.

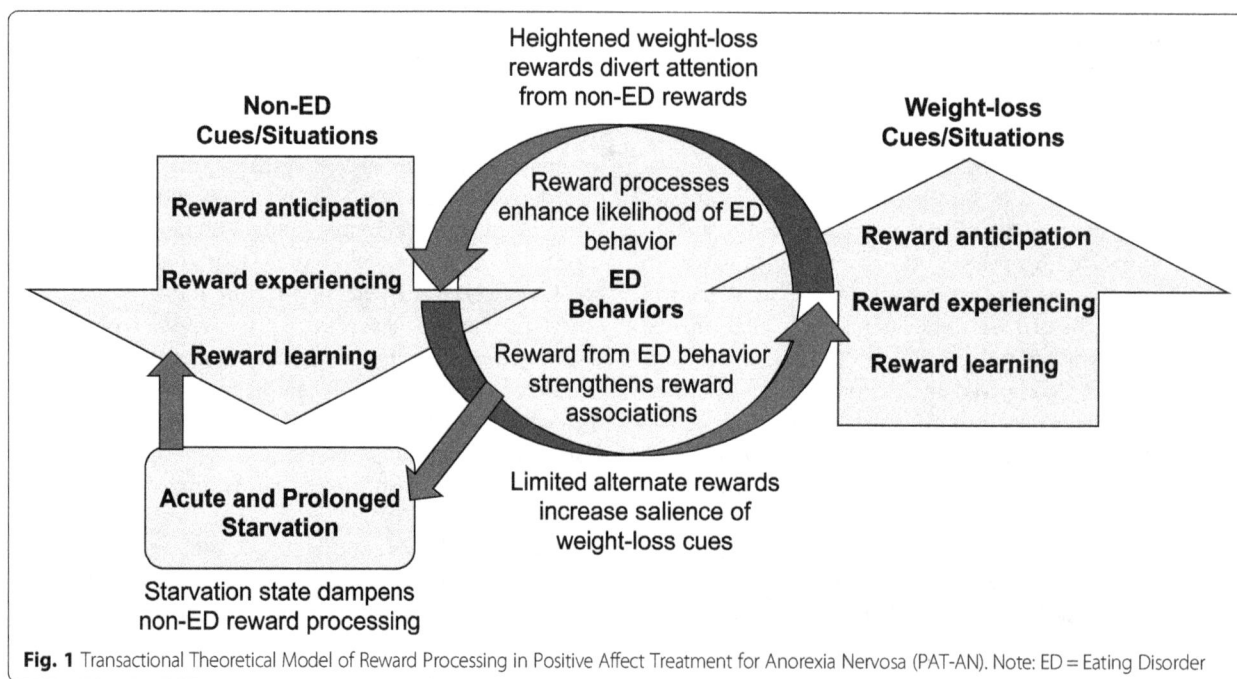

Fig. 1 Transactional Theoretical Model of Reward Processing in Positive Affect Treatment for Anorexia Nervosa (PAT-AN). Note: ED = Eating Disorder

Positive affect treatment: a potential approach to treating reward disturbances in AN

PAT is a treatment that has potential to impact reward abnormalities in AN. PAT is a cognitive-behavioral intervention designed by for the treatment of anhedonia in mood and anxiety disorders [11, 15]. Based on an affective neuroscience model, PAT aims to increase positive affect by engaging the appetitive "approach" system in contrast to the withdrawal "defensive" system that functions to avoid negative outcomes. A primary rationale for the development of PAT was the modest outcomes among existing treatments for depression and anxiety that more typically focus on reducing negative emotions [15]. PAT was specifically developed to target aspects of neurobiological reward processing outlined above: reward anticipation, experiencing, and learning [11]. In a randomized trial in which PAT was compared with a cognitive behaviorally-based negative affect treatment targeting threat sensitivity, PAT was more efficacious in increasing positive emotions and reducing negative emotions, depression, anxiety, stress, and suicidal ideation among individuals with depressive and anxiety disorders [11]. Other trials of this treatment are ongoing (ClinicalTrials.gov: NCT03439748).

The rationale for adapting PAT for AN is based on the above-described research demonstrating neurobiological-based reward and positive affect abnormalities in AN, which suggest that a treatment directly targeting positive affect may be well suited for this population. Below we provide an overview of the components and interventions included in PAT and the proposed adaptations that we suggest to accommodate the symptom presentation and presumed mechanisms of AN. These adaptations are currently being evaluated in an ongoing pilot study (ClinicalTrials.gov: NCT04007900). However, it is important to note that, at this point, the proposed adaptations constitute an idea warranting further investigation, rather than an empirically-supported treatment for AN. Although the scientific basis for PAT-AN is not yet established, the description of this treatment in this manuscript is intended as a launching point for consideration of potential applications of PAT (or alternate reward-based treatments) for AN. As such, we differentiate components that have been empirically tested in mood and anxiety disorders (Standard PAT) and the proposed adaptations to the PAT manual that we are currently testing in AN, for which empirical evidence is forthcoming (Proposed Adaptions for AN).

Overarching proposed adaptions for AN

In our pilot study, we have made three overarching changes to the PAT manual intended to support its application to AN. First, consistent with the original PAT manual [11], our adapted PAT-AN aims to increase positive emotions by using interventions to target global reward anticipation, experiencing, and learning. However, based on the above-described theoretical model (Fig. 1), we have adjusted PAT-AN also to emphasize reducing positive affect and reward associated with eating-disorder symptoms and replacing positive eating-disorder experiences with rewards derived independent of the eating disorder. Thus, the primary targets of treatment are considered: 1) to increase positive affect outside of eating-disorder symptoms; and 2) to decrease positive affect derived from eating-disorder behavior. To facilitate this adaptation to treatment goals, we have added an eating-disorder-specific module to the treatment. Although weight gain is expected and encouraged, it is hypothesized to result as a product of the primary treatment aims, and is not currently targeted separately from positive affect processes.

Second, to accommodate the additional eating-disorder module and to match PAT-AN to more standard eating-disorder treatment durations [59, 60], we extended PAT-AN from 16 [11] to 20 individual psychotherapy sessions, currently delivered in an outpatient setting. Thus, our proposed adaptation of PAT involves six, rather than the original five [11], therapy modules: Psychoeducation (Module 1), Pleasant Events Scheduling (Module 2), Attending to the Positive (Module 3), Cultivating the Positive (Module 4), Replacing Positive Aspects of the Eating Disorder (Module 5); and Relapse Prevention (Module 6) (see Table 1). In the ongoing pilot study of PAT-AN, participants have been permitted to pursue other concurrent treatments and PAT-AN has been delivered either in a standalone or adjunctive manner.

Third, due to the established difficulties accessing reward from social experiences in AN [22, 32, 33], we have proposed an adaptation in PAT-AN to explicitly use the therapeutic relationship as an opportunity to build connections between interpersonal relationships and positive affect. The hypothesis is that a therapeutic stance that is consistently non-judgmental, validating, and strengths-based may establish therapist appreciation of the patient's progress as a motivator for future behavior change [61].

Module 1: Psychoeducation
Standard PAT

PAT begins with an introductory session to establish the treatment rationale and expectations. Patients are provided information about the origin of PAT as a treatment for anxiety and depression, including an overview of initial treatment results in these populations [11]. The treatment introduction also provides psychoeducation about the different components of positive affect targeted in treatment and how increasing positive affect is distinct from decreasing negative

Table 1 Overview of Positive Affect Treatment (PAT) for Anorexia Nervosa (AN)

Module 1: Psychoeducation (Session 1)		
Activity	**Proposed Adaptations for AN**	**Target**
1. Treatment rationale: learning about treatment content, structure, goals, and background	Sharing AN-specific model; discussing how weight and eating goals will be integrated into primary goal of increasing non-eating-disorder-related positive affect	Education
2. Introducing positive mood: learning about positive mood, its importance, and its difference from negative mood	Considering which positive emotions are most closely linked to different eating-disorder behaviors	Education
3. Parts of mood and the mood cycle: learning about the components of mood and how these different parts can cause low positive mood	Discussing the impact of eating-disorder behaviors, starvation, and underweight on positive mood	Education
Module 2: Pleasant Events Scheduling (Sessions 2–7)		
1. Activity planning: identifying events to engage enjoyment, mastery, and/or values	Selecting non-eating-disorder activities that may share a similar function to eating-disorder symptoms; considering how to use exercise as a healthy, rather than disordered, reward (as needed); prioritizing social and long-term rewards; evaluating values	Reward anticipation
2. Activity engagement: executing planned events; recording event-reward associations	Recording link between positive affect, pleasant events, and eating-disorder symptoms; noticing cognitive barriers to positive affect	Reward experiencing and learning
3. Activity recounting: learning and practicing techniques to "savor" past pleasant experiences	Sharing pre-recorded exercise to provide a concrete script; option for socially "co-savoring" if struggling with experiential exercise	Reward experiencing
Module 3: Attending to the Positive (Sessions 8–11)		
1. Finding the silver lining: training to shift attention to positive aspects of daily life and positive stimuli	Noticing the silver lining of difficult aspects of recovery	Reward anticipation
2. Taking ownership: identifying associations between one's own behavior and rewards	Emphasizing the potential importance of taking ownership to increase a sense of self-control and agency in life; identifying and appreciating one's own behavior towards recovery	Reward experiencing and learning
3. Imagining the positive: learning to attend to positive future events	Sharing pre-recorded exercise to provide a concrete script; focusing on goals that will be facilitated through recovery	Reward experiencing and learning
Module 4: Cultivating the Positive (Sessions 12–15)		
1. Loving-kindness and appreciative joy: practicing mental acts of giving	Sharing pre-recorded exercise to provide a concrete script; increasing focus on love, kindness, and appreciation towards oneself to potentially reduce the need for eating-disorder behaviors to boost positive self-referential feelings	Reward experiencing
2. Generosity practice: practicing physical acts of giving	Noting the importance of balance of generosity towards others and towards oneself; increasing focus on generosity towards oneself to potentially reduce the need for eating-disorder behaviors to boost positive self-referential feelings	Reward experiencing
2. Gratitude practice: fostering the ability to appreciate the positive aspects of life	Noticing positive aspects of recovery	Reward experiencing
Module 5: Replacing Positive Aspects of the Eating Disorder (Sessions 16–19)		
1. Monitoring and replacing eating-disorder behavior: diverting attention away from eating-disorder behaviors to healthier alternatives that can elicit positive mood	Skill specific to proposed AN adaptation of PAT	Reward learning
2. Riding the roller coaster: delaying acting on eating-disorder behaviors when positive emotion is low	Skill specific to AN adaptation of PAT	Reward anticipation and learning
3. Counter-conditioning: incorporating positive experiences into situations associated with negative mood, especially surrounding eating-disorder triggers	Skill specific to proposed AN adaptation of PAT	Reward experiencing and learning
4. Breaking the links: removing environmental cues that are associated with positive emotions related to the eating disorder	Skill specific to proposed AN adaptation of PAT	Reward anticipation and learning
Module 6: Relapse Prevention (Session 20)		
1. Check-in: assessing mental health and brainstorming ideas about how to increase the experience of positive emotions	Evaluating progress on weight and eating restoration, as well as cognitive eating-disorder thoughts; planning for future eating-disorder lapses and relapses	Reward experiencing and learning

Note: Adapted from Craske et al., personal communication

affect. As in other treatments [59], an emphasis is placed on making refinements to the model according to the patient's experiences. If a patient is skeptical about the model fit with their personal experience, they are invited to "test" the model throughout treatment by noticing how positive affect affects their life and behavior. The importance of skill practice is emphasized and a workbook is provided to guide homework assignments.

Proposed adaptions for AN

In the pilot adaptation of AN, patients are also described how PAT has been adapted for AN to additionally target putative disorder-specific positive emotions. The proposed theoretical model (Fig. 1) is presented and discussed with the patient, emphasizing that individuals with AN may be prone to low positive affect for many reasons, including trait differences in how their brains process rewards and the impact of malnourishment [10]. The therapist highlights that weight-loss behaviors (e.g., exercise, purging) may lead to short-term increases in positive emotions, possibly contributing to the maintenance of AN, but also long-term decreases in positive emotion [58]. Therefore, they are informed that treatment will emphasize identifying other sources of positive emotion that do not involve engaging in eating-disorder behaviors. The importance of increasing cognitive flexibility around rewards is especially highlighted to individuals with AN, who appear to demonstrate enhanced cognitive control and rigidity surrounding rewards [24, 25, 35–38].

Patients are informed that, although weight and eating-disorder behaviors currently are not targeted as directly in PAT-AN as in other interventions (e.g., through monitoring food logs [59]), normalizing weight and eating are expected goals of treatment. Patients are given the expectation that they will be weighed weekly and that weight patterns will inform intervention (i.e., using the skills to increase weight if it decreases). Patients and therapists collaboratively decide how much the patient should know of their weight depending on the impact of this information upon positive affect. For instance, if the patient believes that learning about weight loss would making them feel good, reinforcing the presumed link between positive affect and eating-disorder symptoms, weighing may be blind and weight change discussed in terms of general patterns. In the current iteration of treatment, there is no formal monitoring of eating behavior built into treatment. However, the patient is informed that the therapist will check in on eating-disorder symptoms briefly at the beginning of each session and adapt skills for use in reducing reliance on eating-disorder behaviors.

Module 2: pleasant event scheduling
Standard PAT

Referred to as "augmented behavioral activation" [11], PAT Module 2 focuses on increasing behaviors that elicit positive affect. Originally described by Lewinsohn [62] the premise of pleasant events scheduling is that avoidance, disengagement, and rigid adherence to routine perpetuates low positive affect. Thus, PAT aims to identify and schedule new activities that elicit positive affect and then monitor the impact on mood. For many patients, small incremental goals are essential to build motivational momentum. Therefore, the variety and novelty of positive affect-eliciting activities gradually increases over treatment. Most critically, behavioral activation is followed by intensive savoring of positive activities through imaginal recounting. In and between sessions, patients are guided to recount the most positive moments of a pleasant activity, including a detailed re-imagining of the sensory and emotional experience, to enhance reward experiencing and learning.

Proposed adaptions for AN

In line with our proposed model of reward processing in AN (Fig. 1), the preliminary adaptation of Module 2 for AN currently focuses on identifying rewarding activities that are independent of or inconsistent with eating-disorder symptoms, especially those that elicit similar positive emotion states (e.g., pride, safety) as the eating-disorder behaviors of interest [55]. Under conditions in which positive affect has been closely linked with eating-disorder behaviors over time, values clarification exercises may be useful in identifying alternate important and fulfilling activities [63]. Because pride, self-control, and long-term rewards are so frequently linked to weight-loss behavior in AN [23, 53–55], we suggest that engaging in other non-eating-disorder activities that involve long-term planning or accomplishment may be especially fruitful for this population. Additionally, because of the noted deficits in social reward experiencing in AN [10], we surmise that goals involving social contact also may be important to encourage. The current manual also provides suggestions for adapting experiential exercise of pleasant event "savoring" to better suit the concrete thinking style characteristic of AN (e.g., re-experiencing in the form of a social conversation, rather than as an imaginal experience) [64].

Module 3: attending to the positive (cognitive training)
Standard PAT

PAT Module 3 emphasizes understanding and altering negative cognitive biases that can perpetuate low positive affect, particularly the tendency to focus only on negative stimuli without noticing neutral and positive stimuli in a situation [11]. In the "Silver Lining" exercise, for example, patients identify positive aspects of experiences initially considered negative. The process of focusing on positive stimuli increases both positive emotion and cognitive flexibility. Through the "Taking Ownership" skill, patients also practice identifying ways that they personally contribute to positive events to increase self-efficacy and reduce negative attributional bias. Additionally, Module 3 includes exercises to practice reward anticipation, in which patients repeatedly focus on imagining specific positive details of an upcoming positive event [65].

Proposed adaptions for AN

Given the evidence suggesting heightened or rigid cognitive control over reward in AN [24, 25, 35–38], increasing cognitive flexibility to enhance positive affect is likely to be an especially important skill in this population. Additionally, because self-conscious positive emotions have been especially linked to eating-disorder behaviors in AN [23, 53–55], the "Taking Ownership" skill may be particularly important to emphasize in order to build a sense of agency disconnected from eating-disorder symptoms. Further, in our current adaptation of PAT-AN, we have attempted to tie the exercises in this module to eating-disorder recovery as often as possible, for example, practicing finding the "silver lining" in eating a difficult meal or taking ownership of progress towards weight restoration.

Module 4: cultivating the positive (compassion training)
Standard PAT

Module 4 includes mindfulness-based exercises that increase reward experiencing [11], including loving kindness, generosity, gratitude, and appreciation practices [66–68]. In the loving kindness meditation, for example, the patient focuses on wishing happiness, safety, and peace towards others and themselves. In gratitude practice, the patient identifies and records things for which they feel grateful daily.

Proposed adaptions for AN

For individuals with AN, the association between eating-disorder symptoms and self-conscious emotions [23, 53–55] suggests that a self-focus in loving kindness, generosity, and gratitude exercises may be especially impactful in replacing the reward functions of eating-disorder behavior. However, it is possible that self-compassion-focused exercises would be challenging if individuals have relied on eating-disorder behaviors to generate positive self-directed feelings. Thus, in the current

iteration of PAT-AN, we provide examples of how to support patients who find self-compassion exercises challenging, such as allowing the patient to generate compassion for themselves in the past (e.g., as a child) or future (e.g., following recovery). As with other experiential exercises, we surmise that making the mindfulness-based exercises in this module as concrete as possible (e.g., with an audio recording) may be helpful for adapting to the cognitive style of many patients with AN [64].

Module 5: replacing positive aspects of the eating disorder
Proposed adaptions for AN

Module 5 was added specifically for the version of PAT-AN under investigation. As such, the utility of this module in the treatment of AN has not yet been determined. In this module, the goal is to decrease the experience of positive emotion associated with eating-disorder symptoms and to shift these positive emotions to contexts independent of the eating disorder, consistent with our theoretical model (Fig. 1). As such, many exercises have been drawn from established therapies that target other positively reinforced problematic patterns (e.g., drug abuse, non-suicidal self-injury) [69, 70]. The module starts with self-monitoring the antecedents and consequences of eating-disorder behavior to determine how eating-disorder behaviors may function to elicit positive affect (e.g., exercise leading to accomplishment). After monitoring, the first goal is to increase and differentially reinforce alternate rewards. Patients are guided towards engaging non-eating-disorder rewards that elicit similar positive emotions (e.g., working on a pride-inducing art project) when eating-disorder urges emerge. Counter-conditioning techniques are also used to increase positive emotions in eating-disorder-relevant situations typically associated with negative emotions (e.g., eating a meal) by pairing these situations with rewards (e.g., talking to a friend during the meal).

A second goal is to decrease the reward salience of eating-disorder behaviors. Patients are introduced the metaphor of "riding the rollercoaster" of positive mood to understand the transience of emotion. Patients practice "riding out" dips in positive emotion without engaging in eating-disorder behaviors. Further, the concept of breaking positive emotion links with eating-disorder behavior is also introduced, in which patients are encouraged to engage in behavior that proactively breaks the positive emotion to eating disorder links (e.g., deleting a calorie counting app, removing underweight pictures from social media).

Module 6: relapse prevention

Standard PAT

The final session of PAT serves as an opportunity to discuss treatment progress and review future strategies for increasing positive affect in order to avoid relapse.

Proposed adaptions for AN

In PAT-AN, further discussion may need to be placed on how patients can use PAT-AN skills to continue to reduce eating-disorder thoughts and behaviors. Because sub-threshold eating-disorder cognitions and behaviors continue to persist following treatment [71] and relapse rates are high in AN [72], it may be helpful for the therapist to normalize symptom fluctuations as signals to use PAT-AN skills, while also encouraging the patient to seek treatment when they are having trouble getting "back on track."

Potential benefits, pitfalls, and future directions of PAT-AN

There are many aspects of PAT that make it a compelling possible treatment for AN. Most strikingly, an approach in which positive affect and reward are primary treatment targets is entirely unique in eating-disorder treatment [8]. The existing literature demonstrating the existence of transdiagnostic reward-based targets and the positive outcomes of PAT for mood and anxiety suggest the potential for PAT-AN to address both AN and common comorbid conditions [73]. Positive affect has an effect on motivational behavior [74] and, therefore, may enhance the treatment motivation that is often lacking in AN [75] and reduce burnout potential among providers [76]. There are also several hypothesized limitations. Placing a primary focus on targeting positive affect may preclude focus on other important targets, including eating-disorder behavior change, or other putative mechanisms of AN, such as negative affect and habit [77, 78]. Certain aspects of the PAT model, particularly those that focus on experiential exercises, may be difficult for those with a more concrete or pragmatic worldview, such as is often described among individuals with AN [64]. Finally, a 20-session treatment length may not be sufficient to achieve symptom remission, especially for individuals with more severe and enduring AN [2]. However, until further data are available about the efficacy of PAT-AN, the potential benefits and pitfalls of the treatment remain hypothetical.

PAT-AN is in nascent stages of development; therefore, research is needed to determine the efficacy of this intervention for AN. Randomized, controlled trials comparing PAT-AN to treatment as usual or other interventions focused on altering eating-disorder symptoms or reward mechanisms will be a first step in understanding the utility of this treatment for AN [59, 63, 79]. Because PAT-AN is intended as a neuroscience-informed treatment, investigating effects of this treatment on putative behavioral and biological maintaining mechanisms of AN (e.g., frontostriatal reward circuitry and reduce frontoparietal control circuit function) may also be informative. Additionally, the initial test of PAT-AN is being conducted among outpatients with AN. Therefore, even following this trial, further information would be needed to determine if PAT-AN could be effective among populations with differing illness presentations (e.g., specific AN subtypes, BMI severities, and stages of illness) or in different treatment settings (e.g., inpatient). Further, it would be clinically useful to determine if PAT-AN can function as a standalone treatment, or how it could be incorporated as an adjunctive treatment in combination with other disorder-focused interventions (e.g., weight monitoring, meal support).

Conclusion

Many individuals who receive treatment for AN do not recover [2]. Therefore, the development and adaptation of innovative, alternative intervention approaches is critical. Recent treatment innovations within the anxiety and mood disorders fields [11] provide an optimal foundation from which to develop novel treatments that target reward-based mechanisms that have been long understudied and rarely addressed in AN treatment. Noting prior research implicating aberrant reward-based processing in individuals with AN, targeting positive affect and reward mechanisms via PAT-AN presents an apt, cutting-edge approach to treating this serious and pernicious disorder.

Abbreviations

AN: Anorexia Nervosa; HC: Healthy Comparison; PAT: Positive Affect Treatment; PAT-AN: Positive Affect Treatment for Anorexia Nervosa

Acknowledgements

The investigators express gratitude to Erin Gallagher and Kaitlin Wright for their contributions to the investigation described in this manuscript.

Authors' contributions

AH was responsible for the conception and primary composition and oversight of the treatment adaptation described herein and the manuscript. AH, LA, CP, and AA contributed to the treatment adaptation and manuscript design and initial drafting. MC provided intellectual consultation regarding all aspects of the treatment adaptation and manuscript. All authors read and approved the final manuscript.

Competing interests

The authors declare that they have no competing interests.

Author details

[1]Department of Psychiatry and Behavioral Sciences, University of Minnesota, 2450 Riverside Ave., Minneapolis, MN 55454, USA. [2]Department of Psychology and Department of Psychiatry and Biobehavioral Sciences, University of California, Los Angeles, Los Angeles, CA, USA.

References

1. Arcelus J, Mitchell AJ, Wales J, Nielsen S. Mortality rates in patients with anorexia nervosa and other eating disorders. A meta-analysis of 36 studies. Arch Gen Psychiatry. 2011;68(7):724–31. https://doi.org/10.1001/archgenpsychiatry.2011.74.

2. Eddy KT, Tabri N, Thomas JJ, Murray HB, Keshaviah A, Hastings E, et al. Recovery from anorexia nervosa and bulimia nervosa at 22-year follow-up. J Clin Psychiatry. 2017;78(2):184–9. https://doi.org/10.4088/JCP.15m10393.

3. Treasure J, Zipfel S, Micali N, Wade T, Stice E, Claudino A, et al. Anorexia nervosa. Nat Rev Dis Primers. 2015;1(1):15074. https://doi.org/10.1038/nrdp.2015.74.

4. Lock J, Le Grange D, Agras WS, Moye A, Bryson SW, Jo B. Randomized clinical trial comparing family-based treatment with adolescent-focused individual therapy for adolescents with anorexia nervosa. Arch Gen Psychiatry. 2010;67(10):1025–32. https://doi.org/10.1001/archgenpsychiatry.2010.128.

5. Brockmeyer T, Friederich HC, Schmidt U. Advances in the treatment of anorexia nervosa: a review of established and emerging interventions. Psychol Med. 2018;48(8):1228–56. https://doi.org/10.1017/S0033291717002604.

6. Glashouwer KA, Brockmeyer T, Cardi V, Jansen A, Murray SB, Blechert J, et al. Time to make a change: a call for more experimental research on key mechanisms in anorexia nervosa. Eur Eat Disord Rev. 2020;28(4):361–7. https://doi.org/10.1002/erv.2754.

7. Walsh BT. The enigmatic persistence of anorexia nervosa. Am J Psychiatry. 2013;170(5):477–84. https://doi.org/10.1176/appi.ajp.2012.12081074.

8. Coniglio KA, Christensen KA, Haynos AF, Rienecke RD, Selby EA. The posited effect of positive affect in anorexia nervosa: advocating for a forgotten piece of a puzzling disease. Int J Eat Disord. 2019;52(9):971–6. https://doi.org/10.1002/eat.23147.

9. O'Hara CB, Campbell IC, Schmidt U. A reward-centred model of anorexia nervosa: a focussed narrative review of the neurological and psychophysiological literature. Neurosci Biobehav Rev. 2015;52:131–52. https://doi.org/10.1016/j.neubiorev.2015.02.012.

10. Haynos AF, Lavender JM, Nelson J, Crow SJ, Peterson CB. Moving towards specificity: a systematic review of cue features associated with reward and punishment in anorexia nervosa. Clin Psychol Rev. 2020;79:101872. https://doi.org/10.1016/j.cpr.2020.101872.

11. Craske MG, Meuret AE, Ritz T, Treanor M, Dour H, Rosenfield D. Positive affect treatment for depression and anxiety: a randomized clinical trial for a core feature of anhedonia. J Consult Clin Psychol. 2019;87(5):457–71. https://doi.org/10.1037/ccp0000396.

12. Frank GK. Altered brain reward circuits in eating disorders: chicken or egg? Curr Psychiatry Rep. 2013;15(10):396. https://doi.org/10.1007/s11920-013-0396-x.

13. Kaye WH, Wierenga CE, Bailer UF, Simmons AN, Bischoff-Grethe A. Nothing tastes as good as skinny feels: the neurobiology of anorexia nervosa. Trends Neurosci. 2013;36(2):110–20. https://doi.org/10.1016/j.tins.2013.01.003.

14. Wierenga CE, Ely A, Bischoff-Grethe A, Bailer UF, Simmons AN, Kaye WH. Are extremes of consumption in eating disorders related to an altered balance between reward and inhibition? Front Behav Neurosci. 2014;8:410. https://doi.org/10.3389/fnbeh.2014.00410.

15. Craske MG, Meuret AE, Ritz T, Treanor M, Dour HJ. Treatment for anhedonia: a neuroscience driven approach. Depress Anxiety. 2016;33(10):927–38. https://doi.org/10.1002/da.22490.

16. Husain M, Roiser JP. Neuroscience of apathy and anhedonia: a transdiagnostic approach. Nat Rev Neurosci. 2018;19(8):470–84. https://doi.org/10.1038/s41583-018-0029-9.

17. Berridge KC, Robinson TE, Aldridge JW. Dissecting components of reward: 'liking', 'wanting', and learning. Curr Opin Pharmacol. 2009;9(1):65–73. https://doi.org/10.1016/j.coph.2008.12.014.

18. Szczypiński JJ, Gola M. Dopamine dysregulation hypothesis: the common basis for motivational anhedonia in major depressive disorder and schizophrenia? Rev Neurosci. 2018 Sep 25;29(7):727–44. https://doi.org/10.1515/revneuro-2017-0091.

19. Atiye M, Miettunen J, Raevuori-Helkamaa A. A meta-analysis of temperament in eating disorders. Eur Eat Disord Rev. 2015;23(2):89–99. https://doi.org/10.1002/erv.2342

20. Cowdrey FA, Finlayson G, Park RJ. Liking compared with wanting for high- and low-calorie foods in anorexia nervosa: aberrant food reward even after weight restoration. Am J Clin Nutr. 2013;97(3):463–70. https://doi.org/10.3945/ajcn.112.046011.

21. Jiang T, Soussignan R, Carrier E, Royet JP. Dysfunction of the mesolimbic circuit to food odors in women with anorexia and bulimia nervosa: a fMRI study. Front Hum Neurosci. 2019;13:117. https://doi.org/10.3389/fnhum.2019.00117.

22. Crucianelli L, Demartini B, Goeta D, Nisticò V, Saramandi A, Bertelli S, et al. The anticipation and perception of affective touch in women with and recovered from anorexia nervosa. Neuroscience. 2020;S0306–4522(20):30579. https://doi.org/10.1016/j.neuroscience.2020.09.013.

23. Lempert KM, Steinglass JE, Pinto A, Kable JW, Simpson HB. Can delay discounting deliver on the promise of RDoC? Psychol Med. 2019;49(2):190–9. https://doi.org/10.1017/S0033291718001770.

24. DeGuzman M, Shott ME, Yang TT, Riederer J, Frank GKW. Association of elevated reward prediction error response with weight gain in adolescent anorexia nervosa. Am J Psychiatry. 2017;174(6):557–65. https://doi.org/10.1176/appi.ajp.2016.16060671.

25. Ehrlich S, Geisler D, Ritschel F, King JA, Seidel M, Boehm I, et al. Elevated cognitive control over reward processing in recovered female patients with anorexia nervosa. J Psychiatry Neurosci. 2015;40(5):307–15. https://doi.org/10.1503/jpn.140249.

26. Wildes JE, Ringham RM, Marcus MD. Emotion avoidance in patients with anorexia nervosa: initial test of a functional model. Int J Eat Disord. 2010;43(5):398–404. https://doi.org/10.1002/eat.20730.

27. Decker JH, Figner B, Steinglass JE. On weight and waiting: delay discounting in anorexia nervosa pretreatment and posttreatment. Biol Psychiatry. 2015;78(9):606–14. https://doi.org/10.1016/j.biopsych.2014.12.016.

28. Anderson LM, Crow SJ, Peterson CB. The impact of meal consumption on emotion among individuals with eating disorders. Eat Weight Disord. 19(3):347–54. https://doi.org/10.1007/s40519-013-0084-1.

29. Soussignan R, Schaal B, Rigaud D, Royet JP, Jiang T. Hedonic reactivity to visual and olfactory cues: rapid facial electromyographic reactions are altered in anorexia nervosa. Biol Psychol. 2011;86(3):265–72. https://doi.org/10.1016/j.biopsycho.2010.12.007.

30. Davies H, Schmidt U, Stahl D, Tchanturia K. Evoked facial emotional expression and emotional experience in people with anorexia nervosa. Int J Eat Disord. 2011;44(6):531–9. https://doi.org/10.1002/eat.20852.

31. Davies H, Schmidt U, Tchanturia K. Emotional facial expression in women recovered from anorexia nervosa. BMC Psychiatry. 2013 Nov 7;13(1):291. https://doi.org/10.1186/1471-244X-13-291.

32. Cardi V, Di Matteo R, Corfield F, Treasure J. Social reward and rejection sensitivity in eating disorders: an investigation of attentional bias and early experiences. World J Biol Psychiatry. 2013;14(8):622–33. https://doi.org/10.3109/15622975.2012.665479.

33. Cserjési R, Vermeulen N, Lénárd L, Luminet O. Reduced capacity in automatic processing of facial expression in restrictive anorexia nervosa and obesity. Psychiatry Res. 2011;188(2):253–7. https://doi.org/10.1016/j.psychres.2010.12.008.

34. Brooks SJ, O'Daly OG, Uher R, Friederich HC, Giampietro V, Brammer M, et al. Differential neural responses to food images in women with bulimia versus anorexia nervosa. PLoS One. 2011;6(7):e22259. https://doi.org/10.1371/journal.pone.0022259.

35. Kerr KL, Moseman SE, Avery JA, Bodurka J, Simmons WK. Influence of visceral interoceptive experience on the brain's response to food images in anorexia nervosa. Psychosom Med. 2017;79(7):777–84. https://doi.org/10.1097/PSY.0000000000000486.

36. Uher R, Brammer MJ, Murphy T, Campbell IC, Ng VW, Williams SC, et al. Recovery and chronicity in anorexia nervosa: brain activity associated with differential outcomes. Biol Psychiatry. 2003;54(9):934–42. https://doi.org/10.1016/s0006-3223(03)00172-0.

37. Uher R, Murphy T, Brammer MJ, Dalgleish T, Phillips ML, Ng VW, et al. Medial prefrontal cortex activity associated with symptom provocation in eating disorders. Am J Psychiatry. 2004;161(7):1238–46. https://doi.org/10.1176/appi.ajp.161.7.1238.

38. Boehm I, King JA, Bernardoni F, Geisler D, Seidel M, Ritschel F, et al. Subliminal and supraliminal processing of reward-related stimuli in anorexia nervosa. Psychol Med. 2018;48(5):790–800. https://doi.org/10.1017/S0033291717002161.

39. Piccolo M, Milos G, Bluemel S, Schumacher S, Müller-Pfeiffer C, Fried M, et al. Food vs money? Effects of hunger on mood and behavioral reactivity to reward in anorexia nervosa. Appetite. 2019;134:26–33. https://doi.org/10.1016/j.appet.2018.12.017.

40. Bailer UF, Narendran R, Frankle WG, Himes ML, Duvvuri V, Mathis CA, et al. Amphetamine induced dopamine release increases anxiety in individuals recovered from anorexia nervosa. Int J Eat Disord. 2012;45(2):263–71. https://doi.org/10.1002/eat.20937.

41. Reville MC, O'Connor L, Frampton I. Literature review of cognitive neuroscience and anorexia nervosa. Curr Psychiatry Rep. 2016;18(2):18. https://doi.org/10.1007/s11920-015-0651-4.

42. Keegan E, Tchanturia K, Wade TD. Central coherence and set-shifting between nonunderweight eating disorders and anorexia nervosa: a systematic review and meta-analysis. Int J Eat Disord. 2020;54(3):229–43. https://doi.org/10.1002/eat.23430.

43. Wagner A, Aizenstein H, Venkatraman VK, Fudge J, May JC, Mazurkewicz L, et al. Altered reward processing in women recovered from anorexia nervosa. Am J Psychiatry. 2007;164(12):1842–9. https://doi.org/10.1176/appi.ajp.2007.07040575.

44. Frank GK, Collier S, Shott ME, O'Reilly RC. Prediction error and somatosensory insula activation in women recovered from anorexia nervosa. J Psychiatry Neurosci. 2016;41(5):304–11. https://doi.org/10.1503/jpn.150103.

45. Klein DA, Schebendach JE, Gershkovich M, Bodell LP, Foltin RW, Walsh BT. Behavioral assessment of the reinforcing effect of exercise in women with anorexia nervosa: further paradigm development and data. Int J Eat Disord. 2010;43(7):611–8. https://doi.org/10.1002/eat.20758.

46. O'Hara CB, Keyes A, Renwick B, Giel KE, Campbell IC, Schmidt U. Evidence that illness-compatible cues are rewarding in women recovered from anorexia nervosa: a study of the effects of dopamine depletion on eye-blink startle responses. PLoS One. 2016;11(10):e0165104. https://doi.org/10.1371/journal.pone.0165104.

47. Scaife JC, Godier LR, Reinecke A, Harmer CJ, Park RJ. Differential activation of the frontal pole to high vs low calorie foods: the neural basis of food preference in anorexia nervosa? Psychiatry Res Neuroimaging. 2016;258:44–53. https://doi.org/10.1016/j.pscychresns.2016.10.004.

48. Stoner SA, Fedoroff IC, Andersen AE, Rolls BJ. Food preferences and desire to eat in anorexia and bulimia nervosa. Int J Eat Disord. 1996 Jan;19(1):13–22. https://doi.org/10.1002/(SICI)1098-108X(199601)19:1<13::AID-EAT3>3.0.CO;2-Z.

49. Giel KE, Kullmann S, Preißl H, Bischoff SC, Thiel A, Schmidt U, et al. Understanding the reward system functioning in anorexia nervosa: crucial role of physical activity. Biol Psychol. 2013;94(3):575–81. https://doi.org/10.1016/j.biopsycho.2013.10.004.

50. Fladung AK, Grön G, Grammer K, Herrnberger B, Schilly E, Grasteit S, et al. A neural signature of anorexia nervosa in the ventral striatal reward system. Am J Psychiatry. 2010;167(2):206–12. https://doi.org/10.1176/appi.ajp.2009.09010071.

51. Horndasch S, Roesch J, Forster C, Dörfler A, Lindsiepe S, Heinrich H, et al. Neural processing of food and emotional stimuli in adolescent and adult anorexia nervosa patients. PLoS One. 2018;13(3):e0191059. https://doi.org/10.1371/journal.pone.0191059.

52. Fitzsimmons-Craft EE, Accurso EC, Ciao AC, Crosby RD, Cao L, Pisetsky EM, et al. Restrictive eating in anorexia nervosa: examining maintenance and consequences in the natural environment. Int J Eat Disord. 2015;48(7):923–31. https://doi.org/10.1002/eat.22439.

53. Ma R, Kelly AC. The fragility of perceived social rank following exercise in anorexia nervosa: an ecological momentary assessment study of shame and pride. Eat Weight Disord. 2020;25(6):1601–7. https://doi.org/10.1007/s40519-019-00797-3.

54. Haynos AF, Berg KC, Cao L, Crosby RD, Lavender JM, Utzinger LM, et al. Trajectories of higher- and lower-order dimensions of negative and positive affect relative to restrictive eating in anorexia nervosa. J Abnorm Psychol. 2017;126(5):495–505. https://doi.org/10.1037/abn0000202.

55. Wang SB, Fox KR, Mair P, Nock MK, Haynos AF. Functional assessment of restrictive eating: a three-study transdiagnostic investigation. J Abnorm Psychol. 2021; In press.

56. Fladung AK, Schulze UM, Schöll F, Bauer K, Grön G. Role of the ventral striatum in developing anorexia nervosa. Transl Psychiatry. 2013;3(10):e315. https://doi.org/10.1038/tp.2013.88.

57. Kullmann S, Giel KE, Hu X, Bischoff SC, Teufel M, Thiel A, et al. Impaired inhibitory control in anorexia nervosa elicited by physical activity stimuli. Soc Cogn Affect Neurosci. 2014;9(7):917–23. https://doi.org/10.1093/scan/nst070.

58. Kaye W. Neurobiology of anorexia and bulimia nervosa. Physiol Behav. 2008; 94(1):121–35. https://doi.org/10.1016/j.physbeh.2007.11.037.

59. Fairburn CG, Cooper Z, Doll HA, O'Connor ME, Bohn K, Hawker DM, et al. Transdiagnostic cognitive-behavioral therapy for patients with eating disorders: a two-site trial with 60-week follow-up. Am J Psychiatry. 2009; 166(3):311–9. https://doi.org/10.1176/appi.ajp.2008.08040608.

60. Peterson CB, Engel SG, Crosby RD, Strauman T, Smith TL, Klein M, et al. Comparing integrative cognitive-affective therapy and guided self-help cognitive-behavioral therapy to treat binge-eating disorder using standard and naturalistic momentary outcome measures: a randomized controlled trial. Int J Eat Disord. 2020;53(9):1418–27. https://doi.org/10.1002/eat.23324.

61. Tsai M, Yard S, Kohlenberg RJ. Functional analytic psychotherapy: a behavioral relational approach to treatment. Psychotherapy (Chic). 2014; 51(3):364–71. https://doi.org/10.1037/a0036506.

62. Lewinsohn PM. A behavioral approach to depression. In: Friedman RJ, Katz MM, editors. Psychology of depression: contemporary theory and research. Oxford: Wiley; 1974. p. 157–78.

63. Hayes SC, Strosahl KD, Wilson KG. Acceptance and commitment therapy, second edition: the process and practice of mindful change. New York: The Guilford Press; 2011.

64. Eichen DM, Matheson BE, Appleton-Knapp SL, Boutelle KN. Neurocognitive treatments for eating disorders and obesity. Curr Psychiatry Rep. 2017;19(9): 62. https://doi.org/10.1007/s11920-017-0813-7.

65. Holmes EA, Mathews A, Mackintosh B, Dalgleish T. The causal effect of mental imagery on emotion assessed using picture-word cues. Emotion. 2008;8(3):395–409. https://doi.org/10.1037/1528-3542.8.3.395.

66. Froh JJ, Kashdan TB, Ozimkowski KM, Miller N. Who benefits the most from a gratitude intervention in children and adolescents? Examining positive affect as a moderator. J Posit Psychol. 2009;4(5):408–22. https://doi.org/10.1080/17439760902992464.

67. Hofmann SG, Grossman P, Hinton DE. Loving-kindness and compassion meditation. Potential for psychological interventions. Clin Psychol Rev. 2011; 31(7):1126–32. https://doi.org/10.1016/j.cpr.2011.07.003.

68. Wood AM, Froh JJ, Geraghty AW. Gratitude and well-being: a review and theoretical integration. Clin Psychol Rev. 2010;30(7):890–905. https://doi.org/10.1016/j.cpr.2010.03.005.

69. Marlatt GA, Donovan DM. Relapse prevention: maintenance strategies in the treatment of addictive behaviors. 2nd ed. New York: Guilford Press; 2004.

70. Linehan M. Cognitive-behavioral treatment of borderline personality disorder. New York: Guilford Press; 1993.

71. Bardone-Cone AM, Harney MB, Maldonado CR, Lawson MA, Robinson DP, Smith R, et al. Defining recovery from an eating disorder: conceptualization, validation, and examination of psychosocial functioning and psychiatric comorbidity. Behav Res Ther. 2010 Mar;48(3):194–202. https://doi.org/10.1016/j.brat.2009.11.001.

72. Pike KM. Long-term course of anorexia nervosa: response, relapse, remission, and recovery. Clin Psychol Rev. 1998;18(4):447–75. https://doi.org/10.1016/s0272-7358(98)00014-2.

73. Hudson JI, Hiripi E, Pope HG Jr, Kessler RC. The prevalence and correlates of eating disorders in the National Comorbidity Survey Replication. Biol Psychiatry. 2007;61(3):348–58. https://doi.org/10.1016/j.biopsych.2006.03.040.

74. Fredrickson BL. The role of positive emotions in positive psychology. The broaden-and-build theory of positive emotions. Am Psychol. 2001;56(3):218–26. https://doi.org/10.1037//0003-066x.56.3.218.

75. Sjogren M. Anorexia nervosa and motivation for behavioral change - Can it be enhanced? J Psychol Clin Psychiatry. 2017;8(4):00489. https://doi.org/10.15406/jpcpy.2017.08.00489.

76. Warren CS, Schafer KJ, Crowley ME, Olivardia R. A qualitative analysis of job burnout in eating disorder treatment providers. Eat Disord. 2012;20(3):175–95. https://doi.org/10.1080/10640266.2012.668476.

77. Haynos AF, Fruzzetti AE. Anorexia nervosa as a disorder of emotion dysregulation: evidence and treatment implications. Clin Psychol. 2011;18(3):183–02. https://doi.org/10.1111/j.1468-2850.2011.01250.x.

78. Steinglass JE, Walsh BT. Neurobiological model of the persistence of anorexia nervosa. J Eat Disord. 2016;4(1):19. https://doi.org/10.1186/s40337-016-0106-2.

79. Martell CR, Dimidjian S, Herman-Dunn R. Behavioral activation for depression: a clinician's guide. New York: Guilford; 2010.

5

The Maudsley Anorexia Nervosa Treatment for Adults (MANTRA): a Feasibility Case Series of an Integrated Group Based Approach

Helen Startup[1]* ⓘ, Mary Franklin-Smith[2], William Barber[1], Nicola Gilbert[1], Yael Brown[3], Danielle Glennon[3], Akira Fukutomi[3] and Ulrike Schmidt[4]

Abstract

Background: Individuals with Anorexia Nervosa (AN) typically struggle in social and emotional contexts. An Integrated Group Based approach for the delivery of MANTRA - The Maudsley Anorexia Nervosa Treatment for Adults – extends current NICE recommended therapy by augmenting treatment with opportunities for experiential practice in a group context. A feasibility case series, delivered across three NHS community services is presented.

Methods: The design was a case series of four Integrated Group MANTRA treatments delivered across three NHS sites ($N = 29$). Feasibility data of: retention, acceptability and effectiveness; alongside the qualitative capture of participant experiences of treatment is presented.

Results: Primary outcomes suggest treatment acceptability. Participants committed to treatment with only 2 dropouts. There was significant change with medium effect sizes for eating disorder cognitions and symptoms (as measured by the global score on EDEQ) and BMI. Core themes emerging from qualitative analysis captured the value of the relational aspect of the treatment, the incorporation of experiential methods, and the opportunity to draw on the support of the group members to reduce shame and stigma.

Conclusions: An Integrated Group based MANTRA approach is a feasible and effective alternative intervention for community Eating Disorder services.

* Correspondence: helen.startup@sussexpartnership.nhs.uk
[1]Sussex Partnership NHS Foundation Trust, Sussex Eating Disorders Service, Brighton, UK
Full list of author information is available at the end of the article

Plain English summary

Treatments for Anorexia Nervosa (AN) are somewhat effective, but there is room for improvement. A core struggle for individuals with Anorexia Nervosa is managing emotions especially in a social context. One of the leading treatments for AN - MANTRA – was adapted to be delivered in a group to provide opportunities for individuals to practice experiencing and managing emotions amongst others. We hoped that being in a group could help tackle the shame and isolation that many people with AN endure. Patients seemed to find value in this approach and there are early signs that it may support people on their journey of recovery from Anorexia Nervosa.

Keywords: Anorexia nervosa, Eating disorders, Group treatment, Emotion regulation

Background

Anorexia Nervosa (AN) characterised by restricted eating, driven by intense fear, in the context of weight, shape and eating concerns [1] has the highest mortality rates of any psychiatric disorder [2, 3]. Incidence is rising; both community service demand and inpatient admissions have increased [NHS Digital, 2017 (digital.nhs.uk)]. AN is not simply a disorder of eating - 60% of individuals have significant personality disorder features (such as emotional dysregulation) and many have anxiety, depression, OCD and other Axis 1 presentations [4, 5]. This routine occurrence of co-morbid difficulties indicates an evidence-based, modularised approach to conceptualisation and treatment.

The Maudsley Anorexia Nervosa Treatment for Adults (MANTRA) offers this [6]. It is NICE recommended and used across UK services and internationally [7]. MANTRA is as effective as the other NICE recommended treatments at improving AN outcomes [8–12]. A Cognitive-Interpersonal Maintenance Model specifies 4 domains of biological and psychological predisposing and maintaining factors: 1) the emotional and social mind, 2) identity, 3) thinking styles, and 4) relationships [13, 14] which map onto intervention targets. MANTRA is a manualised modularised flexible and effective treatment for AN; well liked by patients and therapists [15, 16]. However, outcomes for all 3 leading AN treatments lag behind outcomes for other Axis 1 Presentations [17]. Opportunities are potentially being lost in translation of the known maintenance factors at treatment delivery.

A core MANTRA maintenance loop involves the emotional and social mind. Individuals with AN can struggle with emotional processing, particularly in interpersonal contexts [18, 19]. Difficulties include; identification of emotions, emotional tolerance and integration of emotional material into the self and sense of self in the social world [19–23]. Unfortunately, the starved state achieves emotional bluntness effectively [24], and high levels of worry and rumination can further suppress emotion and worsen ED symptoms [25]. FMRI studies confirm this pattern; individuals with AN who exhibit emotional suppression or distancing show high rumination and worse weight gain outcomes [26]. Individuals are drawn to AN

to cope with limited 'real world' opportunities to update this coping repertoire [19].

A body of work has focused on enhancing emotional processing in the treatment of those with AN (cf. [27]), however, treatments to date underestimate the importance of direct, meaningful interpersonal exposure to maximise change in social and emotional domains. Opportunities to support the emotional regulation of others, as well as receiving emotional support can target affective and interpersonal deficits [18, 28–30]. Furthermore, the Window of Emotional Tolerance (WoT) for those with AN is narrow; intellectualised - or 'paper and pencil' type approaches to therapy can enable patients to remain 'safe' yet emotionally 'cut off' blocking social and emotional processing [31]. Chair work, for example, has shown promise in fostering compassion in relation to the Anorexic Voice [32], and imagery techniques can augment classic CBT when challenging the 'restrictive mode' in AN [33]. Creative approaches with experiential foci, such as drama therapy methods [34, 35], chair work [36, 37], imagery work [38] and play [39] stretch an individual's WoT encouraging new emotional experiences to update old schemata.

Treatment delivery that maximally targets the Emotional and Social Mind mechanism within the MANTRA treatment is important and may be achieved by offering MANTRA within an integrated, group format. The modular arrangement of MANTRA lends itself to a group format whilst more idiosyncratic elements can be delivered within individual sessions. This combination of individual and group formats works well for the Emotional and Social Mind Integrated Bulimia Nervosa treatment [40] and is advocated in the broader psychotherapy literature [41]. The group format provides a supportive live arena for giving and receiving emotional regulation experiences (via attunement, supported social problem solving, safe disclosure of behaviours deemed shameful, as well as self- and other-directed compassion) and for stretching the WoT via the incorporation of in situ experiential methods (such as imagery and chair and role work) which are more likely to enhance emotional connectedness and provide opportunity to update schemata (cf. [36]). It has been highlighted that the group setting serves as an 'interpersonal laboratory' to practice interpersonal skills [42]. Dynamics such as unhelpful competition between group members, sometimes highlighted as a reason against group treatments for AN, can be explored, alongside the elements of group facilitation required to navigate this and turn it to therapeutic use. Individual sessions have a practical focus and foster alliance building. Dips in motivation are discussed, idiosyncratic aspects of an individual's formulation can be addressed and ED relevant goals negotiated and monitored. They provide space to enable any areas that might inhibit the individual to make maximum gain from the group programme to be addressed, therefore guarding against drop out.

This paper describes MANTRA treatment delivery translated into an integrated group-based model, drawing on theories of emotion regulation in context [28], dramatherapy methods [34, 35] and experiential treatments such as schema therapy [36]. Interventions are 'lifted' off the page, encouraging individuals from staying safe yet 'cut off 'and providing opportunities for social and emotional learning and to directly target schemata around shame and isolation. Retention, acceptability and preliminary treatment outcome data is presented regarding this new integrated group-based treatment as delivered across three NHS sites in the UK. Outcomes highlight the potential benefits of an integrated group-based MANTRA approach for patients with Anorexia Nervosa.

Method
Ethical considerations
The UK National Health Service National Research Ethics Service guidance [43] established that this study did not require ethical approval as outcomes were collected as part of routine clinical practice. All participants were aware that their data could be used for evaluation purposes and that all data would be fully anonymised assuring no breaches of confidentiality.

Design
An uncontrolled case series design was used to examine the evidence for an integrated group-based MANTRA intervention. We refer to the treatment as an 'integrated' approach because of the combination of both group and individual sessions. Participants were recruited from three specialist adult eating disorder services between September 2018 to March 2020. Outcomes were reported at assessment, prior to treatment, upon completion of treatment and, for two of the sites, (South London and Sussex), at 6-month follow up. In addition, qualitative group feedback, using semi-structured post intervention questions, was collected from participants and therapists post intervention.

Participants
Participants were recruited from 3 NHS Outpatients ED service sites across England: South London and Maudsley Foundation Trust (Site 1), Sussex Partnership Foundation Trust (Site 2), Leeds and York Partnership Foundation Trusts (Site 3). Consecutive referrals were offered the group if they were; (a) > 18 yrs., and (b) had a DSM-IV diagnosis of anorexia nervosa or Other Specified Feeding Disorder (OSFED), with a body mass index (BMI) < 18.5 kg/m^2. Patients were excluded if they had life-threatening AN requiring intensive treatment, or had insufficient knowledge of English language to engage in the treatment, intellectual disability, severe mental or physical illness needing treatment in its own right (e.g. psychosis), substance dependency or pregnancy.

Outcome measures
Clinical assessments (BMI and the Eating Disorder Examination Questionnaire) took place before and after the group and at 6 months follow up for sites 1 and 2. Group evaluation feedback forms were completed at the final group session.

Body mass index (BMI)
Patient BMI was recorded at each time point.

Eating disorder examination questionnaire (EDE-Q 6.0, [44, 45])
The EDE-Q is a 28-question measure of severity for eating disorders. Items are a combination of open-ended questions requesting frequency of behaviours as well as scoring responses from 0 (no days) to 6 (everyday). Responses are summed into a global score for eating disorder psychopathology by averaging the four EDE-Q subscales: Restraint, eating concern, shape concern and weight concern.

Group evaluation forms
Self-report questionnaires were used to evaluate participants' experience of group-based MANTRA. These were standard service related measures, largely open-ended and focused on the participant experience of the intervention.

Intervention
Group-based MANTRA has been adapted from the standard MANTRA manual [6] with the goal of augmenting change in the social and emotional domain through the use of group processes and live experiential methods [46]. Of note the MANTRA manual is not designed as a 'paper and pencil' workbook, it is a useful guide to supplement collaborative clinical work. The experiential interventions within this integrated group treatment are in line with theoretical goals underpinning

the standard manual, but are of particular relevance and utility to a group setting.

Format of the intervention

Integrated Group MANTRA combines a group delivery format with a number of individual sessions. The group aspect is delivered over twenty, weekly, 90-min group sessions. Two group facilitators each take half of the group members for their individual sessions. Patients are offered 2–8 individual therapy sessions in addition to the group programme, at least two of these being prior to the group starting. The aim is for a group size of 8 to 12 patients. Group facilitators adopt a motivational, curious stance. The group schedule is roughly organised as in Table 1. The session format involves: group check-in, the main event or session topic, and a group check-out, with homework usually from the MANTRA workbook [6] and stemming from the topic of the session.

Individual sessions

Patients have at least two individual sessions prior to the group commencing. If indicated a further two can be spaced out over the course of the intervention. Each individual session is an hour long and practical rather than experiential in foci. The goal of these sessions is: 1) to introduce the manual, to establish baseline motivation and enhance this by drawing on exercises from relevant early MANTRA workbook sessions, including formulation 2) to psycho-educate in regard weight, nutrition and links to the putative maintenance factors and to set initial weight and nutrition targets, 3) to provide time for questions and to work through any worries or practicalities around joining the group. Ongoing individual sessions are used flexibly alongside the group programme. Addition individual sessions were used to problem solve idiosyncratic concerns that arose as the treatment progressed that were not fully addressed in the group. Examples included provision of psycho-education and guidance around managing binge/purge cycles, discussing interpersonal worries

triggered outside of the group, or for one individual considering the role of increased flashbacks as weight increased.

Management of Risk

Prior to each group session patients were weighed by a clinician; they arrived 15 mins ahead of the group so that this could be done without impacting on group time. Where possible their allocated therapist was also the person who weighed them and weighing took place in a clinic room away from other group members. Time was allowed for a brief check-in around weight and nutrition goals, as well as exploring the emotional impact of any weight change directly within the group setting. If further specific clinical support was needed, such as time to discuss a boost to nutrition goals or involvement of a family member, additional individual sessions would be scheduled (in line with the protocol). Where additional stepped up care was indicated this was managed in the usual way by the service.

Key apparatus

Communicube. This is used to support check-ins and outs (www.communicube.co.uk). A Communicube is a clear structure of shelves with 5 levels, for the purposes of the group we tend to work with these levels as symbolic of levels of conscious awareness, but they can also be used to think about' levels' present within our bodies, our families and the group itself. Group participants are invited to select an object or card (objects were gathered via charity shops as well as an email request around the departments to bring in any small objects, toys, pictorial cards etc.) to reflect their emotional state and the level of awareness they had of their current emotional world. Common emotional themes often fed into the main topic of discussion. At the check-out patients are invited again to reflect on the session using the Communicube. Reflections do not need to be verbalised and can be represented using an object, sometimes other group members put voice to the feeling state.

Table 1 Key features of the integrated group MANTRA programme

Module (workbook chapter)		Number of sessions	Content
5	Formulation	1–4	1:1 vicious flower formulation, preparing for working in a group, working with loved ones in their support network and SMART goal setting.
7	Social and Emotional Mind	6	Understanding of emotions/feelings, range of emotions, feelings and behaviours towards loved ones, externalising the inner critic, reflecting and responding to emotions.
8	Thinking Styles	4	Identifying thinking style, how thinking styles perpetuates AN, and alternative thinking styles.
9	Identity	4–6	Sense of identity with and without ED, personal values and interests/hobbies, practicing the healthy flourishing self, challenging ED rules.
4	Nutrition	3–4	Each module has an attached nutrition model to link course learning and diet. Module 1) Link between food and mood; Module 2) how diet impacts/influences thinking style; Module 3) how their sense of self is affected by nutritional needs. There is one additional session which focuses on relapse prevention and nutritional needs post discharge.

Session focus and delivery methods

The main event changes by module and session. Each session aims to target one of the putative maintenance factors and there are a range of delivery methods for achieving this. Some of these methods are drawn directly from the MANTRA manual and some were specific in delivery to the group format. Therapists flexibility choose from a range of different ways of working, some of which are listed in Table 1 and full details are in Franklin-Smith (2019).

Treatment fidelity

All therapists had been trained and were experienced in delivering individual MANTRA, training in the group model was provided by one of the authors, MFS. The three sites met regularly to assure adherence to the therapist manual [46] for the group intervention as well as to share ongoing practice and supervisory reflections and learnings.

Data analysis

Quantitative data were analysed using IBM SPSS Statistics Version 26. Demographic data is presented as means, standard deviation and frequency where appropriate. Paired sample t-tests were used to compare means at assessment with post-group for BMI, and because of insufficient EDEQ data at assessment, means were compared for this variable at baseline and post-group. Effect sizes are reported using Pearson's r correlation coefficients. Follow up data were available for two participating sites and therefore an additional repeated measures one-way ANOVA was run comparing BMI and timepoint.

Qualitative

The open-ended questions on the group evaluation forms were analysed using framework analysis methodology [47]. Authors HS, NG and WB familiarised themselves with the data and through regular discussion developed a framework consisting of five overarching themes from issues originating in the familiarisation stage, as well as a priori concerns about the adaptation of MANTRA for a group setting. Data were then indexed onto this framework and summarised, following which authors HS, NG, and WB collectively mapped and interpreted the data, discussing alternative explanations and inconsistent findings.

Results

Participants

Figure 1 documents patient flow through the case series. Twenty-nine participants were recruited to Group Based MANTRA. Of those who took part in treatment, 27 (93.1%) were considered 'completers' by attending 70%

of the programme. Participant age ranged from 18 to 54 yr (M = 29.83; SD = 10.21) and they were primarily female (89.7%). The average BMI at assessment was 16.79 (SD = 1.2) and 93.1% had a diagnosis of AN – restriction subtype.[1] Average duration of eating disorder was 9.26 years (SD = 9.9) with mean age of onset 22.04 years (SD = 8.71). In regard treatment history; 44.8% had received previous outpatient treatment, and 13.8% a previous ED inpatient admission. Full demographics are presented in Table 2.

Groups

In total, four groups took place across 3 sites with a median attendance of 7 participants per group session (Range = 6 to 9). Average number of group sessions attended was 15.17 (SD = 3.86) alongside 7.3 individual sessions (SD = 3.85).

Paired samples t-test

Following completion of group-based MANTRA, there was a significant increase in BMI with a medium effect size from assessment to post treatment, $N = 27$, $p = .013$, $r = -.293$. There were insufficient data to explore EDE-Q scores at assessment, however, there was a significant decrease in EDE-Q Global score between start and end of treatment with a medium effect size, $N = 15$, $p = .006$, $r = .366$. See Table 3.

Follow up data

Where follow-up data were available (Site 1 $n = 10$, Site 2 $n = 7$) comparisons were made across all times points (assessment, baseline, post-treatment, 6-month follow-up) for BMI.

Differences in BMI scores had an average change of 1.4 (SD = 1.13) from assessment to follow-up. The full-factorial model found significant differences between mean BMI score across timepoints, F (1.65, 26.39) = 15.32, $p < .001$, MSE = .78, $\eta p2 = .995$. Bonferroni post-hoc analysis revealed BMI to significantly increase between assessment (M = 16.91, SD = 1.20) and post-treatment (M = 17.98, SD = 1.59, CI [– 2.03, –.13], $p < .03$) and assessment and follow up (M = 18.3, SD = 1.44, CI [– 2.22, –.57], $p < .001$). Furthermore, significant differences were observed from baseline (M = 17.39, SD = 1.37, CI [– 1.15, –.03], $p < .04$) to post-treatment but there was no significant difference between assessment and baseline or post-treatment and follow-up, $p > .05$.

---

[1] Of available data ($n = 27$), 3 participants engaged in regular purging and 4 in regular bingeing, defined as at least once per week over the past 28 days [48].

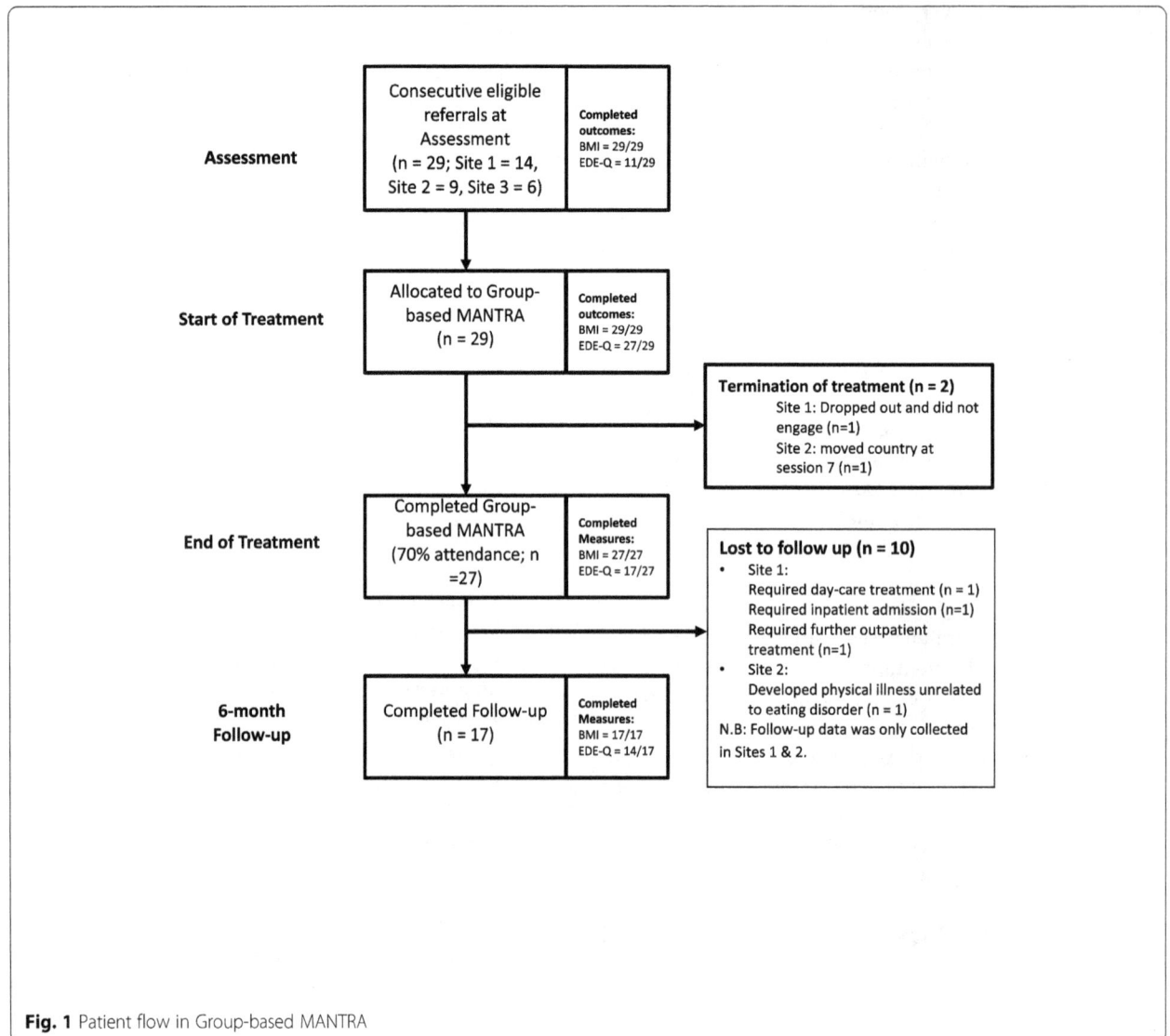

Fig. 1 Patient flow in Group-based MANTRA

Thematic analysis

Eleven participants completed five open-ended questions regarding their personal experience of the Integrated Group Treatment. Analysis is presented under five themes: 1) The group in context, 2) Bringing MANTRA concepts to life, 3) A space to be authentic, vulnerable and understood, 4) Support, empathy and care in the group setting and 5) Others as a motivator for change.

The group in context

Participants highlighted elements of the environmental, organisational, social and personal context in which group-based MANTRA occurred that impeded or enhanced their experience.

For example, participants tended to find the duration of the group (90 mins) acceptable; longer than 90 mins was predicted to have taxed concentration. Morning sessions were liked. Sitting on floor cushions were viewed particularly positively as they made the group feel more "informal" and as a result contributed to it being "easier to share things with the group."

Several participants raised issues relating to the mix of people in the group; one mentioned that she was the only young person in the group and another that he was the only man. However, both felt that this did not negatively affect their experience of the group, or how supportive they found it:

"I know all too well society's awareness and acceptance that men also face the challenge of eating disorders is not where I would like it to be. What I can genuinely say is that the support from my therapists and the group was equal to all with gender having no bearing on the level of empathy and understanding of my situation."

Table 2 Participant demographics, full sample (n = 29)

Variable	Frequency (%)
Females	26 (89.7%)
Age, m (sd)	29.83 (10.21)
Diagnosis	
Anorexia Nervosa – Restricting subtype	27 (93.1%)
Anorexia Nervosa – Binge/Purge subtype	2 (6.9%)
Body Mass Index (kg/m²), m (sd)	
Assessment	16.78 (1.2)
Weight (kg), m (sd)	
Assessment	47.26 (7.03)
Age of Onset, m (sd)	22.04 (8.71)
Duration of illness (years), m (sd)	9.26 (9.9)
Previous ED treatment	
Outpatient	13 (44.8%)
Inpatient	4 (13.8%)
Day-care	0

Participants expressed challenges linked to fitting group-based MANTRA into their lives. However, many participants found the regular slot a helpful addition to their life which extended beyond the time spent in the group:

"Having a dedicated time slot in the week to think about all this, whether I wanted to or not. It was a useful thing to hold on to in weeks which felt like I have a lot to say ("Hold on till Friday, talk it through then") and a reminder not to ignore/pretend/forget in weeks where I was burying my head in the sand."

Bringing MANTRA concepts to life

Participants had largely positive responses to the 'creative exercises' used in group-based MANTRA, including 'chairwork', the value/identity box, using objects, music, movement, space, the body and literature to connect to emotions, letter-writing and pictorial cards. The over-arching theme in participant responses was that they were helpful in enabling participants to express difficult emotions or thoughts to the group, making the

process "less daunting" particularly if they were struggling to put feelings into words:

"I found [the Communicube] very helpful as quite often it helped me speak about things I was bottling up and express and receive support on issues troubling me."

Participants valued exercises where core aspects of the MANTRA programme could be realised either spatially or relationally with other group members. These included use of 'chairwork' as a tool for gaining a new perspective on their eating disorder, getting other group members to act out compassionate voices, and use of objects in order to stimulate reflection on values and identity. Overall participants felt that these activities were interactive and engaging and 'helped bring the concepts to life':

"when talking about perspectives we actually changed our positions in the room/stood on chairs and looked at our ED thoughts from different angles to encourage us to always do this when battling with them".

"There was one when we were in groups and trying to answer each other questions/be the compassionate voice the partner couldn't hear. I remember coming away feeling a bit more settled".

The values box exercise was highlighted as a strong tool and there was a request that this is introduced at an early point to accompany the treatment journey. Participants were overwhelmingly positive about the course content and supporting materials, finding the structured approach helpful and valuing the workbook as a resource to look through. There was a wide-range of course components that participants rated as being most useful (with no single component standing out in analysis), suggesting that the diversity of modules was important in catering to differing needs in the group. Some suggestions to improve course content were to tie it more into the MANTRA book with specific things to read alongside each module, and to set weekly challenges.

Table 3 Paired samples t-test for primary outcome measures

Variable	Timepoint						95% CI for Mean Difference	t	df	r
	1			2						
	M	SD	n	M	SD	n				
BMI[a]	16.78	1.21	27	17.74	1.84	27	−1.69, −.22	−2.67*	26	.293
EDE-Q[b]	3.23	1.49	15	2.15	1.24	15	.34, 1.8	3.21**	14	.366

* $p < .05$, ** $p < .01$
[a]Assessment to post-intervention; [b]Baseline to post-intervention

Participants particularly valued some of the adaptations made to the MANTRA programme in order to integrate it with the group dynamic and use other group-participants to bring MANTRA concepts to life in novel and therapeutically effective ways:

> *"Engaging with thinking styles and relationships with others exercise and discussing these as a group because it bought it to life and helped to apply the new strategies during the rest of the week."*

A space to be authentic, vulnerable and understood

A core component of the group-based MANTRA programme valued by participants was the creation of a safe space where they were able to be open and vulnerable with others who shared a diagnosis of AN. This was felt to increase connection with their own emotions and reduce shame and isolation, however it required careful management from therapists in order to reduce the negative consequences of being 'triggered' by others in the group setting.

Participants consistently emphasised the therapeutic importance of being open, honest and expressing themselves in the group. Participants reported that the MANTRA groups were "safe spaces to express [your]-self", free from shame, judgment or criticism, which facilitated this process. Being vulnerable in this way not only enabled participants to feel 'valued as an individual' but also, through connections to others, helped them connect with their own emotions:

> *"Open up as much as possible sharing vulnerabilities helps others and is an important part in connecting with emotions."*

Significantly, as a result of listening to others' experiences of AN and sharing their own, participants reported that they felt less ashamed about their eating disorder. Listening to others voice similar thoughts and feelings was a powerful tool for overcoming this:

> *"Being able to say how I really felt and have other people: a) agree that they felt like that or thought like that; b) understood and didn't judge me. It was reassuring to know that some of the ways I used to think (which I thought were horrible and was ashamed of) other people thought as well."*

> *"The value this brings is a feeling that maybe you're not insane, not alone, and this is simply a challenge in life to slowly work through."*

The challenge of ensuring the group was not damaging to participants was also recognised in their feedback.

Participants had worries prior to the group commencing about it being potentially 'triggering', and during the group programme participants reported that listening to other's struggles and making comparisons too often gave substance to their "ED critics". However, alongside this, participants also recognised that engaging with others in the group was a necessary means to engage with their own emotions. Being able to discuss, reflect on and cope with the often distressing feelings that had arisen as a result of others' contributions to the group has the potential to be an important mechanism by which group treatment for AN could be effective, if managed sensitively.

"We really rooted for each other": support, empathy and care in the group setting

Participants also valued the support they received from the group, and the opportunity to support others. Within the therapy group it was felt that participants really "rooted for each other", with a reduced sense of aloneness or isolation being the common cited helpful element of the approach. Support from other group members was particularly valued, although several participants commented on valuing "supportive and encouraging" therapists as well:

> *"It's enlightening hearing others with similar feelings and you'll be surprised how similar they are and how support and a simple smile or understanding nod from a stranger can make the world of difference."*

Equally, giving support and comfort to others through the process was important to participants: *"The opportunity to share our struggles & go some way to helping others has been invaluable."*

> *"Meeting new people and comforting them with my own experience".*

Others as a motivator for change

Participants reported being encouraged by listening to others' experiences of recovery. Offering a sense that change was possible, with a suggestion that it would be helpful for people who had benefited from previous groups to come back and talk about their experiences to enhance this aspect of group-based MANTRA. Furthermore, others' accounts broadened participants' conception of what recovery could mean, not just in terms of being better able to step away from anorexic thoughts and behaviours, but in rediscovering an authentic self, separate from the illness:

["Until then I had always believed I would just always think like an anorexic but just at a higher weight. A clinician could have told me I won't have believed them because I'd think, 'how do you know?' 'I've always thought like this, I don't believe you that I could stop believing that (i.e. that I have to exercise every day, I can't eat nice food because I don't deserve to). But to hear X someone who has had anorexia and has recovered say "I used to believe xxxxxx but now I can honestly say I don't" gave me huge encouragement. It helped me believe that it was my ED, and not me underneath, that believed that thought pattern and that there was therefore hope that the me underneath didn't believe it."

Another key source of motivation was the process of empathising with others in the group stimulating self-empathy, and self kindness. This was connected to a recognition (often less possible in a solely self-directed way) that AN was something which caused huge loss of value in people's lives. This recognition often helped participants make radical changes in their own lives:

"It was the push I needed to give myself over to inpatient treatment as I saw what the ED was taking away from me and that it was not my friend and how it was tearing down the wonderful ladies in front of me. I couldn't believe that they didn't see the worth or all of their wonderful qualities."

Discussion

This paper describes a feasibility case series of the integrated group-based delivery of MANTRA, where group processes and experiential techniques were used to target social and emotional processing. Quantitative and qualitative methods were used in analysis. Our primary goal explored feasibility questions including treatment retention, drop out, acceptability and preliminary treatment outcomes as delivered across three NHS sites in the UK. We were also interested in learning about what was valuable and what could be improved regarding the treatment experience.

Preliminary findings suggest that an integrated group-based MANTRA approach (Franklin-Smith, 2019) was acceptable. Of those who took part ($n = 29$), only two dropped out (7%), one who was engaged well but had to move country. Preliminary signs of effectiveness were seen, with medium effect size (pre vs post intervention) changes in regard eating disorder cognitions and behaviours (as measured by the EDEQ) and in terms of weight and BMI (from assessment to post intervention). This is encouraging given our sample of AN patients were as unwell as patients in recent large trials – [11, 12, 49], but with longer-lasting illness [50]. These findings

provide preliminary feasibility data for an Integrated Group Based MANTRA approach. A randomised controlled trial (RCT) (group vs individual MANTRA) exploring postulated mechanisms of change (social and emotional processing) on core outcome (EDEQ and BMI) with a comprehensive follow up period, would enable comprehensive exploration.

The qualitative component is valuable in regard the potential of this adaptation to an already evidence-based treatment. Framework analysis methodology was used [47] to explore themes arising from semi-structured questions completed by participants at the end of treatment. The first theme: 'The group in context', largely validated the practical arrangements such as the length of the group, the importance of 'creature comforts' such as cushions, and spoke to how hard people fought to prioritise time for the treatment. As therapists securing room space was difficult. These comments remind us of the importance of the environment in enabling people to feel safe and valued.

The three remaining themes were relational and highlighted the value of the group element of the treatment and the experiential techniques. Theme two: 'Bringing MANTRA concepts to life', suggested that participants valued the experiential techniques to enable them to express feelings that were difficult to articulate (i.e. via the communicube), to augment perspective shifting and emotional processing (via movement in the room and chair work) and to 'bring body and life to aspects of the self', such as via the identity box. This theme speaks to the value of experiential methods to 'lift' tasks 'off the page' when targeting the social and emotional domain within the MANTRA treatment [30, 34, 35]. The third and fourth themes, i.e. 'A space to be authentic, vulnerable and understood' and 'We really rooted for each other', underscored the value of the group in providing a safe setting for self-expression, and to receive and offer compassion and encouragement, targeting the shame, isolation and stigma often reported by individuals with AN [51]. The fifth theme 'Others as a motivator for change' suggested a value in group members coming from different stages of the illness. Seeing others making changes, even after decades of being unwell, afforded a shift in perspective that enhanced personal motivation to change, creating an atmosphere of hope. Important too was the way in which offering empathy to others, prompted self-empathy. Of note, negative competitive dynamics did not take hold at any point. These were an unwell, chronic group of individuals with AN who cared for and supported each other, via effective and skilled group facilitation to empower each other and themselves to make good clinical progress. These are powerful examples of social and emotional change realised within a relational context [18, 29, 30].

This feasibility case series of an integrated group-based approach to delivering MANTRA provides preliminary indications that a group setting with an experiential focus is a useful arena for targeting emotional and social difficulties in those with Anorexia Nervosa, whilst also achieving improvements in broader outcomes. However, the freedoms and creativity of a 'real world' case series naturally afford some limitations. The study is underpowered, particularly in regard the follow up data, to draw conclusions about the effectiveness of the intervention or about its generalizability to specific ED presentations, such as AN binge/purge sub-types. There are a number of confounding variables that make it difficult to disentangle active ingredients of change. Of note, the study took place across three different NHS sites, with different therapists at each base and of course we describe a treatment approach that necessitated both an individual and group component. Furthermore, there was also a flexibility afforded to therapists in the treatment delivery which may hinder replication. An RCT of group vs individual MANTRA could provide a useful next step to assess AN patients' willingness to be randomly allocated to these different treatment modalities and to use a broader range of outcome measures. Future trials should also focus on questions of cost and cost-effectiveness of using group versus individual MANTRA in AN. Clear in the feedback was the power of the group in minimising shame, loneliness and stigma around having an eating disorder. Therapists said they were honored to accompany their patients on this journey.

"After so many years living with anorexia, I really feel now as though I am finally moving on and standing on my own" (group member).

Conclusion

This case series suggests that delivering MANTRA in an integrated group format is a feasible and effective intervention for individuals with severe and enduring Anorexia Nervosa. Opportunities for live social and emotional experiences within the group arena were maximized to reduce shame and encourage alternative ways of managing emotion. Future research is needed to confirm the effectiveness and mechanisms of change of this Integrated Group based approach.

Abbreviations
AN: Anorexia Nervosa; MANTRA: Maudsley Anorexia Nervosa Treatment for Adults; WoT: Window of Emotional Tolerance

Acknowledgements
US is supported by a National Institute for Health Research (NIHR) Senior Investigator Award and receives salary support from the NIHR Biomedical Research Centre (BRC) at South London and Maudsley NHS Foundation Trust and King's College London. The views expressed in this publication are those of the authors and not necessarily those of the National Health Service, the NIHR or the UK Department of Health.

Authors' contributions
HS lead on the write up of the case series, along with MFS and all authors read and contributed to drafts. WB supported the collection of data across sites and initial data analysis, which was overseen by HS. MFS contributed to the write up, designed and authored the Group Treatment Manual, ran groups and contributed thought the trial in regard assuring our treatment adherence and supervision. MFS, YB, HS, NG and AF were all involved in running the groups within this case series. US was involved in the design and conception of the ideas within the evolution of the Group treatment and this case series. The authors read and approved the final manuscript.

Competing interests
HS and US are authors of the MANTRA individual workbook. MFS is the author of the MANTRA group workbook.

Author details
Sussex Partnership NHS Foundation Trust, Sussex Eating Disorders Service, Brighton, UK. [2]Leeds Partnership NHS Foundation Trust, CONNECT: The West Yorkshire Adult Eating Disorder Service, Leeds, UK. [3]South London and Maudsley NHS Foundation Trust, Eating Disorders Outpatient Service, London, UK. [4]Department of Psychological Medicine, King's College London, Institute of Psychiatry, London, UK.

References
1. American Psychiatric Association. Diagnostic and statistical manual of mental disorders. 5th ed. Arlington: APA; 2013. https://doi.org/10.1176/appi.books.9780890425596.
2. Arcelus J, Mitchell AJ, Wales J, Nielsen S. Mortality rates in patients with anorexia nervosa and other eating disorders: a meta-analysis of 36 studies. Arch Gen Psychiatry. 2011;68(7):724–31. https://doi.org/10.1001/archgenpsychiatry.2011.74.
3. Smink FR, van Hoeken D, Hoek HW. Epidemiology, course, and outcome of eating disorders. Curr Opin Psychiatry. 2013;26(6):543–8. https://doi.org/10.1097/YCO.0b013e328365a24f.
4. Link TM, Beermann U, Mestel R, Gander M. Treatment outcome in female in-patients with anorexia nervosa and comorbid personality disorders prevalence-therapy drop out and weight gain. Psychother Psychosom Med Psychol. 2017;67(9 10):420–30.
5. Miller AE, Racine SE, Klonsky ED. Symptoms of anorexia nervosa and bulimia nervosa have differential relationships to borderline personality disorder symptoms. Eat Disord. 2019:1–14. https://doi.org/10.1080/10640266.2019.1642034.
6. Schmidt U, Startup H, Treasure J. A cognitive-interpersonal therapy workbook for treating anorexia nervosa: the Maudsley model. London: Routledge; 2018. https://doi.org/10.4324/9781315728483.
7. NICE. Eating disorders: recognition and treatment. London: National Institute for Health and Care Excellence; 2017. Retrieved from https://www.nice.org.uk/guidance/ng69/evidence/full-guideline-pdf-161214767896
8. Byrne S, Wade T, Hay P, Touyz S, Fairburn CG, Treasure J, et al. A randomised controlled trial of three psychological treatments for anorexia nervosa. Psychol Med. 2017;47(16):2823–33.
9. Schmidt U, Oldershaw A, Jichi F, Sternheim L, Startup H, McIntosh V, et al. Out-patient psychological therapies for adults with anorexia nervosa: randomised controlled trial. Br J Psychiatry. 2012;201(5):392–9.
10. Schmidt U, Renwick B, Lose A, Kenyon M, DeJong H, Broadbent H, et al. The MOSAIC study-comparison of the Maudsley model of treatment for adults with anorexia nervosa (MANTRA) with specialist supportive clinical management (SSCM) in outpatients with anorexia nervosa or eating disorder not otherwise specified, anorexia nervos. Trials. 2013;14(1):1–10.
11. Schmidt U, Magill N, Renwick B, Keyes A, Kenyon M, Dejong H, et al. The Maudsley outpatient study of treatments for anorexia nervosa and related conditions (MOSAIC): comparison of the Maudsley model of anorexia nervosa treatment for adults (MANTRA) with specialist supportive clinical management (SSCM) in outpatients with. J Consult Clin Psychol. 2015;83(4):796–807. https://doi.org/10.1037/ccp0000019.
12. Schmidt U, Ryan EG, Bartholdy S, Renwick B, Keyes A, O'Hara C, et al. Two-year follow-up of the MOSAIC trial: a multicenter randomized controlled trial comparing two psychological treatments in adult outpatients with

broadly defined anorexia nervosa. Int J Eat Disord. 2016;49(8):793–800. https://doi.org/10.1002/eat.22523.

13. Schmidt U, Treasure J. Anorexia nervosa: valued and visible. A cognitive-interpersonal maintenance model and its implications for research and practice. Br J Clin Psychol. 2006;45(3):343–66. https://doi.org/10.1348/0144 66505X53902.

14. Treasure J, Schmidt U. The cognitive-interpersonal maintenance model of anorexia nervosa revisited: a summary of the evidence for cognitive, socio-emotional and interpersonal predisposing and perpetuating factors. J Eat Disord. 2013;1(13):1–13.

15. Lose A, Davies C, Renwick B, Kenyon M, Treasure J, Schmidt U, et al. Process evaluation of the maudsley model for treatment of adults with anorexia nervosa trial. Part II: patient experiences of two psychological therapies for treatment of anorexia nervosa. Eur Eat Disord Rev. 2014;22(2):131–9. https://doi.org/10.1002/erv.2279.

16. Waterman-Collins D, Renwick B, Lose A, Kenyon M, Serpell L, Richards L, et al. Process evaluation of the MOSAIC trial, part I: therapist experiences of delivering two psychological therapies for treatment of anorexia nervosa. Eur Eat Disord Rev. 2014;22(2):122–30. https://doi.org/10.1002/erv.2278.

17. Bulik CM, Berkman ND, Brownley KA, Sedway JA, Lohr KN. Anorexia nervosa treatment: a systematic review of randomized controlled trials. Int J Eat Disord. 2007;40(4):310–20. https://doi.org/10.1002/eat.20367.

18. Christensen KA, Haynos AF. A theoretical review of interpersonal emotion regulation in eating disorders: enhancing knowledge by bridging interpersonal and affective dysfunction. J Eat Disord. 2020;8:1–10.

19. Oldershaw A, Lavender T, Sallis H, Stahl D, Schmidt U. Emotion generation and regulation in anorexia nervosa: a systematic review and meta-analysis of self-report data. Clin Psychol Rev. 2015;39:83–95. https://doi.org/10.1016/j.cpr.2015.04.005.

20. Caglar-Nazali HP, Corfield F, Cardi V, Ambwani S, Leppanen J, Olabintan O, et al. A systematic review and meta-analysis of 'Systems for Social Processes' in eating disorders. Neurosci Biobehav Rev. 2014;42:55–92. https://doi.org/10.1016/j.neubiorev.2013.12.002.

21. Oldershaw A, Lavender T, Schmidt U. Are socio-emotional and neurocognitive functioning predictors of therapeutic outcomes for adults with anorexia nervosa? Eur Eat Disord Rev. 2018;26(4):346–59. https://doi.org/10.1002/erv.2602.

22. Oldershaw A, Startup H, Lavender T. Anorexia nervosa and a lost emotional self: a psychological formulation of the development, maintenance, and treatment of anorexia nervosa. Front Psychol. 2019;10:219. https://doi.org/10.3389/fpsyg.2019.00219.

23. Oldershaw A, Startup H. 18 building the healthy adult in eating disorders. Creat Methods Schema Ther. 2020. https://doi.org/10.4324/9781351171847-18.

24. Brockmeyer T, Friederich HC, Küppers C, Chowdhury S, Harms L, Simmonds J, et al. Approach bias modification training in bulimia nervosa and binge-eating disorder: a pilot randomized controlled trial. Int J Eat Disord. 2019; 52(5):520–9. https://doi.org/10.1002/eat.23024.

25. Startup H, Lavender A, Oldershaw A, Stott R, Tchanturia K, Treasure J, et al. Worry and rumination in anorexia nervosa. Behav Cogn Psychother. 2013; 41(3):301–16. https://doi.org/10.1017/S1352465812000847.

26. Seidel M, King JA, Ritschel F, Boehm I, Geisler D, Bernardoni F, et al. The real-life costs of emotion regulation in anorexia nervosa: a combined ecological momentary assessment and fMRI study. Transl Psychiatry. 2018; 8(1):1–11.

27. Adamson J, Leppanen J, Murin M, Tchanturia K. Effectiveness of emotional skills training for patients with anorexia nervosa with autistic symptoms in group and individual format. Eur Eat Disord Rev. 2018;26(4):367–75. https://doi.org/10.1002/erv.2594.

28. Doré BP, Silvers JA, Ochsner KN. Toward a personalized science of emotion regulation. Soc Personal Psychol Compass. 2016;10(4):171–87. https://doi.org/10.1111/spc3.12240.

29. Reeck C, Ames DR, Ochsner KN. The social regulation of emotion: an integrative, cross-disciplinary model. Trends Cogn Sci. 2016;20(1):47–63. https://doi.org/10.1016/j.tics.2015.09.003

30. Doré BP, Morris RR, Burr DA, Picard RW, Ochsner KN. Helping others regulate emotion predicts increased regulation of one's own emotions and decreased symptoms of depression. Personal Soc Psychol Bull. 2017;43(5): 729–39. https://doi.org/10.1177/0146167217695558.

31. Ogden, P., Minton, K., & Pain, C. (2006). Trauma and the body: a sensorimotor approach to psychotherapy (Norton series on interpersonal neurobiology). WW Norton & Company.

32. Hibbs R, Pugh M, Fox JR. Applying emotion-focused therapy to work with the "anorexic voice" within anorexia nervosa: a brief intervention. J Psychother Integr. 2020. https://doi.org/10.1037/int0000252.

33. Mountford V, Waller G. Using imagery in cognitive-behavioral treatment for eating disorders: tackling the restrictive mode. Int J Eat Disord. 2006;39(7): 533–43. https://doi.org/10.1002/eat.20329.

34. Dokter D. Arts therapies and clients with eating disorders: fragile board. London and Bristol: Jessica Kingsley Publishers; 1995.

35. Wood LL, Schneider C. Setting the stage for self-attunement: Drama therapy as a guide for neural integration in the treatment of eating disorders. Drama Therapy Review. 2015;1(1):55–70. https://doi.org/10.1386/dtr.1.1.55_1.

36. Heath G, Startup H. Creative methods in Schema therapy: advances and innovation in clinical practice. London: Routledge; 2020. https://doi.org/10.4324/9781351171847.

37. Pugh M. Cognitive behavioural chairwork: distinctive features: Routledge; 2019. https://doi.org/10.4324/9780429023927.

38. Simpson S, Arntz A. Core principles of imagery (chapter 5). In: G. Heath, & H. Startup, creative methods in Schema therapy: advances and innovation in clinical practice (p. 15). London: Routledge; 2020.

39. Shaw I. Spontaneity and play in Schema therapy (chapter 10). In: G. Heath, & H. Startup, creative methods in Schema therapy: advances and innovation in clinical practice (p. 11). London; 2020. -Routledge.

40. Lavender A, Startup H, Naumann U, Samarawickrema N, DeJong H, Kenyon M, et al. Emotional and social mind training: a randomised controlled trial of a new group-based treatment for bulimia nervosa. PLoS One. 2012;7(10): e46047. https://doi.org/10.1371/journal.pone.0046047.

41. Bernard H, Burlingame G, Flores P, Greene L, Joyce A, Kobos JC, et al. Clinical practice guidelines for group psychotherapy. Int J Group Psychother. 2008;58(4):455–542. https://doi.org/10.1521/ijgp.2008.58.4.455.

42. Wilfley D, Shore A. Interpersonal psychotherapy. International encyclopedia of the Social & Behavioral Sciences, 631-636. 2015. https://doi.org/10.1016/b978-0-08-097086-8.21065-9.

43. National Health Service Health Research Authority. (2011). National research ethics service guidance: does my project require review by a research ethics committee? Retrieved from Downloaded from: http://www.hra.nhs.uk/documents/2013/09/does-my-project-require-rec-review.pdf

44. Fairburn CG, Beglin SJ. Assessment of eating disorder psychopathology: interview or self-report questionnaire? Int J Eat Disord. 1994;16(4):363–70.

45. Fairburn CG, Beglin S. Eating disorder examination questionnaire. In: Fairburn CG, editor. Cognitive behavior therapy and eating disorders. New York: Guilford Press; 2008. p. 309–13.

46. Franklin-Smith, M. (2019). MANTRA outpatients group guide manual. Unpublished.

47. Ritchie J, Spencer L. Qualitative data analysis for applied policy research. In: Bryman A, Burgess RG, editors. Analysing qualitative data. London: Routledge; 1994. p. 173–94. https://doi.org/10.4324/9780203413081_chapter_9.

48. Luce KH, Crowther JH, Pole M. Eating disorder examination questionnaire (EDE-Q): norms for undergraduate women. Int J Eat Disord. 2008;41(3):273–6. https://doi.org/10.1002/eat.20504.

49. Ambwani S, Cardi V, Albano G, Cao L, Crosby RD, Macdonald P, et al. A multicenter audit of outpatient care for adult anorexia nervosa: symptom trajectory, service use, and evidence in support of "early stage" versus "severe and enduring" classification. Int J Eat Disord. 2020;53(8):1337–48. https://doi.org/10.1002/eat.23246.

50. Wonderlich SA, Bulik CM, Schmidt U, Steiger H, Hoek HW. Severe and enduring anorexia nervosa: update and observations about the current clinical reality. Int J Eat Disord. 2020;53(8):1303–12. https://doi.org/10.1002/eat.23283.

51. Troop NA, Allan S, Serpell L, Treasure JL. Shame in women with a history of eating disorders. Eur Eat Disord Rev. 2008;16(6):480–8. https://doi.org/10.1002/erv.858.

6

How and Why does the Disease Progress? A Qualitative Investigation of the Transition into Long-standing Anorexia Nervosa

Catherine Broomfield[1][*] [iD], Paul Rhodes[1] and Stephen Touyz[2]

Abstract

Objective: Despite an increased interest in understanding characteristics of long-standing anorexia nervosa (AN), there is a lack of knowledge into the processes that occur with the development and maintenance of the disease. This has impeded the development of novel treatment approaches that may prove more effective than traditional medical models of therapy. To improve the prognosis of these long-standing presentations, an understanding as to how and why the AN disease progresses is required. It was therefore the aim of the current study to investigate the transition of AN from earlier to later stages.

Method: The study adopted a narrative inquiry approach and a total of 11 women with long-standing AN participated in an interview. The newly developed photovoice method assisted in data collection with typologies of chronic illness facilitating the emergence of salient themes.

Results: The qualitative analysis resulted in the identification of five themes: (a) transition, (b) trauma, (c) functionality, (d) identity, and (e) failure of current models of treatment.

Conclusions: Together with identifying key themes, the study provides insight into some possible reasons why current treatment models are failing to promote recovery. Future research examining the effectiveness of treatment that targets underlying causes and maintaining factors of the illness are suggested. Additional education for health professionals is also recommended in order to reduce the trauma that is currently being experienced by some patients with a long-standing illness.

Keywords: Anorexia nervosa, Long-standing, Transition, Progression, Trauma, Functionality, Identity, Treatment

Plain English summary

Anorexia nervosa (AN) is a complex illness that has the potential to develop into a long-term presentation. When this occurs, the best way of treating this stage of the disease is currently being debated with new models of care being investigated and compared to more traditional approaches to treatment. One of the difficulties in developing more effective treatment is the lack of understanding into how and why the AN illness transitions from an earlier to later stage. It was the aim of the current study to discover the changes that occur as the AN illness progresses. A total of 11 women were interviewed to discuss their experience of AN as it progressed into a long-term illness. It was discovered

*Correspondence: catebroomfield@hotmail.com
[1] School of Psychology, Griffith Taylor Building, The University of Sydney, Sydney, NSW 2006, Australia
Full list of author information is available at the end of the article

that across participants, five themes emerged: (a) transition, (b) trauma, (c) functionality, (d) identity, and (e) failure of current models of treatment. Possible reasons as to why current treatment approaches are not working for long-term AN are discussed. Recommendations are made for improving education for health professionals so as to reduce the trauma that is currently being experienced by some individuals with a long-standing illness.

Background

Anorexia nervosa (AN) is a complex illness that manifests in various ways making the eating disorder difficult to treat and the recovery process slow [1, 2]. Interest into later stages of the illness has corresponded with an increased focus on understanding these presentations in order to ascertain more effective treatment options [3–5]. One barrier to developing effective treatment includes limited information regarding how and why the disease progresses. This lack of knowledge limits the ability of researchers and health professionals to understand why AN can become so resistant and what aspects of the disease are not being adequately addressed in current treatment models.

With an estimated twenty per cent of patients developing a longer-term presentation [6], quantitative [7–9] and qualitative [10, 11] research methods have been utilised in order to better understand the characteristics of long-standing AN. Despite these efforts, there is still a limited understanding of this complex stage of the illness, especially in relation to how and why this presentation develops. In a qualitative study investigating the personal meaning of symptoms and treatment approaches, Stockford et al. [12] identified that a lack of early identification and implementation of interventions was a theme that emerged from a severe and enduring AN sample. A contribution to the development of a protracted course of AN may be the absence of parental support and lengthy waiting lists at treatment facilities [12]. Social support systems also emerged as part of the 15 themes identified by Robinson et al. [13] whilst investigating the management of patients with an AN illness duration of 20 years. Based on the findings from this study [13], psychological and social functioning were determined to be the most negatively impacted domains by this long-standing eating disorder.

In a study investigating the recovery of patients with severe and enduring AN, Dawson et al. [14] described motivation, support, self-efficacy and hope to be fundamental aspects in treating these presentations. This was in contrast to previous methods that resulted in unsuccessful treatment attempts with participants reporting an external locus of control that prevented autonomy over their own recovery [14]. Although research efforts have attempted to understand characteristics of the illness [9, 12, 13], there has been a greater overall focus to date on understanding the development of the acute stage of AN [15–17] and recovery from the illness [14, 18, 19]. What

is missing in the field is an understanding as to the development of the later stage of the illness—as well as its maintenance over a long period of time—which is essential when developing more effective and targeted treatment options for these presentations.

It was crucial in the current study to adopt a qualitative research approach given underlying experiences can be missed when using quantitative methods [20, 21]. This approach would allow first-hand knowledge to be acquired as to these experiences from the perspective of affected individuals [22]. Narrative inquiry as a qualitative research method captures and analyses life stories, allowing for rich detail to be gathered on topics that are human centred and complex [23]. By illuminating the lived experience, this technique facilitated the investigation as to how and why the illness perseveres. It was the aim of the current study to track processes that occur as the AN illness progresses.

Method

Participants

Participants were required to meet the following self-reported criteria: (a) be at least 18 years of age; (b) currently or previously have met the Diagnostic and Statistical Manual of Mental Disorders, fifth edition (DSM-5) criteria for AN [24]; and (c) currently or previously have experienced the AN illness for a duration of seven or more years [25]. The decision to recruit participants using illness duration was based on this criterion being the most frequently cited definition in the literature for the later stage of AN as indicated in a systematic review by Broomfield et al. [25]. By adopting the same inclusion criteria, the findings in the current study were comparable to other research that has been dedicated to this subpopulation. Recruitment took place through snowball sampling (method of detecting participants through social networks) [26], social media and clinician recommendation in Sydney, Australia. Participants were assessed and included if they consented and met the inclusion criteria. This study was approved by the Human Research Ethics Committee at the University of Sydney.

Research design, data collection and procedure

The research design included a narrative inquiry approach with the use of the newly developed photovoice method. Narrative inquiry is advantageous when

Table 1 Interview questions

Can you tell me what your AN means to you?
How do you experience AN?
How long have you been experiencing AN?
Were there any time periods during your life where the experience of AN was particularly consuming, important or had a major impact on your life?
Were there any time periods where the opposite was found, in that the illness had little impact on you and your life?
Was there a specific time where you noticed or realised that the AN you were experiencing was going to be enduring?
Can you tell me the journey you have had with AN?
Is there anything that you would like health professionals and the research community to know about your experience of AN?

Note AN Anorexia Nervosa

researching a process that occurs over a period of time, which is particularly relevant when considering illness transition that can span many years [27]. For the current study, personal processes and the meaning behind lived experiences was prioritised in the construction of narratives.

Photovoice as a method allows participants to communicate aspects of their lives through the use of photographs [28]. This facilitates the development of an affective response and allows the story to become real for both the participant and the researcher [28, 29]. Shaped by feminist theory, this method of data collection is guided by participants allowing for a deep exploration of the often taken-for-granted lived experience of women [30, 31]. Participants were instructed to provide up to 10 photographs related to their lived experience with AN. This allowed participants to symbolise the most salient aspects of their journey, with experiences outside of these photographs discussed in order to extrapolate a timeline of events. Along with the photographs, participants were asked to record: (1) what was in each photograph, (2) what each photograph meant to the participant and (3) why each photograph was taken [32].

Limitations of the photovoice method include ethical considerations regarding consent of individuals appearing in photographs, as well as the possibility of meaning in photographs being misconstrued [33]. To overcome these limitations, participants were instructed to only include individuals in photographs who had provided written consent with consent forms provided to participants at the beginning of the study (consent forms were approved by the Human Research Ethics Committee at the University of Sydney). Photographs were explored in interviews to avoid the researcher misinterpreting the meaning of images. Data collection took place through face-to-face interviews or via Skype and was audio-recorded. The first two thirds of the interview was focused on an examination of the selected photographs with the final third used to extrapolate and explore potential underlying meanings. Prompting for further

details was at times required in order to co-produce a descriptive timeline of the participant's experience (see Table 1 for Interview Questions).

The interview was then transcribed verbatim so as to capture and preserve the "voice" of participants by using their own words as much as possible. Similar to the method used by Dawson et al. [14], identified processes were placed in a temporal order to examine commonalities across narratives. The interview took approximately two hours to complete with additional time for member checking (a process whereby the analysis is checked by participants with any requested changes made to increase precision) [22].

Data analysis

After member checking was complete, an inductive analytic process took place whereby data relating to the experiences of the illness were studied for emerging themes [34]. Typologies proposed by medical sociologist Arthur Frank [27, 35] were used as a guide to help make meaning out of the emerging concepts, with this model allowing for chronic illness to be represented through a variety of lenses. This included stories of chaos, quest, restitution and illness-as-normality, with these typologies present to varying degrees across the narratives of participants. The type of story told through each narrative was found to be changeable, with some stages of the AN illness representing one lens, which would later transform to another lens with the progression of the disorder. Through an exploration of these four lenses [27, 35] a greater understanding of the ways in which AN transitioned in the experiences told by participants became clear. After each narrative was investigated using these typologies as a guide [27, 35], commonalities across the experience of long-standing AN became salient. Links were established between the raw data and the aim of this research (i.e., to determine the transition of AN from earlier to later stages of the illness) [36], which further highlighted similarities across narratives. Overarching themes were discovered

Table 2 Participant demographics

Characteristic	n (proportion)	Mean (SD; years)	Range (years)
Age		41.6 (11.5)	29–66
Duration of illness[a]		26.2 (13.2)	7–53
Stage of illness			
Currently ill	6 (54.55%)	–	–
Recovering	3 (27.27%)	–	–
Recovered[b]	2 (18.18%)	–	–
AN subtype			
Restricting	9 (81.82%)	–	–
Binge-eating/purging	2 (18.18%)	–	–
Employment status			
Unemployed	4 (36.36%)	–	–
Casual	2 (18.18%)	–	–
Part-time	1 (9.09%)	–	–
Full-time	4 (36.36%)	–	–
Marital status			
Single	8 (72.73%)	–	–
De-facto/married	3 (27.27%)	–	–
Children			
No	8 (72.73%)	–	–
Yes	3 (27.27%)	–	–
Language spoken at home			
English	11 (100%)	–	–

Note AN Anorexia Nervosa. BMI was not collected as irrelevant for the current study

[a] Each participant provided their own indication of when their illness began. The decision to have women decide the illness starting point was in line with the current research method of working with lived-experience participants who are regarded as the expert on their experience. The majority of participants regarded the starting point of their illness to be when they themselves first noticed symptoms of AN (*n* = 10), with some of these women (*n* = 2) also receiving a diagnosis by a health professional the same year symptoms began. The remaining participant (*n* = 1) regarded the illness starting point to be when family and friends first noticed symptoms

[b] Although classified as recovered, participants (*n* = 2) still experienced cognitive symptoms related to AN

with evidence of these higher-order conceptualisations investigated in the data until a "best fit" model was reached [37]. Inductive thematic saturation was adopted in the current study, a process whereby no new information can be generated by additional data as demonstrated by no new themes emerging from the analysis [38].

Methodological rigor

The methodology was evaluated based on criteria relating to credibility, fittingness and auditability [39]. Credibility was maintained by using direct quotes when possible to construct narratives. To ensure accuracy, participants were offered the opportunity to member check their narratives. Participant characteristics were described in order to facilitate an understanding of fittingness. Auditability was demonstrated by a thorough audit trail kept in order to ensure analytic transparency [39]. To reduce bias, narratives were cross-coded by two authors with any disagreements resolved through discussion.

Results

A total of 11 women participated in the study. As required, all participants self-reported meeting the DSM-5 criteria at some point during their seven or more year experience with AN [24, 25]. For participant demographics, see Table 2.

Photographs provided by participants varied in content. Images consisted of significant individuals, triggers of illness, physical activities and hobbies.

Themes

There were a total of five themes that emerged from the data during analysis: (a) transition, (b) trauma, (c) functionality, (d) identity, and (e) the failure of current treatment models.

Theme 1: Transition

All participants (*n* = 11) described transitional periods throughout their illness. The most common transition related to the progression from an acute to a later stage of the disease with the manner of in which this transition occurred varying across experiences. Some of the women ($n=8$) experienced distinct shifts when the illness progressed into long-standing AN with the remaining women ($n=3$) experiencing a more linear progression with no distinct turning points.

When a distinct turning point was experienced, some of the women ($n=5$) identified this to have occurred when their life had become completely consumed by the illness:

> "When I was younger, I could have periods of time where I was a bit better or, you know, it wasn't 24 hours a day. I wasn't dreaming about it, you know, but then when I got older, there was no, nothing outside the eating disorder. Nothing escaped that filter; it was like it was enclosed in your head. There was nothing else." – Participant 3

This consumption of their life by the illness was often paired with an overwhelming sense of grief when there was a realisation that recovery might be harder to achieve than originally hoped:

> "It was horrible in that sense of grief...that's what I would, would call 'severe and enduring' as when it's become such a huge part of your life, it's become more of your life than your life itself and so, that's why I think that it's harder to recover from..." – Participant 9

For some women ($n=2$), the transition into long-standing AN was paired with a life-changing experience that brought a sense of acceptance of the illness, which propelled them towards recovery. This included being confronted by life-threatening consequences if failing to address the disorder ($n=1$) and an unsuccessful suicide attempt ($n=1$). In another experience ($n=1$), the turning point came after all available treatment models were attempted with little success:

> "At that moment it was huge grief, huge grief, uhmm, which I still feel sometimes right, because part of, part of what letting go of the idea of getting better and recovering means is letting go of all the things I had hoped to do and hoped to be able to do with ease. Uhmm and as you can see that still makes me sad, uhmm cause there are always going to be things that are inaccessible to me and that's both okay and tragic." – Participant 5

Other transitional periods included turning points towards recovery ($n=5$), the ability to contribute towards society through work ($n=3$), or in contrast, being unable to continue work as a result of health complications ($n=4$). Entering into new roles was another transition for some participants including becoming a mother ($n=3$). These experiences required participants to shift their relationship with the eating disorder in order to meet the demands of new roles, which at times involved recovery, periods of remission or continuing along the trajectory of their long-standing eating disorder.

Theme 2: Trauma

Trauma was present across narratives during different times of the illness with all participants ($n=11$) reporting to experience some form of trauma that pre-dated the development of the eating disorder. In most cases ($n=8$), the trauma immediately preceded the development of symptoms relating to AN. The more common forms of trauma developed from witnessing abuse or tension in the family home ($n=3$), being sexually abused by a family friend ($n=2$) or date ($n=1$) and being physically abused by a parent ($n=1$) or sibling ($n=1$):

> "I think it was just a loaded gun...probably the main trigger for my anorexia was the abuse." – Participant 6
> "I found very complicated ways of trying to manage what had happened [rape] and just made things worse... in that sense my life did get out of control, because I was trying to undo something that had happened by doing other things, that ended up making it worse..." – Participant 8

Disconnected relationships with family ($n=5$), friends ($n=2$) or both ($n=2$) was reported as traumatic with the ensuing isolation preventing other people from intervening in the progression of the illness. In some circumstances ($n=5$), this left AN to go undetected for long periods of time.

The embodiment of trauma occurred for many of the women ($n=7$) after feeling pressure from family ($n=1$), peers ($n=1$) or both ($n=1$) to lose weight. Other women ($n=4$) experienced a sense of competition with themselves.

> "...I think it [AN] had a lot to do with being really traumatised in my body." – Participant 9

When other people communicated displeasure over the participant's body ($n=3$), the impact of their criticism manifested in numerous ways. Adopting dieting techniques from parents ($n=1$) or being placed on a diet ($n=2$) were some of the ways participants began their difficult relationship with food, which for one woman occurred as early as four years of age.

Theme 3: Functionality

The theme of functionality related to the way in which the illness served a purpose in the lives of the women, which ultimately made recovery difficult to achieve. Although there were multiple reasons for the illness having a prolonged trajectory, all of the women ($n=11$) described the fundamental purpose of AN as a way to regain a sense of control over certain aspects of their lives. For most participants ($n=9$), this was in relation to the body itself with a loss of control through physical development and puberty ($n=3$), becoming victimised through sexual ($n=3$) or physical abuse ($n=2$) and the loss of bodily functions through the symptoms of another chronic health condition ($n=1$).

As AN transitioned into a later stage, the function of the illness also transitioned for most participants ($n=8$). With the illness initially functioning as a way to regain control, AN eventually became a way to manage subsequent distressing emotions such as grief ($n=3$), maintaining an idealised body shape ($n=2$), forming part of the individual's identity ($n=2$) and encompassing a perspective for experiencing the world ($n=1$).

The use of the illness to avoid experiencing distressing emotions ($n=10$) acted as an original function of AN for some participants ($n=7$) and developed as the illness progressed for other participants ($n=3$). For individuals who were experiencing symptoms of post-traumatic stress as a result of sexual ($n=3$) or physical abuse ($n=2$), AN was used as a method to drown out distressing emotions and focus attention on pain inflicted upon themselves:

> "I wanted the physical pain as opposed to the emotional because that made sense. I could recognise that, that's what was wrong whereas emotionally it was just too, you know, too hard to identify it." – Participant 9
>
> "...nothing can harm you because of the way you're harming yourself, basically." – Participant 1

Other incidents that caused social isolation ($n=3$) and stress ($n=2$) were often paired with difficult emotions that some of the women felt incapable of managing without the illness:

> "...as long as I'm in the anorexic range I can cope with life. The second I'm not, I can't." – Participant 6

By removing complications in life and assisting in the management of distressing emotions, AN offered participants ($n=11$) safety:

> "Anorexia offered this really clean, pure, serene, space that really contrasted to all that messy, ugly, nasty, out of control stuff...it's a safer place to be." – Participant 8

Theme 4: Identity

Although identity was a theme that emerged throughout most of the experiences ($n=10$), there was a clear division in the way that women identified with the illness. There was an even split in the experiences involving identity with half of the women ($n=5$) identifying with the illness and the other half ($n=5$) rejecting a personal interconnection. The degree of illness identity also changed as the disease progressed. Some of the women ($n=5$) who previously identified with AN re-formed their identity during recovery ($n=3$) or shifted their perspective away from the problematic features of the disease ($n=2$):

> "I think part of the reason that I maybe still identify with the term [AN] is I tend not think of it as an illness." – Participant 8

Given the typical development of AN occurs during adolescence and then progresses into adulthood for longstanding presentations, women reported a consistent and dependable aspect of their lives to have become the disease:

> "It [AN] just gets into everything and particularly over time...it just seeps into every part of your life..." – Participant 8

At times, the illness needed to be grieved in order to reach a point of recovery ($n=1$):

> "...why I think a lot of people with 'severe and enduring' have 'severe and enduring', cause the acceptance of grief and losing a part of yourself, what's been a part of yourself for so long becomes even harder... It's not that I loved my eating disorder but it had become a part of me and my life, so letting go of something, that was so now engrained was a huge thing uhmm, for me it was like losing a child." – Participant 9

The reasons for women rejecting an identification with AN ($n=5$), included the illness interfering with their values ($n=2$), violating professional ($n=1$) or personal ($n=1$) goals as well as regarding their illness as not being severe enough in their life to associate with personally ($n=1$).

> "I was very, very aware of the two selves that were happening, you know, the crazy self and the sane self that was watching, which sounds awful doesn't it? Uhmm and it was a bit scary at the time actually of being driven by something you didn't understand and you didn't think was necessarily part of you..." – Participant 7

Theme 5: Failure of current models of treatment

The failure of current models of treatment was found in the experience of almost all women ($n = 10$), except for one participant who avoided the health care system. There were commonalities identified across the majority of participants ($n = 10$), which included a lack of success in long-term recovery following the attempt of evidence-based treatment approaches offered between 1960 and 2018. This often involved attempting different models of treatment that were available during the time of their illness:

> "I tried everything, all the different three letter acronym-types of therapy, uhmm, different day programs, bunch of clinical trials, uhmm, yeah and in-patient was the only thing I hadn't done and I did that, and it didn't help." – Participant 5

The second most common failure of treatment included a general lack of understanding about long-standing AN from treating staff ($n = 8$). Protocols used in treatment facilities revealed a lack of awareness by clinicians of fundamental aspects of the illness. By denying a patient their sense of autonomy through the process of treatment, attempts at recovery were often ineffective and left the participant feeling more traumatised than before they were admitted into therapy. For some participants ($n = 5$), this involved treating staff using threats in order to persuade patients to increase their food intake, a method reported by the current sample to have occurred between 1980 and 2016. This included threats to ban visits from family and friends ($n = 3$), withholding hospital leave ($n = 1$), phone calls ($n = 1$), personal clothing items ($n = 1$) and blankets ($n = 1$) if patients did not comply:

> "In the in-patient it was very much that idea of, 'If you eat your food you can have visitors, if you eat your food you can have a blanket, if you don't you can't'. Uhmm, again, I'm not really entirely sure what they were hoping that would achieve, uhmm it didn't really achieve very much other than I got very cold and very miserable." – Participant 8

Treatment facilities also threatened patients with involuntary tube feeding ($n = 2$; between 1998 and 2018), scheduling ($n = 1$; between 2000 and 2010) and being tied to a bed ($n = 1$; between 2008 and 2018) if they did not comply with treatment guidelines. For some participants ($n = 4$) who presented to facilities, there was also rejection by staff. Reasons for rejection included their illness being too complex ($n = 2$; between 1998 and 2018), not severe enough ($n = 1$; between 2000 and -2010) and the individuals being too disengaged/avoidant during previous admissions ($n = 1$; between 2008 and 2018):

> "...I know there are like hundreds of people who fall through the cracks for being too thin or self-harming...like the system is so broken in that sense. Uhmm but that is such an awful feeling to be asking people to help you and them saying, 'Well, prove to us why we should.'" – Participant 5

Abuse and adverse experiences were also reported ($n = 3$), which included treating staff sexually assaulting patients ($n = 1$; between 2000 and 2010), force-feeding and incorrectly placing feeding tubes ($n = 1$; between 2008 and 2018) as well as unsupported treatment methods for AN being recommended, such as a lobotomy and deep sleep therapy ($n = 1$; between 1960 and 1970):

> "I think the treatments probably done more harm than good you know, I need to recover from the treatment more than I need to recover from the disorder. Uhmm yeah if you ask me, you know, the most damaging thing in my life, I'm not going to say anorexia, I'm going to say treatment for anorexia" – Participant 11

Discussion

Five themes were identified whilst investigating the progression of AN. The theme of transition was a common experience and a distinct turning point was described by most participants during their development of long-standing AN. Given this was often described in the context of a realisation that most of their lives had become permeated by the disease, incorporating this indicator into an assessment tool could assist in identifying these presentations. Additionally, targeting the associated grief that was often paired with this transition may be important to address during therapy.

The finding that trauma pre-dated the development of AN was consistent with previous research that has identified trauma as a risk factor [40, 41]. When trauma[1] was described to result from the breakdown of close relationships, it is worthwhile to determine this influence on a prolonged illness trajectory through further research. With early intervention shown to improve outcomes from AN [42], limited social support during the onset of the illness may have prevented recognition of AN symptoms and reduced any corresponding encouragement by social networks to seek treatment during earlier stages of the disease. A lack of early identification and implementation of interventions was a theme identified by Stockford et al. [12] in their severe and enduring AN sample, which was similarly suggested to perhaps be contributed

---

[1] In the current study, the definition of trauma by Herman [43] was adopted, which describes psychological trauma as the experience of powerlessness that disrupts an individual's sense of control, connection and meaning.

to by the absence of parental support during the early stages of the illness. Although not all participants in the current study described this form of trauma, further investigation into the effect of a disrupted social network on the likelihood of transitioning into long-standing AN is warranted.

With all participants in the current study describing a loss of control as contributing towards the aetiology of their illness, these findings are consistent with earlier models of AN, which suggested that the disease developed as a method to compensate for loss of control [44]. A unique finding in the current study was how the function of AN changed over time for some participants. In terms of improving current treatment methods, ensuring that underlying causes of the illness are addressed may be important given the potential link between functionality and maintenance of the disease. Targeting symptoms alone may be insufficient for patients who have used AN as a method for coping with challenges over a substantial period of time. It is therefore important that the functionality of the disease is continuously assessed during treatment.

Stockford et al. [12] described identity to be a major theme in their sample of severe and enduring AN, which is consistent with the findings of the current study. It is recommended that assessments include an investigation into the role of the illness in the identity formation of patients, and that this be addressed in treatment. For patients who identify with AN, it may be beneficial for therapy to assist in the formation of new identities outside of the illness in order to provide hope for a future free of the disorder. For patients who deny AN as forming part of their identity, this variable could potentially be used as a tool in therapy. Utilising strategies such as cognitive challenging may promote recovery by highlighting the incongruence of the illness from how the patient identifies themselves as an individual.

The ineffectiveness of current treatment models was not surprising given the lack of knowledge of long-standing AN and the corresponding limited evidence-based treatments available. However, a significant finding to have emerged from this research was the participants' report of coercive methods in some treatment facilities that left them feeling miserable and at times, stripped of their basic human rights. This may relate to the findings by Dawson et al. [14] with participants identifying unhelpful treatment to include 'scare tactics' and punishments as forms of motivation. Perhaps this was similar to the coercion described by participants in the current study who reported the ineffectiveness of these methods in facilitating recovery. This may be the reason why some individuals experiencing AN disengage from services [45].

Another surprising discovery was that help-seeking individuals were occasionally turned away from treatment facilities. As previously mentioned, early intervention has been found to be a predictor of better outcomes for patients [42]. This raises concerns as to whether this finding may be a contributing factor in the persistence of some cases of AN. Further research is essential in determining why health professionals are denying treatment to some patients, as is better education for staff on the potential consequences. Furthermore, the effectiveness of traditional 'therapeutic' strategies outlined in the current study and described in the findings of Dawson et al. [14], such as withholding personal items as forms of punishment, need to be evaluated against more novel treatment options.

A more recently applied model to presentations that persist into the later stage of AN is recovery-based models. The basis of recovery-based models is a shift in the focus of treatment from symptom elimination to improving quality of life and general wellbeing [46]. Calugi et al. [47] recommend adopting a recovery-based approach when treating patients with severe and enduring AN with findings from a longitudinal outcome study suggesting this is well tolerated and a viable option for individuals experiencing this illness. Although it was beyond the scope of the current paper to investigate whether recovery-based models prove more effective in treatment than traditional medical models, it is hoped the current findings will inspire research into discovering what approaches are most effective for long-standing AN. The authors recommend the use of mixed research methods when continuing to investigate transitions between the stages of AN with prospective research particularly beneficial for studying the development of illness over time. Furthermore, a comparison between the processes that occur in the long-standing illness with individuals who recover from AN may provide a greater understanding of the factors that differentiate these experiences from those with a better outcome.

The current study had several limitations including being unable to confirm causality with additional research required for this purpose. The convenience sampling method of the snowball technique may have biased recruitment [26]. With this being a retrospective study requiring participants to recall details from early childhood as well as at times when they were severely unwell, it is possible that there may have been recall bias, limiting the accuracy of findings. Additionally, a limitation of all qualitative research particularly from a narrative inquiry framework is the inevitability of some interpretive efforts. Although the intention is to extract meaning made by participants, narrative research involves a degree of interpretation by the researcher and an understanding of the participant differently to how they may perceive themselves [48]. To address this limitation, member checking was offered but only optional with some participants completing this process ($n = 6$), others returning incomplete edits ($n = 3$) or requesting to not be involved ($n = 2$). Although this may have affected the accuracy and validity of the data, it was important to allow participants autonomy over this process. Despite keeping recruitment open to all genders, only females participated, which limited the generalizability of these findings to other genders. Additionally, the recruitment of participants based on the inclusion criterion of illness duration may be argued as a limitation in terms of the theme that emerged in the data analysis of failure of current models of treatment. Individuals were required to have a long-term illness to participate and so the emergence of this theme was not an altogether surprising finding. However, this theme was important and directly addressed the aim of the current study to investigate how and why the AN illness transitions from an early to late stage. Furthermore, there was initial interest expressed in the current study by 26 individuals, with 15 people deciding against participation. This may be argued to reflect a potential bias in recruitment with the final sample perhaps only including individuals who had more time available to participate.

A narrative inquiry approach strengthened the findings in the current study by facilitating an understanding of underlying elements of the stories told by participants, which may have otherwise remained undiscovered [49]. Another strength was achieving thematic saturation, which was identified during data analysis after recruiting a particularly large sample of participants. Previous qualitative research on long-term AN has featured up to eight participants [12–14]. Accordingly, a strength of the current study could be argued to be that it achieved one of the largest sample sizes for this topic, which was required for this research to achieve thematic saturation. Additional strengths included recruiting individuals with large variability in duration of illness and at different points in their experience of long-standing AN, which meant that the findings encapsulated the variability of this disease as it manifests over time.

Conclusion

It was the aim of the current study to provide a greater understanding of the processes that occur when AN progresses from earlier to later stages. Along with identifying the key themes of transition, trauma, functionality and identity, this research provides insight into how current models of treatment have failed these individuals. In terms of the practical implications, findings from the current study suggest that periods of transition occur along the trajectory of these long-standing presentations with the function of the illness likely to change throughout the experience. Trauma may be a common experience with disrupted social networks potentially acting as a barrier to early interventions with further research required to confirm the existence of a relationship. Identity may be an important aspect to consider when managing patients with these presentations, and potentially provide a technique for use in therapy based on the degree of association between the individual and their illness. The finding of currently ineffective and in some circumstances, harmful treatment approaches, requires further investigation. It is imperative that practices involving the mistreatment and abuse of some of these patients disguised under forms of 'treatment' are abolished. There is a need to employ both qualitative and quantitative methods when exploring more effective treatment approaches.

Abbreviations
AN: Anorexia Nervosa; DSM-5: Diagnostic and Statistical Manual of Mental Disorders, Fifth Edition [24].

Acknowledgements
No funding source or acknowledgements.

Authors' contributions
The first author (CB) conducted interviews, analysed the data and was involved in writing the manuscript. The second author (PR) assisted with data analysis and provided guidance on writing the manuscript. The second author (PR) and third author (ST) provided supervision to the first author (CB) and assisted with editing the manuscript. All authors read and approved the final manuscript.

Competing interests
The authors have no conflict or competing interests to declare.

Author details
[1]School of Psychology, Griffith Taylor Building, The University of Sydney, Sydney, NSW 2006, Australia. [2]InsideOut Institute, Charles Perkins Centre, The University of Sydney, Sydney, NSW 2006, Australia.

References

1. Fairburn CG, Harrison PJ. Eating disorders. Lancet (London, England). 2003;361:407–16.
2. Tierney S, Fox JRE. Chronic anorexia nervosa: a Delphi study to explore practitioners' views. Int J Eat Disord. 2009;42:62–7.
3. Elbaky GBA, Hay PJ, Le Grange D, Lacey H, Crosby RD, Touyz S. Pre-treatment predictors of attrition in a randomised controlled trial of psychological therapy for severe and enduring anorexia nervosa. BMC Psychiatry. 2014. https://doi.org/10.1186/1471-244X-14-69.
4. Touyz S, Hay P. Severe and enduring anorexia nervosa (SE-AN): In search of a new paradigm. J Eat Disord. 2015. https://doi.org/10.1186/s40337-015-0065-z.
5. Touyz S, Le Grange D, Lacey H, Hay P, Smith R, Maguire S, et al. Treating severe and enduring anorexia nervosa: a randomized controlled trial. Psychol Med. 2013;43:2501–11.
6. Steinhausen H. The outcome of anorexia nervosa in the 20th century. Am J Psychiatry. 2002;159:1284–93.
7. Ambwani S, Cardi V, Albano G, Cao L, Crosby RD, Macdonald P, et al. A multicenter audit of outpatient care for adult anorexia nervosa: Symptom trajectory, service use, and evidence in support of "early stage" versus "severe and enduring" classification. Int J Eat Disord. 2020;53:1337–48.
8. Noordenbos G, Oldenhave A, Muschter J, Terpstra N. Characteristics and treatment of patients with chronic eating disorders. Eat Disord. 2002;10:15–29.
9. Wildes JE, Forbush KT, Hagan KE, Marcus MD, Attia E, Gianini M, et al. Characterizing severe and enduring anorexia nervosa: an empirical approach. Int J Eat Disord. 2017;50:389–97.
10. Fox JRE, Diab P. An exploration of the perceptions and experiences of living with chronic anorexia nervosa while an inpatient on an eating disorders unit: an interpretative phenomenological analysis (IPA) study. J Health Psychol. 2015;20:27–36.
11. Musolino CM, Warin M, Gilchrist P. Embodiment as a paradigm for understanding and treating SE-AN: locating the self in culture. Front Psych. 2020. https://doi.org/10.3389/fpsyt.2020.00534.
12. Stockford C, Kroese BS, Beesley A, Leung N. Severe and enduring anorexia nervosa: the personal meaning of symptoms and treatment. Women's Stud Int Forum. 2018;68:129–38.
13. Robinson PH, Kukucska R, Guidetti G, Leavey G. Severe and enduring anorexia nervosa (SEED-AN): a qualitative study of patients with 20+ years of anorexia nervosa. Eur Eat Disord Rev. 2015;23:318–26.
14. Dawson L, Rhodes P, Touyz S. "Doing the impossible": the process of recovery from chronic anorexia nervosa. Qual Health Res. 2014;24:494–505.
15. Machado BC, Goncalves SF, Martins C, Hoek HW, Machado HW. Risk factors and antecedent life events in the development of anorexia nervosa: A Portuguese case-control study. Eur Eating Disord Rev. 2014;22:243–51.
16. Nevonen L, Broberg AG. The emergence of eating disorders: an exploratory study. Eur Eat Disord Rev. 2000;8:279–92.
17. Pike KM, Hilburt A, Wilfley DE, Fairburn CG, Dohm FA, Walsh BT, et al. Toward an understanding of risk factors for anorexia nervosa: a case–control study. Psychol Med. 2008;38:1443–53.
18. Hsu LK, Crisp AH, Callender JS. Recovery in anorexia nervosa—the patient's perspective. Int J Eat Disord. 1992;11:341–50.
19. Zerwas S, Lund BC, Von Holle A, Thornton LM, Berrettini WH, Brandt H. Factors associated with recovery from anorexia nervosa. J Psychiatr Res. 2013;47:972–9.
20. Conti J, Rhodes P, Adams H. Listening in the dark: Why we need stories of people living with severe and enduring anorexia nervosa. J Eat Disord. 2016. https://doi.org/10.1186/s40337-016-0117-z.
21. Rogers WS, Willig C. The SAGE handbook of qualitative research in psychology. London: SAGE Publications Ltd; 2017.
22. Willig C. Introducing qualitative research in psychology. 3rd ed. New York: Open University Press; 2013.
23. Mertova P, Webster L. Using narrative inquiry as a research method: an introduction to critical event narrative analysis in research, training and professional practice. New York: Routledge; 2020.
24. American Psychiatric Association. Diagnostic and statistical manual of mental disorders: DSM-5. 5th ed. Arlington: American Psychiatric Association; 2013.
25. Broomfield CL, Stedal K, Touyz S, Rhodes P. Labeling and defining severe and enduring anorexia nervosa: a systematic review and critical analysis. Int J Eat Disord. 2017;50:611–23.
26. Noy C. Sampling knowledge: the hermeneutics of snowball sampling in qualitative research. Int J Soc Res Methodol. 2008;11:327–44.
27. Frank A. The wounded storyteller: body, illness, and ethics. 2nd ed. Chicago: The University of Chicago Press; 2013.
28. Wang CC. Photovoice: a participatory action research strategy applied to women's health. J Women's Health. 1999;8:185–92.
29. Sackett CR, Granberg EM, Jenkins AM. An exploration of adolescent girls' perspectives of childhood obesity through photovoice: a call for counsellor advocacy. J Humanist Couns. 2016;55:215–33.
30. Liebenberg L. Thinking critically about photovoice: achieving empowerment and social change. Int J Qual Methods. 2018. https://doi.org/10.1177/1609406918757631.
31. Wang C, Burris MA. Empowerment through photo novella: portraits of participation. Health Educ Q. 1994;21:171–86.
32. Novek S, Morris-Oswald T, Menec V. Using photovoice with older adults: some methodological strengths and issues. Ageing Soc. 2012;32:451–70.
33. Jarldorn M. Photovoice handbook for social workers: method, practicalities and possibilities for social change. Cham: Springer; 2018.
34. Azungah T. Qualitative research: deductive and inductive approaches to data analysis. Qual Res J. 2018;18:383–400.
35. Frank A. Letting stories breathe: a socio-narratology. Chicago: The University of Chicago Press; 2010.
36. Thomas DR. A general inductive approach for analyzing qualitative evaluation data. The American Journal of Evaluation. 2006;27:237–46.
37. Polkinghorne D. Narrative configuration in qualitative analysis. Int J Qual Stud Educ. 1995;8:5–23.
38. Saunders B, Sim J, Kingstone T, Baker S, Waterfield J, Bartlam B, et al. Saturation in qualitative research: exploring its conceptualization and operationalization. Qual Quant. 2018;52:1893–907.
39. Beck CT. Qualitative research: the evaluation of its credibility, fittingness, and auditability. West J Nurs Res. 1993;15:263–6.
40. Jaite C, Schneider N, Hilbert A, Pfeiffer E, Lehmkuhl U, Salbach-Andrae H. Etiological role of childhood emotional trauma and neglect in adolescent anorexia nervosa: a cross-sectional questionnaire analysis. Psychopathology. 2012;45:61–6.
41. Monteleone AM, Monteleone P, Serino I, Scognamiglio P, Genio M, Maj M. Childhood trauma and cortisol awakening response in symptomatic patients with anorexia nervosa and bulimia nervosa. Int J Eat Disord. 2015;48:615–21.
42. Treasure J, Russell G. The case for early intervention in anorexia nervosa: theoretical exploration of maintaining factors. Br J Psychiatry J Ment Sci. 2011;199:5–7.
43. Herman JL. Trauma and recovery. New York: BasicBooks; 1992.
44. Bruch H. The golden cage: the enigma of anorexia nervosa. Cambridge: Harvard University Press; 1978.
45. DeJong H, Broadbent H, Schmidt U. A systematic review of dropout from treatment in outpatients with anorexia nervosa. Int J Eat Disord. 2011;45:635–47.
46. Cruwys T, Stewart B, Buckley L, Gumley J, Scholz B. The recovery model in chronic mental health: a community-based investigation of social identity processes. Psychiatry Res. 2020. https://doi.org/10.1016/j.psychres.2020.113241.
47. Calugi S, El Ghoch M, Dalle GR. Intensive enhanced cognitive behavioural therapy for severe and enduring anorexia nervosa: a longitudinal outcome study. Behav Res Ther. 2017;89:41–8.
48. Josselson R. The ethical attitude in narrative research: principles and practicalities. In: Clandinin DJ, editor. Handbook of narrative inquiry: mapping a methodology. Thousand Oaks: Sage Publications; 2007. p. 537–66.
49. Wang CC, Geale SK. The power of story: Narrative inquiry as a methodology in nursing research. Int J Nurs Sci. 2015;2:195–8.

7

Structural Brain Differences in Recovering and Weight-recovered Adult Outpatient Women with Anorexia Nervosa

Brooks B. Brodrick[1,2], Adrienne L. Adler-Neal[1], Jayme M. Palka[1], Virendra Mishra[3], Sina Aslan[1,3] and Carrie J. McAdams[1]* ⓘ

Abstract

Background: Anorexia nervosa is a complex psychiatric illness that includes severe low body weight with cognitive distortions and altered eating behaviors. Brain structures, including cortical thicknesses in many regions, are reduced in underweight patients who are acutely ill with anorexia nervosa. However, few studies have examined adult outpatients in the process of recovering from anorexia nervosa. Evaluating neurobiological problems at different physiological stages of anorexia nervosa may facilitate our understanding of the recovery process.

Methods: Magnetic resonance imaging (MRI) images from 37 partially weight-restored women with anorexia nervosa (pwAN), 32 women with a history of anorexia nervosa maintaining weight restoration (wrAN), and 41 healthy control women were analyzed using FreeSurfer. Group differences in brain structure, including cortical thickness, areas, and volumes, were compared using a series of factorial f-tests, including age as a covariate, and correcting for multiple comparisons with the False Discovery Rate method.

Results: The pwAN and wrAN cohorts differed from each other in body mass index, eating disorder symptoms, and social problem solving orientations, but not depression or self-esteem. Relative to the HC cohort, eight cortical thicknesses were thinner for the pwAN cohort; these regions were predominately right-sided and in the cingulate and frontal lobe. One of these regions, the right pars orbitalis, was also thinner for the wrAN cohort. One region, the right parahippocampal gyrus, was thicker in the pwAN cohort. One volume, the right cerebellar white matter, was reduced in the pwAN cohort. There were no differences in global white matter, gray matter, or subcortical volumes across the cohorts.

Conclusions: Many regional structural differences were observed in the pwAN cohort with minimal differences in the wrAN cohort. These data support a treatment focus on achieving and sustaining full weight restoration to mitigate possible neurobiological sequela of AN. In addition, the regions showing cortical thinning are similar to structural changes reported elsewhere for suicide attempts, anxiety disorders, and autistic spectrum disorder. Understanding how brain structure and function are related to clinical symptoms expressed during the course of recovering from AN is needed.

*Correspondence: carrie.mcadams@utsouthwestern.edu
[1] Department of Psychiatry, University of Texas Southwestern Medical Center, 5323 Harry Hines Blvd., Suite BL6.110, Dallas, TX 75390-9070, USA
Full list of author information is available at the end of the article

Plain English summary

Anorexia nervosa is a life-threatening mental illness defined in part by an inability to maintain a body weight in the normal range. Malnutrition and low weight are factors typically present in the anorexia nervosa and can affect brain structure. We conducted a detailed analysis of brain structure using Freesurfer, focusing on regional cortical thicknesses, areas, and volumes, in adult outpatient women with anorexia nervosa. The study included both a partially weight-restored cohort with anorexia nervosa, a cohort sustaining a healthy body weight with history of anorexia nervosa, and a healthy comparison cohort. Reduced cortical thicknesses were observed in eight regions, primarily in the frontal lobe and cingulate for the cohort recently with anorexia nervosa but only one frontal region in the weight-maintained cohort. These data emphasize the importance of sustained weight-restoration for adult women with anorexia nervosa. Further, the impacted neural regions have been associated with impulsivity, attention, self-regulation, and social interactions in other clinical cohorts, suggesting that these neuropsychological processes may warrant study in patients recovering from anorexia nervosa. Future work should consider whether these factors have clinical relevance in the outpatient treatment of adults with anorexia nervosa.

Keywords: Eating disorders, Social cognition, Anorexia nervosa, Autism, Depression, Anxiety, Bulimia nervosa, Self-perception, Gray matter

Introduction

Anorexia nervosa (AN) is a life-threatening mental illness characterized by low body weight and impaired sense of self-worth, with an over emphasis placed that one's body shape and size determines one's value as a person. Recovery from AN often takes years and 5–10% of individuals with AN will die [1] due to its severe medical complications or suicide [2]. Even after intensive treatment and restoration of normal body weight, relapse is common in adults with AN [3]. Avoidance of weight loss immediately following treatment was associated with long-term weight maintenance [4]; whereas psychological measures at discharge were not predictive of clinical course [5]. A critical gap in AN research has been difficulty identifying psychological and cognitive factors that enable successful weight maintenance after acute weight restoration. As such, improving our understanding of neurobiological changes that occur during this critical time period could contribute to our understanding of the course of illness, and potentially elucidate treatment targets important during recovery from AN.

Structural brain analyses can measure gray and white matter volumes, cortical thicknesses and areas, as well as subcortical volumes for regions and structures within the brain. In one meta-analysis of global brain structure in AN, Seitz and colleagues [6] characterized changes in gray matter volumes, white matter volumes, and cerebrospinal fluid volume while considering acutely ill AN, short-term weight-recovered AN, and long-term recovered AN. All measures were reduced in the acutely ill group, reductions in gray matter and cerebrospinal fluid were observed in the short-term weight recovered cohort, and no significant differences were observed in the long-term weight restored cohort. In considering regional differences in brain structure, many studies have compared underweight AN cohorts early or even before beginning treatment to a healthy comparison group [7–12], generally reporting reductions in cortical thickness in some regions in AN. Some studies have considered both underweight AN as well as weight-restored individuals, with most differences resolved after weight-restoration [13–16], with one machine-learning study suggesting increases in orbitofrontal and insula as well as decreases in superior frontal regions might be a state biomarker of AN [17]. Considered as a whole, the literature strongly supports the hypothesis that structural brain differences in AN are closely tied to weight.

Importantly, as AN is defined by alterations in eating behaviors and changes in body mass index (BMI), weight and the disorder are always confounded [18]. Because acute malnutrition alters brain volumes [19], examination of partially-weight restored individuals with AN may reduce the impact of acute malnutrition and provide a better understanding of neurobiological processes relevant during the early stages of recovering. Clinically, the greatest risk of weight loss and resumption of eating disorder behaviors occurs in the first year after intensive treatment [3], supporting a need to better understand individuals at this stage of illness. Regional brain differences have only been analyzed for a single cohort of young, partially-weight restored participants with AN responding well to recent intensive treatment. This cohort showed normalization of cortical thinning [14] and improvement in most local gyrification indices [20] in relation to a healthy comparison cohort. These two studies shared participants, and deployed a longitudinal design such that only those individuals achieving marked weight-restoration in a short time period were included. Thus, there remains a gap in our knowledge, as there are no studies that have evaluated regional brain structure for adult outpatients in the process of recovering from AN.

There is a clinical need to develop a better understanding of neuropsychological factors during partial weight restoration as many patients spend substantial time in this state. In a recent 5-year annual follow-up study of adult patients with AN following intensive weight rehabilitation, only 46% maintained a BMI greater than 18.5 throughout follow-up, with only 17% sustaining both a BMI greater than 18.5 and normalization of EDE-Q scores [5]. These data are consistent with that from several naturalistic studies that have followed outpatients with AN, reporting remission rates from 39 to 42% [21–23]. One large cohort study of adults with AN has found that 31% were recovered after 9 years and 62% recovered at 22 years [24]. In a clinical trial reporting on time-to-relapse after acute weight-restoration for adults with AN, less than 30% maintained a BMI over 18.5 for twelve months [25], with relapse most common in the first two months [26]. In concert, these data suggest that maintaining weight-restoration and achieving recovery is a slow and unpredictable process for adults with AN. Developing a better neurobiological understanding at this stage of the illness may help in designing and targeting treatments to improve outcomes.

Given this need to identify neuropsychological factor that may impact illness course, we compared cortical thicknesses, areas, and volumes in 37 partially weight-restored women with anorexia nervosa (pwAN), 32 adult women with a history of AN and maintaining weight-restoration (wrAN), and 41 healthy comparison (HC) adult women. The goal of this study is to increase our understanding of neuropsychological problems present during outpatient treatment of adult women with AN. We anticipated that clinical symptoms (BMI, depression, eating, self-esteem) would be worse in the pwAN relative to the wrAN and HC cohorts. Based on the extant eating disorder literature in structural brain analyses, we hypothesized that frontal and cingulate regions would show reduced cortical thickness in the pwAN cohort relative to the HC cohort, and expected normalization for all cortical regions in the wrAN cohort.

Methods

Participants

The participants for this study were drawn from two separate IRB-approved neuroimaging protocols that included different functional brain imaging tasks [27–31]; this is the first publication examining structural brain data collected from these protocols. For this study, all participants were required to be female, and between age 18 and 46 years. The HC cohort was required to have no current DSM-IV psychiatric illnesses, with a BMI

between 19 and 30. Substance use disorders, bipolar disorder, and psychotic disorders were exclusionary for all cohorts; participants with major depressive disorder and anxiety disorders were permitted. Current use of mood stabilizers and antipsychotic medications were exclusionary but antidepressants were permitted.

For the AN cohorts, participants with AN from the earlier studies were classified into two cohorts based on both BMI at the time of the scan, as well as the duration at which the person had sustained a BMI greater than 18.5. This study defined partially weight restored AN (pwAN) as individuals whose body mass index (BMI) had been less than 18.5 in prior six months, but were at a stable or increasing weight over the last month, and whose BMI at the time of the scan remained under 19.5. Most of the pwAN cohort were recruited from and scanned soon after completion of intensive treatment programs, including inpatient, residential, partial hospital, and intensive outpatient; all individuals whose BMI was under 17.5 were scanned within a month of discharge, and continued to show a stable or increasing BMI over that period. To qualify for the weight-restored cohort (wrAN), participants had a lifetime-diagnosis of AN, a BMI greater than 19.5, and had not had a BMI under 18.5 at any time in at least six months.

Clinical measures

Both protocols used the Structured Clinical Interview for DSM-IV (SCID) psychiatric disorders to establish eating disorder diagnosis and comorbidities. The timeline from the SCID provided an age of onset for both AN cohorts and age of recovery for the wrAN cohort. The clinical assessments common to both protocols included Eating Attitudes Test-26 (EAT) and its three subscales dieting (EAT-D), bulimia and food preoccupation (EAT-B) and oral control (EAT-O) [32], and the Quick Inventory of Depressive Symptoms [33]. Self-esteem was assessed with the Self-Liking and Self-Competence (SLSC) Questionnaire [34] and social problem-solving with the short version of the Social Problem Solving Inventory-R Short (SPSI-R [35], which provides five subscales that include positive problem orientation (PPO), negative problem orientation (NPO), rational problem solving (RPS), impulsivity/carelessness style (ICS), and avoidance style (AS).

MRI methods

Structural brain scans were acquired using a 3 T Philips Achieva MRI scanner. A high-resolution T1-weighted image called Magnetization Prepared Rapid Acquisition of Gradient-Echo (MPRAGE) sequence was collected with the following parameters: FOV $= 256 \times 256 \times 160$ mm^3, TR/TE $= 8.1$ ms/3.7 ms, flip angle $= 12$, 160 sagittal slices, voxel size $= 1 \times 1 \times 1$ mm^3 and duration of 4 min. The cortical surface was reconstructed for each subject using the FreeSurfer 6.0.1 pipeline [36, 37]. Briefly, each T1-weighted image was spatially and intensity normalized to Talairach Atlas. Volumetric segmentation and subcortical labelling were then performed on the normalized images. The gray matter (GM) and white matter (WM) boundaries were then automatically identified and reconstructed into a mesh of over 150,000 tessellated vertices for surface measures. Gyral anatomy was then aligned to a standard spherical template using surface convexity and curvature measures.

An estimate of contrast to noise ratio (CNR) in white matter was computed for every subject using the Free-Surfer's QA tools (https://surfer.nmr.mgh.harvard.edu/fswiki/QATools). Only data with a CNR > 15 were utilized for further analysis. Furthermore, the datasets that passed the CNR threshold but had a poorly reconstructed surface, we performed manual correction following the guidelines of the FreeSurfer developers. Thickness (mm) and area (mm^2) measures were extracted for all cortical regions identified in Desikan-Killiany atlas [38] along with default volume (mm^3) measures for all cortical and subcortical regions were extracted for all participants, using the FreeSurfer tools, aparcstats2table and asegstats2table, respectively.

Statistical analyses

Prior to conducting statistical analyses, data were examined for the presence of outliers and subjected to assumption testing. For demographic (i.e., race, ethnicity, age, years of education and clinical outcomes (i.e., BMI, QIDS total score, EAT-D score, EAT-B score, EAT-O score, and EAT total score), group differences were examined using chi-squared analyses (for categorical variables) or a one-way ANOVA (for continuous variables). For models that did not meet homogeneity of variance assumptions (i.e., QIDS, EAT-D, EAT-B, EAT-O, and EAT total), Welch's robust ANOVA was used. Tukey post-hoc tests were conducted on statistically significant results. These analyses were conducted using IBM SPSS Statistics version 25.0 (Armonk, NY: IBM Corp.).

To determine group differences in thickness, area, and volumes, a series of factorial F-tests were completed. All models included a group factor (i.e., HC, pwAN, wrAN), with HC as the reference group, while age was entered as a covariate. Results were considered statistically significant at $p < 0.05$. To correct for multiple comparisons among the 166 factorial F-tests, the Benjamini and Hochberg (1995) false discovery rate (FDR) method was applied [39]. An FDR Q-value of 0.15 was chosen in order to remain conservative yet still detect true positives. Six

families of comparisons were identified based upon the type of structural data (i.e. thickness, area, and volume) as well as hemisphere (left, right); FDR corrections were conducted within each family separately. Models with omnibus p-values that passed FDR correction with a statistically significant group effect at $p < 0.05$ were retained. Finally, Cohen's d values were calculated for models that remained statistically significant after applying FDR corrections. The FDR analyses were conducted in R [40] using the lm and p.adjust functions.

Statistically significant models obtained with the analytic sample ($n = 110$) used in the primary analyses, were analyzed a second time using a new analytic sample ($n = 103$) with those having a BMI < 17 removed. This was to ensure that the findings derived from the primary analyses were not driven by the seven individuals in the pwAN cohort with a BMI < 17 at the time of the scan.

Results

Demographic and clinical measures

Participants in the study from the first study protocol included 12 pwAN, 8 wrAN, and 13 healthy comparison (HC) women, and from the second protocol included 25 pwAN, 24 wrAN, and 28 HC women. The full sample includes 37 pwAN, 32 wrAN, and 41 HC women. Antidepressants were permitted, with 16 in the pwAN cohort, 11 in the wrAN, and 1 in the HC cohort. For comorbidities, 13 from the pwAN and 15 from the wrAN had recurrent major depressive disorder; and, eight each from the pwAN and wrAN cohort had a comorbid anxiety disorder (generalized anxiety disorder, panic disorder, or agoraphobia). None of the HC sample met criteria for a eating disorders (lifetime), current anxiety disorders, or had a current episode of major depressive disorder; one HC had a history of recurrent major depressive disorder. Participants were largely non-Hispanic ($n = 101$) and Caucasian ($n = 91$), although there were a few Native American ($n = 2$), Asian ($n = 13$) and Black ($n = 4$) participants; no differences in race ($X^2(4, 110) = 1.189$, $p = 0.888$) or ethnicity ($X^2(2, 110) = 0.102$, p > 0.99) were observed in the comparisons across the three cohorts. Age and education did not differ across the three groups (Table 1).

Clinically, results from the one-way ANOVA (Table 1) revealed statistically significant group differences in BMI with the pwAN cohort lower than the other two groups (HC vs. pwAN: $p < 0.001$, $d = 2.266$; wrAN vs. pwAN: $p < 0.001$, $d = 2.311$). There were no differences in the age of onset of anorexia nervosa across the pwAN and wrAN cohorts, with both groups developing the illness in late adolescence (Age of Onset, years, pwAN 17.0 [3.57], wrAN 16.4 [5.92], F(1,67) = 0.290, $p = 0.592$). A similar proportion of both cohorts had the restricting

Table 1 Demographic and clinical measures by cohort

		Clinical cohort						Statistical comparisons		
		pwAN (n = 37)		wrAN (n = 32)		HC (n = 41)				
		Mean	SD	Mean	SD	Mean	SD	F	df (b/w)	p
Age (years)		25.4	6.75	29.4	8.27	26.7	6.20	2.908	2/107	.059
Education (years)		15.08	2.23	15.44	2.36	15.76	2.29	0.846	2/107	.432
Body mass index		**17.83**[a]	1.17	22.09	2.33	23.17	3.12	82.138	2/59.827	**<.001**
Quick inventory of depression		**6.92**[a]	4.68	**6.53**[a]	5.15	2.22	2.20	22.026	2/56.078	**<.001**
Eating attitudes test (EAT) total		**31.41**[a]	19.80	**23.78**[a]	14.69	3.78	3.93	59.504	2/48.294	**<.001**
EAT	Dieting subscale	**16.89**[a]	11.81	**14.56**[a]	9.07	2.29	3.13	49.189	2/50.754	**<.001**
EAT	Bulimia and food subscale	**7.22**[ab]	5.32	**4.81**[ab]	3.14	0.41	0.81	56.898	2/47.564	**<.001**
EAT	Oral control subcale	**6.81**[ab]	5.16	**4.16**[ab]	4.52	1.12	1.44	25.875	2/50.407	**<.001**
Self-esteem (SLSC)										
SLSC	Self-liking	**17.89**[a]	6.68	**17.44**[a]	6.49	31.41	6.55	54.54	2/107	**<0.001**
SLSC	Self-competence	**22.97**[a]	6.29	**23.47**[a]	3.93	28.90	4.98	15.10	2/107	**<0.001**
Social problem solving inventory-revised (SPSI-R)		**11.54**[a]	2.84	**12.27**[a]	2.43	14.66	2.58	13.91	2/104	**<0.001**
SPSI-R	Positive problem orientation	**9.30**[ab]	3.62	**11.28**[ab]	3.55	13.24	2.43	13.62	2/104	**<0.001**
SPSI-R	Negative problem orientation	**11.54**[ab]	4.39	**8.81**[ab]	3.57	4.66	3.62	28.95	2/104	**<0.001**
SPSI-R	Rational problem solving	10.41	3.45	10.41	3.62	12	3.49	2.45	2/104	.091
SPSI-R	Impulsivity/carelessness style	3.03	3.15	5.03	3.88	3.66	3.13	3.03	2/104	.053
SPSI-R	Avoidance style	7.43[a]	4.76	6.44[a]	4.39	3.63	4.45	6.84	2/104	**.002**

Bold values indicate statistically significant Tukey post hoc comparisons at $p < .05$ with [a]different from HC and [b]differences between pwAN and wrAN cohorts

and binge-purge subtypes of AN (pwAN, 21 restrict, 16 binge-purge; wrAN 19 restrict, 13 binge-purge; $X^2(1,69) = 0.048$, $p = 0.826$). The age of recovery for the wrAN cohort averaged 26.4 [7.1] years. Ten individuals in the pwAN cohort and two individuals in the wrAN cohort had BMIs between 18.5 and 19.5; the individuals in pwAN cohort who reported maintaining a BMI over 18.5 had done so for 2.6 [1.35] months while the two in the wrAN cohort had BMIs over 18.5 for an average of 7.5 [0.5] months.

Many differences in the self-report measures of depression, eating, self-esteem, and social problem solving were observed across the three groups (Table 1). Statistically significant group differences were present in the EAT, with the pwAN group having the highest scores on the EAT and all its subscales: EAT total score (HC vs. pwAN: $p < 0.001$, $d = -1.936$; HC vs. wrAN: $p < 0.001$, $d = -1.861$). Of note, the pwAN and wrAN also differed from each other on the bulimia subscale of the EAT (EAT-B; pwAN vs. wrAN: $p = 0.016$, $d = 0.552$), and the oral control subscale of the EAT (EAT-O; pwAN vs. wrAN: $p = 0.017$, $d = 0.547$). Both the pwAN and wrAN cohorts had elevated depression scores relative to the HC cohort, and did not differ from each other (QIDS; HC vs. pwAN: $p < 0.001$, $d = -1.285$; HC vs. wrAN: $p < 0.001$, $d = -1.089$). Similarly, both the pwAN and wrAN cohorts had lower self-esteem measures than the HC

cohort, including self-liking (SL; HC vs. pwAN: $p < 0.001$, $d = 13.32$; HC vs. wrAN: $p < 0.001$, $d = 13.98$) and self-competence (SC; HC vs. pwAN: $p < 0.001$, $d = 5.93$; HC vs. wrAN: $p < 0.001$, $d = 5.43$), but did not differ from each other. Although the total SPSI-R scores were lower for both pwAN and wrAN relative to HC (SPSI-R; HC vs. pwAN: $p < 0.001$, $d = 3.11$; HC vs. wrAN: $p = 0.001$, $d = 2.39$) they did not differ for each other. However, on both the positive problem orientation (PPO) and the negative problem orientation (NPO) subscales of the SPSI-R, all three groups differed from each other (PPO: HC vs. pwAN: $p < 0.001$, $d = 3.94$; HC vs. wrAN: $p < 0.038$, $d = 1.96$; wrAN vs. pwAN $p < 0.036$, $d = 1.984$; NPO: HC vs. pwAN: $p < 0.001$, $d = -6.88$; HC vs. wrAN: $p < 0.001$, $d = -4.16$; wrAN vs. pwAN $p < 0.014$, $d = -2.73$). No other differences in the SPSI-R were significant across cohorts.

Brain structure

No statistically significant differences were observed in cerebral white matter volume (CWM, pwAN 290,777 mm³, wrAN 299,594 mm³, HC 300,015 mm³; $F[3, 104] = 1.796$; $p = 0.153$), total gray matter volume (TGM, pwAN 442,391 mm³, wrAN 452,821 mm³, HC 458,506 mm³; $F[3, 104] = 0.882$; $p = 0.453$) or subcortical gray matter volume (SGM pwAN 39,351 mm³, wrAN 40,233 mm³, HC 40,517 mm³; $F[3, 104] = 0.534$; $p = 0.660$).

Group differences survived FDR corrections for nine cortical thicknesses and one volume difference (Fig. 1; Table 2). These regions included: right bank SSTS (pwAN: $\beta = -0.075$, $p = 0.021$), right caudal anterior cingulate (pwAN: $\beta = -0.131$, $p < 0.001$), right parahippocampal (pwAN: $\beta = 0.109$, $p = 0.036$), right pars opercularis (pwAN: $\beta = -0.057$, $p = 0.035$), right pars orbitalis (wrAN: $\beta = -0.081$, $p = 0.036$; pwAN: $\beta = -0.079$, $p = 0.034$), right posterior cingulate (pwAN: $\beta = -0.082$, $p = 0.002$), left posterior cingulate (pwAN: $\beta = -0.092$, $p = 0.006$), left rostral middle frontal (pwAN: $\beta = -0.059$, $p = 0.022$), right superior frontal (pwAN: $\beta = -0.077$, $p = 0.002$), and right cerebellar white matter (pwAN: $\beta = -848.929$, $p = 0.034$). The effect sizes associated with these differences were medium to large, with the smallest difference in the right pars opercularis (Cohen's $d = 0.400$) and the largest difference in the right caudal anterior cingulate (Cohen's $d = 0.799$).

The majority of the cortical thickness differences were in the right hemisphere (7/9), and in the frontal lobe [5]. One region, the right pars orbitalis, was thinner in both the pwAN and wrAN cohorts. Seven regions were thinner in the pwAN cohort than the HC, with two of these regions, the left and right posterior cingulate, also thinner in the pwAN cohort compared to the wrAN cohort. One region, the right parahippocampal gyrus, was thicker in the pwAN cohort than the HC cohort. The right cerebellar white matter was smaller in the pwAN than the other two cohorts (Right Cerebellum White Matter mm³, pwAN 9139(1417) wAN 10,239(1986) HC 10,045(1788),

$F[3,104] = 4.060$, $p = 0.009$; pwAN vs. HC, $d = -0.562$; pwAN vs. wrAN, $d = -0.638$; wrAN vs. HC, $d = 0.102$).

To confirm that results from the primary analyses were not driven by the $n = 7$ individuals with a BMI < 17, f-tests were repeated for the above mentioned statistically significant models, after removing $n = 7$ from the analytic sample (Additional file 1: Table S1). The group effect in six models remained statistically significant with an analytic $n = 103$: right bank SSTS (pwAN: $\beta = -0.081$, $p = 0.020$), right caudal anterior cingulate (pwAN: $\beta = -0.146$, $p < 0.001$), right parahippocampal (pwAN: $\beta = 0.109$, $p = 0.037$), right pars orbitalis (wrAN: $\beta = -0.081$, $p = 0.042$; pwAN: $\beta = -0.091$, $p = 0.024$), right posterior cingulate (pwAN: $\beta = -0.084$, $p = 0.003$), and right superior frontal (pwAN: $\beta = -0.066$, $p = 0.010$).

Discussion

Clinical, psychological and structural differences in the brain were compared across three groups: women partially weight-restored and appropriate for outpatient treatment of AN (pwAN), women with history of AN but currently weight-restored (wrAN), and women without EDs (HC). The pwAN and wrAN cohorts both had significantly more depression, eating symptoms, and lower self-esteem scores than the HC cohort; in addition, the pwAN cohort had higher levels of disordered eating, as well as more negative (NPO on SPSI-R) and less positive (PPO on SPSI-R) orientations in social problem solving than the wrAN cohort. Several structural neural differences were observed in group comparisons, including

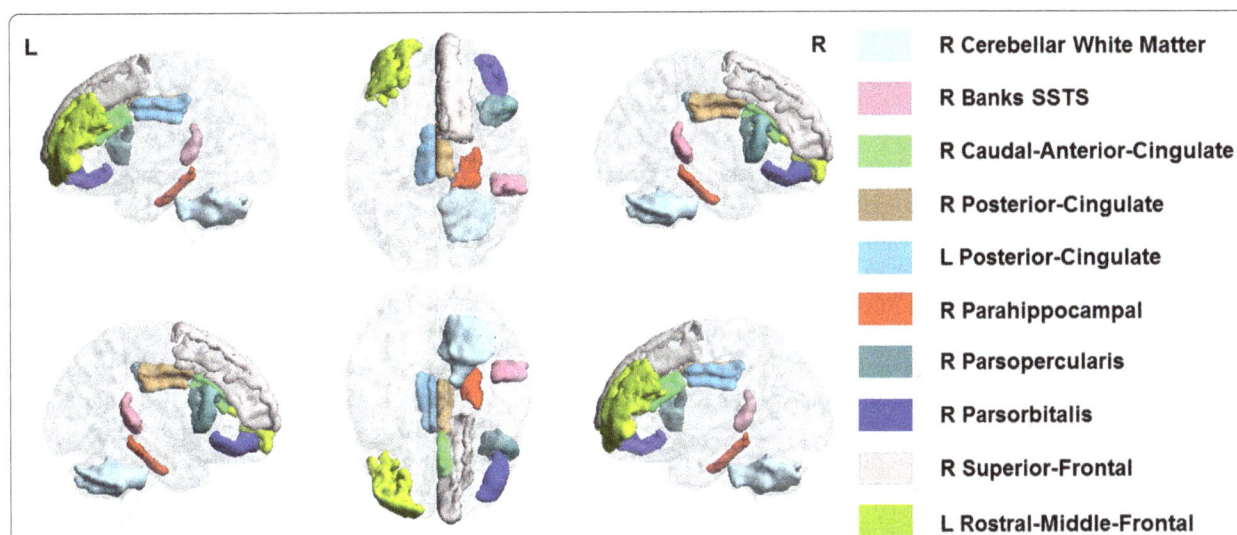

Fig. 1 Nine cortical thicknesses and one volume showed significant differences across the three cohorts. Each region is colored slightly differently. Of note, the R parahippocampal gyrus (red) was thicker in the pwAN cohort relative to the HC cohort; the R pars orbitalis (blue) was thinner in both the pwAN and wrAN relative to the HC cohort; the posterior cingulate thicknesses were thinner in the pwAN cohort relative to both the wrAN and HC cohorts; the remaining cortical thicknesses were thinner for the pwAN cohort relative to the HC cohort

Table 2 Cortical thickness differences in cohorts

	Clinical group						Statistical comparisons				
	pwAN (n = 37)		wrAN (n = 32)		HC (n = 41)				Pairwise effect sizes		
	Mean	SD	Mean	SD	Mean	SD	F	p	Comparison		Cohen's d
R Bank SSTS	2.65[a]	0.15	2.69	0.15	2.72	0.12	3.192	.027	pwAN	wrAN	−0.267
										HC	**−0.515**
									wrAN	HC	−0.221
R Caudal Anterior Cingulate	2.50[a]	0.13	2.57	0.18	2.63	0.19	5.979	<.001	pwAN	wrAN	−0.446
										HC	**−0.799**
									wrAN	HC	−0.324
R Parahippocampal	2.82[a]	0.22	2.76	0.22	2.70	0.25	4.987	.003	pwAN	wrAN	0.273
										HC	**0.510**
									wrAN	HC	0.255
R Parsopercularis	2.77[a]	0.13	2.78	0.12	2.82	0.12	5.763	.001	pwAN	wrAN	−0.080
										HC	**−0.400**
									wrAN	HC	−0.333
R Parsorbitalis	2.83[a]	0.18	2.80[a]	0.17	2.90	0.15	5.398	.002	pwAN	wrAN	0.171
										HC	**−0.423**
									wrAN	HC	**−0.624**
R Posterior Cingulate	2.49[ab]	0.10	2.57	0.12	2.57	0.12	5.324	.002	pwAN	wAN	**−0.724**
										HC	**−0.724**
									wrAN	HC	0.000
L Posterior Cingulate	2.48[ab]	0.16	2.57	0.13	2.57	0.14	3.374	.021	pwAN	wrAN	**−0.617**
										HC	**−0.599**
									wrAN	HC	0.000
L Rostral Middle Frontal	2.53[a]	0.12	2.55	0.12	2.58	0.10	3.866	.011	pwAN	wrAN	−0.167
										HC	**−0.453**
									wrAN	HC	−0.272
R Superior Frontal	2.83[a]	0.11	2.86	0.10	2.90	0.10	7.935	<.001	pwAN	wrAN	−0.285
										HC	**−0.666**
									wrAN	HC	−0.400

Bold values indicate statistically significant comparisons at p < .05, with [a]different from HC and [b]differences between pwAN and wrAN cohorts. For all F-tests, df(b/w) = 3/104

eight neural regions with reduced cortical thickness in the pwAN cohort relative to the HC cohort, with one of these regions, the right pars orbitalis, also showing reduced cortical thickness in the wrAN cohort. No differences in cortical surface areas were observed, and only one volume measure, the right cerebellar white matter volume, was reduced in the pwAN cohort compared to the other groups. The effect sizes for all observed cortical differences were medium to large.

The differences in cortical thinning observed in the pwAN cohort are more pronounced than those observed in the only other study that has evaluated a cohort of partially weight restored AN. That cohort was younger (average age 15.5 years), assessed on average three months after beginning an intensive weight restoration program

from a low starting weight, and restricted to participants able to gain substantial weight during the treatment [14]. Nevertheless, differences in local gyrification index were observed after weight-restoration for this younger cohort, and those differences were in right-sided frontal and temporal regions [20]; the same areas we report to be thinner in our pwAN cohort. Considering that our sample was about 10 years older, these data support a hypothesis that frontal and temporal regions may be slow to recover following an acute episode of AN.

The first step in recovery from AN is weight-restoration and requires sufficient caloric intake to maintain an individual at a healthy body weight. Most previous studies examining weight-recovered cohorts with AN suggest structural brain differences resolve after sustained weight restoration [13–16]. Unfortunately, clinical studies have shown that achieving and maintaining weight restoration is quite difficult for adult women with AN [5, 21, 24–26]. Clinical differences are seldom reported for comparisons of both pharmacological and psychological outpatient treatments for adults with AN [41, 42], suggesting a critical need to better understand treatments that are effective at this stage of AN. In this discussion, we consider the differences observed in the pwAN and wrAN cohorts, in relation to both common roles for these regions in healthy individuals, and prior studies of these areas in eating disorder and other psychiatric illnesses that can be comorbid with AN. These comparisons may be helpful in guiding future research to improve our understanding of the neuropsychological changes involved in the recovery process for adult outpatients with AN.

Only one cortical thickness, the right pars orbitalis, differed in both pwAN and wrAN. In studies of healthy human behaviors, this area has been associated with impulse-control [43], emotional communication [44, 45], and social exclusion [46]. Numerous studies have observed functional brain differences in the inferior frontal gyrus and insula in both AN and BN, a region anatomically close and overlapping with this area [47, 48]. Previously, from a subset of this sample, we reported that reduced activations of the right inferior frontal gyrus were observed in an AN cohort relative to a HC cohort when participants were engaged in evaluation of social interactions relative to conducting a non-social, physical evaluation about interactions [27]. In adolescents with bulimia nervosa, reduction in cortical thickness of the right inferior frontal gyrus was previously hypothesized to be a potential trait marker of bulimia nervosa, as more pronounced reduction correlated with increased frequency of purging episodes [49]. The observed cortical thinning in this region for both the pwAN and wrAN cohorts lend additional credence to consideration of this area as a potential trait marker important in eating disorders.

Here, we also observed social cognitive differences between the pwAN and wrAN cohorts in two subscales of the social problem solving inventory, with more negative and less positive problem-solving orientations, as assessed with the NPO and PPO subscales of the SPSI-R, for the pwAN cohort relative to wrAN, and both cohorts relative to HC. Clinically, problems with mentalization and non-verbal social communication have been observed in patients with AN [50–52], and interventions that target social-emotional function are being explored in anorexia nervosa. Cognitive remediation and emotional skill training (CREST) augments treatment of severe AN, addressing social anhedonia, alexithymia, and quality of life [53, 54]. Improvements in eating disorder

symptoms, anxiety, and depression were observed with a brief group therapy intervention targeting self-attributions and perspective-taking for outpatients with eating disorders [55]. Since these social cognitive processes (PPO and NPO) differ both in relation to illness (both pwAN and wrAN differ from HC), and the degree of difference is impacted by illness state (pwAN is worse than wrAN), these data support a hypothesis that social cognition is altered during the course of recovering from AN.

Many of the structural differences observed in the pwAN cohort, including reduced cortical thickness in the right banks of the superior temporal gyrus, right pars opercularis, right pars orbitalis, right superior frontal gyrus, bilateral posterior cingulate, and diminished right cerebellar volume, are in areas frequently linked to social cognitive behaviors and emotional reasoning. The right pars opercularis is closely tied to reasoning and social cognition [56]. Both the inferior frontal gyrus (includes pars opercularis and orbitalis) and the superior temporal sulcus are engaged during tasks that involve empathy, imitation, and theory of mind in healthy participants [57]. When self-relevant information is attributed to another person, both the superior frontal gyrus and posterior cingulate are activated [58]. In previously published functional MRI studies from subsets of participants from this sample, altered activations during social self-evaluations were reported for the posterior cingulate, precuneus and dorsal anterior cingulate [28, 30], while diminished responses were observed in the temporoparietal junctions in AN during both a social attribution task [27] and a social neuroeconomic game [29].

Cerebellar volume deficits have been amongst the most consistent regional volume differences present in AN [6]. Reduced cerebellar volume has been associated with duration of illness in AN [59]. Reduced right cerebellum volume has also been associated with autistic behaviors in both animal models and humans with autistic spectrum disorders, with the right cerebellar crus showing strong functionally connectivity with both the superior frontal gyrus and posterior cingulate in neurotypical adults [60]. Recently, the cerebellum has been hypothesized to be essential for the adaptations and learning required for social behaviors [61].

Three regions in the cingulate were also thinner in pwAN including the right caudal anterior cingulate as well as the right and left posterior cingulate. Reduced cortical thickness in the cingulate has been one of the most common regional changes reported in AN [6]. The anterior cingulate is involved in value-based decision-making including social motivation and reward-based behaviors [62]. The posterior cingulate is a key node in the default mode network, and associated with arousal, activities that require internally-directed attention and consideration of oneself in relation to others [63–65]. Problems in self-regulation, both regarding recognition of internal emotional as well as physical states, are well-established in AN [66]. Also potentially relevant to AN, thinning of the cingulate cortex has been associated with low vitamin D in normal aging [67]. Of note, both posterior cingulate cortical thicknesses were the only regions for which the pwAN cohort differed from both the wrAN and HC cohorts, further supporting a hypothesis that the cingulate may be particularly vulnerable to malnutrition.

One of only two differences on the left side of the brain was a thinner left rostral middle frontal region, an area associated with emotional stress [68]. Cortical thickness in this area also mediates the relationship between expressed neuroticism and polygenic risk score for the trait of neuroticism [69]. This area has previously been reported as thinner in panic disorder [70] as well as in suicide attempts [71]. In the Sarkinaite's examination of suicidality, cortical thicknesses were compared for both single attempt and multiple attempt patients, finding three regions that were thinner than the healthy comparison cohort in single attempt individuals and seventeen regions that were thinner in the multiple attempt individuals [71]. Several regions from both suicidality cohorts overlap with regions observed to be thinner in the pwAN cohort here. Suicidality is common in anorexia nervosa, with most deaths from the illness due to suicide [2].

Finally, one area, the right parahippocampal gyrus, was larger in the pwAN cohort relative to the other two cohorts. The parahippocampal gyrus has been associated with memory formation, exercise, and emotional regulation The exercise data may be most relevant to this sample, as the parahippocampal gyrus shows increased cortical thickness in relation to increased exercise in many different types of studies in both human and animal models (for review [72]). One study assessed hippocampal volume in women with AN in relation to excessive exercise, observing a larger hippocampal volume in women with AN engaged in excessive exercise that normalized after weight restoration [73]. Another potentially relevant study examined individuals with anxiety disorders undergoing cognitive behavioral therapy, finding reduced activations in the right parahippocampal gyrus were associated with improved clinical symptoms after treatment, with those authors proposing that this area may be involved in maintaining negative emotional states [74]. Both overexercise [75] and maintaining negative emotional states [76] are also common in AN.

There are many limitations to this study. First, this study combined structural data obtained from two different functional imaging studies to increase sample size, and relatively few clinical measures overlapped across the studies or differed in the pwAN and wrAN

cohorts, preventing examination of whether structural changes could be directly related to clinical assessments. The clinical course of AN in adult patients is complex, and some factors that may be related to nutrition and the brain structure including duration at low body weight were not available. The study is moderately-sized, larger than most structural studies in the literature for AN, but not as large as many studies of other psychiatric illnesses. The limited sample size prevents consideration of the impact of antidepressant use or comorbid diagnoses on the results. Neither cohort included severely underweight individuals, so questions about the brain structure present in more severely malnourished individuals cannot be answered. This is a cross-sectional study of only adult women, so results should not be generalized to younger ages that are also common in AN, and its cross-sectional nature prevents assigning function and symptoms changes to the brain differences.

Conclusions

These structural brain imaging data from outpatients recovering and recovered from AN provide new information about brain structure during the later stages of weight restoration and weight maintenance. Most importantly, nearly all of the structural changes were resolved in the wrAN cohort, supporting the importance of keeping a focus in treatment of AN on both achieving and maintaining a BMI greater than 19.5, approximately the third percentile for adult women in the United States. Even after excluding the lowest weight individuals (BMI < 17, 19% of the pwAN cohort), many structural differences remained, suggesting the neurobiological impact of AN resolves slowly. Areas showing cortical thinning in the pwAN cohort share similarities with structural changes previously reported in suicide attempts, anxiety disorders, and autistic spectrum disorder; more research evaluating these types of symptoms over time in patients with AN in concert with structural and functional neural data is needed. A broader set of neural, clinical and psychological symptom data may be helpful to establish how neurophysiological changes are related to clinical problems experienced by individuals recovering from AN.

Abbreviations

AN: Anorexia nervosa; pwAN: Partially-weight restored cohort with anorexia nervosa; wrAN: A 6-month minimum weight-restored cohort with lifetime history of AN; HC: The healthy comparison cohort; IRB: Institutional review board.

Acknowledgements

Appreciation to all of the study participants and research assistants involved in generating this dataset.

Authors' contributions

BBB conceptualized study, reviewed literature, and edited manuscript; AALN wrote first draft of introduction and reviewed literature; JMP conducted statistical analyses, wrote statistical methods and edited manuscript; VM and SA completed Freesurfer analysis, and edited manuscript; CJM conceptualized study, edited manuscript, collected data, and acquired funding. All authors read and approved the final manuscript.

Competing interests

The authors declare that there are no potential conflicts of interest with respect to the research, authorship and publication of this article.

Author details

¹Department of Psychiatry, University of Texas Southwestern Medical Center, 5323 Harry Hines Blvd., Suite BL6.110, Dallas, TX 75390-9070, USA. ²Department of Internal Medicine, University of Texas Southwestern Medical Center, 5323 Harry Hines Blvd., Dallas, TX 75390-9070, USA. ³Advance MRI LLC, Frisco, TX 75034, USA.

References

1. Arcelus J, Mitchell AJ, Wales J, Nielsen S. Mortality rates in patients with anorexia nervosa and other eating disorders: a meta-analysis of 36 studies. Arch Gen Psychiatry. 2011;68(7):724–31.
2. Goldstein A, Gvion Y. Socio-demographic and psychological risk factors for suicidal behavior among individuals with anorexia and bulimia nervosa: a systematic review. J Affect Disord. 2019;245:1149–67.
3. Khalsa SS, Portnoff LC, McCurdy-McKinnon D, Feusner JD. What happens after treatment? A systematic review of relapse, remission, and recovery in anorexia nervosa. J Eat Disord. 2017;5:20.
4. Kaplan AS, Walsh BT, Olmsted M, Attia E, Carter JC, Devlin MJ, et al. The slippery slope: prediction of successful weight maintenance in anorexia nervosa. Psychol Med. 2009;39(6):1037–45.
5. Glasofer DR, Muratore AF, Attia E, Wu P, Wang Y, Minkoff H, et al. Predictors of illness course and health maintenance following inpatient treatment among patients with anorexia nervosa. J Eat Disord. 2020;8(1):69.
6. Seitz J, Herpertz-Dahlmann B, Konrad K. Brain morphological changes in adolescent and adult patients with anorexia nervosa. J Neural Transm (Vienna). 2016;123(8):949–59.
7. Seitz J, Walter M, Mainz V, Herpertz-Dahlmann B, Konrad K, von Polier G. Brain volume reduction predicts weight development in adolescent patients with anorexia nervosa. J Psychiatr Res. 2015;68:228–37.
8. Lavagnino L, Amianto F, Mwangi B, D'Agata F, Spalatro A, Zunta-Soares GB, et al. Identifying neuroanatomical signatures of anorexia nervosa: a multivariate machine learning approach. Psychol Med. 2015;45(13):2805–12.
9. Lavagnino L, Amianto F, Mwangi B, D'Agata F, Spalatro A, Zunta Soares GB, et al. The relationship between cortical thickness and body mass index differs between women with anorexia nervosa and healthy controls. Psychiatry Res Neuroimaging. 2016;248:105–9.
10. Fuglset TS, Endestad T, Hilland E, Bang L, Tamnes CK, Landro NI, et al. Brain volumes and regional cortical thickness in young females with anorexia nervosa. BMC Psychiatry. 2016;16(1):404.
11. Yue L, Wang Y, Kaye WH, Kang Q, Huang JB, Cheung EFC, et al. Structural alterations in the caudate nucleus and precuneus in un-medicated anorexia nervosa patients. Psychiatry Res Neuroimaging. 2018;281:12–8.
12. Leppanen J, Sedgewick F, Cardi V, Treasure J, Tchanturia K. Cortical morphometry in anorexia nervosa: an out-of-sample replication study. Eur Eat Disord Rev J Eat Disord Assoc. 2019;27(5):507–20.
13. King JA, Geisler D, Ritschel F, Boehm I, Seidel M, Roschinski B, et al. Global cortical thinning in acute anorexia nervosa normalizes following long-term weight restoration. Biol Psychiatry. 2015;77(7):624–32.
14. Bernardoni F, King JA, Geisler D, Stein E, Jaite C, Natsch D, et al. Weight restoration therapy rapidly reverses cortical thinning in anorexia nervosa: a longitudinal study. Neuroimage. 2016;130:214–22.
15. Miles AE, Voineskos AN, French L, Kaplan AS. Subcortical volume and cortical surface architecture in women with acute and remitted anorexia nervosa: an exploratory neuroimaging study. J Psychiatr Res. 2018;102:179–85.
16. Cascino G, Canna A, Monteleone AM, Russo AG, Prinster A, Aiello M, et al. Cortical thickness, local gyrification index and fractal dimensionality in people with acute and recovered Anorexia Nervosa and in people with Bulimia Nervosa. Psychiatry Res Neuroimaging. 2020;299:111069.
17. Lavagnino L, Mwangi B, Cao B, Shott ME, Soares JC, Frank GKW. Cortical thickness patterns as state biomarker of anorexia nervosa. Int J Eat Disord. 2018;51(3):241–9.
18. King JA, Frank GKW, Thompson PM, Ehrlich S. Structural neuroimaging of anorexia nervosa: future directions in the quest for mechanisms underlying dynamic alterations. Biol Psychiatry. 2018;83(3):224–34.
19. Frintrop L, Trinh S, Liesbrock J, Leunissen C, Kempermann J, Etdoger S, et al. The reduction of astrocytes and brain volume loss in anorexia nervosa-the impact of starvation and refeeding in a rodent model. Transl Psychiatry. 2019;9(1):159.
20. Bernardoni F, King JA, Geisler D, Birkenstock J, Tam FI, Weidner K, et al. Nutritional status affects cortical folding: lessons learned from anorexia nervosa. Biol Psychiatry. 2018;84(9):692–701.
21. Amianto F, Spalatro A, Ottone L, Abbate Daga G, Fassino S. Naturalistic follow-up of subjects affected with anorexia nervosa 8 years after multimodal treatment: personality and psychopathology changes and predictors of outcome. Eur Psychiatry J Assoc Eur Psychiatr. 2017;45:198–206.
22. Brodrick B, Harper JA, Van Enkevort E, McAdams CJ. Treatment utilization and medical problems in a community sample of adult women with anorexia nervosa. Front Psychol. 2019;10:981.
23. Danielsen M, Bjornelv S, Weider S, Myklebust TA, Lundh H, Ro O. The outcome at follow-up after inpatient eating disorder treatment: a naturalistic study. J Eat Disord. 2020;8(1):67.
24. Eddy KT, Tabri N, Thomas JJ, Murray HB, Keshaviah A, Hastings E, et al. Recovery from anorexia nervosa and bulimia nervosa at 22-year follow-up. J Clin Psychiatry. 2017;78(2):184–9.
25. Walsh BT, Kaplan AS, Attia E, Olmsted M, Parides M, Carter JC, et al. Fluoxetine after weight restoration in anorexia nervosa: a randomized controlled trial. JAMA. 2006;295(22):2605–12.
26. Walsh BT, Xu T, Wang Y, Attia E, Kaplan AS. Time course of relapse following acute treatment for anorexia nervosa. Am J Psychiatry. 2021:appiajp202121010026.
27. McAdams CJ, Krawczyk DC. Impaired neural processing of social attribution in anorexia nervosa. Psychiatry Res. 2011;194(1):54–63.
28. McAdams CJ, Krawczyk DC. Who am I? How do I look? Neural differences in self-identity in anorexia nervosa. Soc Cognit Affect Neurosci. 2014;9(1):12–21.
29. McAdams CJ, Lohrenz T, Montague PR. Neural responses to kindness and malevolence differ in illness and recovery in women with anorexia nervosa. Hum Brain Mapp. 2015;36(12):5207–19.
30. McAdams CJ, Jeon-Slaughter H, Evans S, Lohrenz T, Montague PR, Krawczyk DC. Neural differences in self-perception during illness and after weight-recovery in anorexia nervosa. Soc Cognit Affect Neurosci. 2016;11(11):1823–31.
31. Xu J, Harper JA, Van Enkevort EA, Latimer K, Kelley U, McAdams CJ. Neural activations are related to body-shape, anxiety, and outcomes in adolescent anorexia nervosa. J Psychiatr Res. 2017;87:1–7.
32. Berland NW, Thompson JK, Linton PH. Correlation between the eat-26 and the eat-40, the eating disorders inventory, and the restrained eating inventory. Int J Eat Disord. 1986;5(3):569–74.
33. Bernstein IH, Rush AJ, Stegman D, Macleod L, Witte B, Trivedi MH. A Comparison of the QIDS-C16, QIDS-SR16, and the MADRS in an adult outpatient clinical sample. CNS Spectr. 2010;15(7):458–68.
34. Tafarodi RW, Swann WB Jr. Self-linking and self-competence as dimensions of global self-esteem: initial validation of a measure. J Pers Assess. 1995;65(2):322–42.

35. D'Zurilla TJ, Nezu AM, Maydeu-Olivares A. Social problem-solving inventory-revised (SPSI-R): technical manual. North Tonawanda: Multi-Health Systems Inc; 2002.

36. Fischl B, Dale AM. Measuring the thickness of the human cerebral cortex from magnetic resonance images. Proc Natl Acad Sci U S A. 2000;97(20):11050–5.

37. Fischl B, van der Kouwe A, Destrieux C, Halgren E, Segonne F, Salat DH, et al. Automatically parcellating the human cerebral cortex. Cereb Cortex. 2004;14(1):11–22.

38. Desikan RS, Segonne F, Fischl B, Quinn BT, Dickerson BC, Blacker D, et al. An automated labeling system for subdividing the human cerebral cortex on MRI scans into gyral based regions of interest. Neuroimage. 2006;31(3):968–80.

39. Benjamini Y, Hochberg Y. Controlling the false discovery rate: a practical and powerful approach to multiple testing. J R Stat Soc Ser B. 1995;57(1):289–300.

40. Team RC. R: A language and environment for statistical computing. Vienna: R Foundation for Statistical Computing; 2020.

41. Solmi M, Wade TD, Byrne S, Del Giovane C, Fairburn CG, Ostinelli EG, et al. Comparative efficacy and acceptability of psychological interventions for the treatment of adult outpatients with anorexia nervosa: a systematic review and network meta-analysis. Lancet Psychiatry. 2021;8(3):215–24.

42. Byrne S, Wade T, Hay P, Touyz S, Fairburn CG, Treasure J, et al. A randomised controlled trial of three psychological treatments for anorexia nervosa. Psychol Med. 2017;47(16):2823–33.

43. Aron AR, Robbins TW, Poldrack RA. Inhibition and the right inferior frontal cortex: one decade on. Trends Cogn Sci. 2014;18(4):177–85.

44. Seydell-Greenwald A, Chambers CE, Ferrara K, Newport EL. What you say versus how you say it: comparing sentence comprehension and emotional prosody processing using fMRI. Neuroimage. 2020;209:116509.

45. Krautheim JT, Steines M, Dannlowski U, Neziroglu G, Acosta H, Sommer J, et al. Emotion specific neural activation for the production and perception of facial expressions. Cortex. 2020;127:17–28.

46. Mwilambwe-Tshilobo L, Spreng RN. Social exclusion reliably engages the default network: a meta-analysis of cyberball. Neuroimage. 2021;227:117666.

47. Donnelly B, Touyz S, Hay P, Burton A, Russell J, Caterson I. Neuroimaging in bulimia nervosa and binge eating disorder: a systematic review. J Eat Disord. 2018;6:3.

48. Frank GK. Advances from neuroimaging studies in eating disorders. CNS Spectr. 2015;20(4):391–400.

49. Cyr M, Kopala-Sibley DC, Lee S, Chen C, Stefan M, Fontaine M, et al. Reduced inferior and orbital frontal thickness in adolescent bulimia nervosa persists over two-year follow-up. J Am Acad Child Adolesc Psychiatry. 2017;56(10):866–74.

50. Kuipers GS, Bekker M. Attachment, mentalization, and eating disorders: a review of studies using the adult attachment interview. Curr Psychiatry Rep. 2012;8:326–36.

51. Kerr-Gaffney J, Mason L, Jones E, Hayward H, Harrison A, Murphy D, et al. Autistic traits mediate reductions in social attention in adults with anorexia nervosa. J Autism Dev Disord. 2020;51:2077–90.

52. Harrison A. Experimental investigation of non-verbal communication in eating disorders. Psychiatry Res. 2021;297:113732.

53. Tchanturia K, Doris E, Mountford V, Fleming C. Cognitive Remediation and Emotion Skills Training (CREST) for anorexia nervosa in individual format: self-reported outcomes. BMC Psychiatry. 2015;15:53.

54. Harrison A, Stavri P, Tchanturia K. Individual and group format adjunct therapy on social emotional skills for adolescent inpatients with severe and complex eating disorders (CREST-A). Neuropsychiatrie. 2020.

55. Hunt B, Hagan WS, Pelfrey S, Mericle S, Harper JA, Palka JM, et al. Pilot data from the self-blame and perspective-taking intervention for eating disorders. J Behav Cogn Therapy. 2021;31:57–66.

56. Hartwigsen G, Neef NE, Camilleri JA, Margulies DS, Eickhoff SB. Functional segregation of the right inferior frontal gyrus: evidence from coactivation-based parcellation. Cereb Cortex. 2019;29(4):1532–46.

57. Schmidt SNL, Hass J, Kirsch P, Mier D. The human mirror neuron system-a common neural basis for social cognition? Psychophysiology. 2021;58:e13781.

58. Schindler S, Kruse O, Stark R, Kissler J. Attributed social context and emotional content recruit frontal and limbic brain regions during virtual feedback processing. Cogn Affect Behav Neurosci. 2019;19(2):239–52.

59. Fonville L, Giampietro V, Williams SC, Simmons A, Tchanturia K. Alterations in brain structure in adults with anorexia nervosa and the impact of illness duration. Psychol Med. 2014;44(9):1965–75.

60. Stoodley CJ, D'Mello AM, Ellegood J, Jakkamsetti V, Liu P, Nebel MB, et al. Altered cerebellar connectivity in autism and cerebellar-mediated rescue of autism-related behaviors in mice. Nat Neurosci. 2017;20(12):1744–51.

61. Stoodley CJ, Tsai PT. Adaptive prediction for social contexts: the cerebellar contribution to typical and atypical social behaviors. Annu Rev Neurosci. 2021;44:475–93.

62. Apps MA, Rushworth MF, Chang SW. The anterior cingulate gyrus and social cognition: tracking the motivation of others. Neuron. 2016;90(4):692–707.

63. Leech R, Sharp DJ. The role of the posterior cingulate cortex in cognition and disease. Brain. 2014;137(Pt 1):12–32.

64. Bellucci G, Camilleri JA, Eickhoff SB, Krueger F. Neural signatures of prosocial behaviors. Neurosci Biobehav Rev. 2020;118:186–95.

65. Koban L, Gianaros PJ, Kober H, Wager TD. The self in context: brain systems linking mental and physical health. Nat Rev Neurosci. 2021;22(5):309–22.

66. Prefit AB, Candea DM, Szentagotai-Tatar A. Emotion regulation across eating pathology: a meta-analysis. Appetite. 2019;143:104438.

67. Foucault G, Duval GT, Simon R, Beauchet O, Dinomais M, Annweiler C, et al. Serum vitamin D and cingulate cortex thickness in older adults: quantitative MRI of the brain. Curr Alzheimer Res. 2019;16(11):1063–71.

68. Michalski LJ, Demers CH, Baranger DAA, Barch DM, Harms MP, Burgess GC, et al. Perceived stress is associated with increased rostral middle frontal gyrus cortical thickness: a family-based and discordant-sibling investigation. Genes Brain Behav. 2017;16(8):781–9.

69. Song L, Zhou Z, Meng J, Zhu X, Wang K, Wei D, et al. Rostral middle frontal gyrus thickness mediates the relationship between genetic risk and neuroticism trait. Psychophysiology. 2021;58(2):e13728.

70. Asami T, Takaishi M, Nakamura R, Yoshida H, Yoshimi A, Whitford TJ, et al. Cortical thickness reductions in the middle frontal cortex in patients with panic disorder. J Affect Disord. 2018;240:199–202.

71. Sarkinaite M, Gleizniene R, Adomaitiene V, Dambrauskiene K, Raskauskiene N, Steibliene V. Volumetric MRI analysis of brain structures in patients with history of first and repeated suicide attempts: a cross sectional study. Diagnostics (Basel). 2021;11(3):488.

72. Loprinzi PD. The effects of physical exercise on parahippocampal function. Physiol Int. 2019;106(2):114–27.

73. Beadle JN, Paradiso S, Brumm M, Voss M, Halmi K, McCormick LM. Larger hippocampus size in women with anorexia nervosa who exercise excessively than healthy women. Psychiatry Res. 2015;232(2):193–9.

74. Bomyea J, Ball TM, Simmons AN, Campbell-Sills L, Paulus MP, Stein MB. Change in neural response during emotion regulation is associated with symptom reduction in cognitive behavioral therapy for anxiety disorders. J Affect Disord. 2020;271:207–14.

75. Melissa R, Lama M, Laurence K, Sylvie B, Jeanne D, Odile V, et al. Physical activity in eating disorders: a systematic review. Nutrients. 2020;12(1):183.

76. Castellon P, Sudres JL, Voltzenlogel V. Self-defining memories in female patients with anorexia nervosa. Eur Eat Disord Rev J Eat Disord Assoc. 2020;28(5):513–24.

8

Exploring the Experience of Being Viewed as "not sick enough": a Qualitative Study of Women Recovered from Anorexia Nervosa or Atypical Anorexia Nervosa

Kari Eiring[1], Trine Wiig Hage[2] and Deborah Lynn Reas[2]* [ID]

Abstract

Background: Despite common misconceptions, an individual may be seriously ill with a restrictive eating disorder without an outwardly recognizable physical sign of the illness. The aim of this qualitative study was to investigate the perspectives of individuals who have previously battled a restrictive eating disorder who were considered "not sick enough" by others (e.g., peers, families, healthcare professionals) at some point during their illness, and to understand the perceived impact on the illness and recovery. Such misconceptions are potentially damaging, and have been previously linked with delayed help-seeking and poorer clinical outcomes.

Methods: Seven women who had recovered from anorexia nervosa or atypical anorexia nervosa participated in semi-structured interviews. Interviews were transcribed and interpretive phenomenological analysis was used.

Results: Three main themes emerged: (1) dealing with the focus upon one's physical appearance while battling a mental illness, (2) "project perfect": feeling pressure to prove oneself, and (3) the importance of being seen and understood. Participants reported that their symptoms were occasionally met with trivialization or disbelief, leading to shame, confusion, despair, and for some, deterioration in eating disorder symptoms which drove further weight loss. In contrast, social support and being understood were viewed as essential for recovery.

Conclusion: To facilitate treatment seeking and engagement, and to optimize chances of recovery, greater awareness of diverse, non-stereotypical presentations of restrictive eating disorders is needed which challenge the myth that weight is the sole indicator of the presence or severity of illness.

Plain English Summary

A persistent myth is that restrictive eating disorders are outwardly recognizable due to severely low body weight or emaciation. Atypical anorexia nervosa (AAN) and anorexia nervosa (AN) are both characterized by restrictive eating behavior. Individuals with AAN do not have current low body weight, although some research suggests they have higher levels of impairment and eating disorder pathology than their peers with AN, and their physical health may be equally compromised. Despite this, individuals with AAN are more likely to have a longer duration of illness and

*Correspondence: deborah.lynn.reas@ous-hf.no
[2] Regional Department of Eating Disorders, Division of Mental Health and Addiction, Oslo University Hospital-Ullevål, P.O. Box 4956, 0424 Nydalen Oslo, Norway
Full list of author information is available at the end of the article

less likely to receive inpatient care, suggesting their illness is not always recognized by others. Additionally, thinness is highly valued in today's society and restrictive eating behavior or "dieting" is commonplace, which may promote trivialization, or even reinforcement, of initial weight loss by friends or family. With this in mind, our study aimed to explore the experiences of seven recovered individuals recovered from AN or AAN who were directly or indirectly told by peers, families, or healthcare professionals that they were "not sick enough" at some point during their course of illness. We explored the perceived effects on symptoms, motivation for treatment, mental health and well-being. Participants reported their symptoms were occasionally trivialized or dismissed, leading to shame, confusion, and self-doubt regarding the seriousness of their symptoms. For some, a deterioration in eating disorder symptoms ensued that led to additional weight loss, sometimes in a competitive or perfectionist pursuit to "succeed" at eating restrictively. Findings demonstrated the value of being seen and understood, as well as the potential damage of being considered as "not sick enough" by others when battling a restrictive eating disorder.

Keywords: Eating disorders, Anorexia nervosa, Atypical anorexia nervosa, The thin ideal, Not sick enough

Introduction

A prevailing misconception is that an eating disorder, particularly those marked by restrictive eating, is always outwardly recognizable due to malnutrition or emaciation [1]. In reality, restrictive eating disorders occur across a range of body weights [2, 3]. For instance, Atypical Anorexia Nervosa (AAN), currently categorized as an Other Specified Feeding and Eating Disorder in the DSM-5 (OSFED) [4] and formerly categorized under ED Not Otherwise Specified in the DSM-IV (EDNOS) [5], shares the same criteria as AN, but individuals are within or above normal body mass index range (BMI) despite undergoing significant weight loss. This group is diverse, inclusive of boys and men, persons who are overweight or obese prior to illness [6], or those in a prodromal or residual phase of AN. Despite normal weight status, individuals with atypical AN are at risk for medical instability and malnourishment, with a similar array of medical comorbidities similar to AN, including low bone mineral density, bradycardia and hypotension [7–10]. Moreover, some evidence suggests that individuals with atypical AN have even higher levels of eating disorder psychopathology than AN, including greater distress related to body image concerns [6].

Delays in treatment attributable to trivialization of symptoms by healthcare professionals, or stringent weight-based criteria to access treatment, have been previously identified as barriers to early intervention [11, 12]. Early detection and early intervention are key to making a full recovery [13, 14], yet individuals with atypical presentations often endure a longer duration of illness [15–17] and are less likely to receive inpatient care [18], suggesting underrecognition. Furthermore, sociocultural environments in which thinness is highly valued, restrictive eating behavior or "dieting" is normative [19] and weight-based stigma is pervasive [20] may promote trivialization, or even reinforcement, of initial weight loss by peers, family, and healthcare providers.

Eating disorders are typically furtive illnesses, and treatment seeking overall is strikingly low, with as few as 17–31% of persons in the community with a diagnosable eating disorder seeking treatment [21]. While the number of individuals with atypical presentations seeking treatment is increasing, i.e., up five-fold in five years at one acute inpatient adolescent setting [3], a recent systematic review found that AAN remains underrepresented in clinical samples compared to epidemiological samples [22]. One study investigating treatment-seeking characteristics amongst a sample of US adolescents estimated that only 20% of their sample sought treatment for their illness, and individuals with "counter-stereotypical" symptoms were the least likely to seek treatment [23]. Although the vast majority of clinical studies have included predominantly white female adolescents with limited diversity [22], atypical AN presentations are also not uncommon among adults in diverse population samples [24], such as military Veterans [25], yet active help-seeking is similarly low. Anecdotal evidence from clinical observations and personal accounts in "Almost Anorexic" by Thomas and Schaefer [26] suggest that individuals struggling from eating problems may forego seeking help due to fears of not being "sick" or "thin" enough to deserve or warrant treatment. While some individuals may indeed present with less severity or impairment than full-criteria AN resulting in less frequent referral or admission, those who are actively seeking treatment are likely experiencing a significant level of distress or concern over their eating difficulties, and would benefit from clinical attention.

Little is known regarding the experiences of individuals who have actively sought help for a restrictive eating disorder and the perceived impact of delayed, denied, or diminished treatment opportunities due to others perceiving them as "not sick or thin enough." Some research has found that former patients had experienced referral and admission criteria to be exceedingly weight-based, setting "a threshold that appeared to *promote* weight loss as a means of accessing support..." [27]. Similarly, a qualitative study undertaken by the Academy of Eating Disorders reported that some service users perceived the necessity of being "physically on death's door" in order to gain access to treatment [28], and this may remain a salient issue across all phases of the illness and recovery. Relying upon physical measures of illness to determine discharge readiness, for instance, may result in relapse if not accompanied by improvements in other domains. Additionally, waiting until significant weight loss occurs prior to resumption of treatment　readmission may undermine patient motivation, leaving individuals unsupported in their efforts to manage a relapse.

The aim for this qualitative study was to understand the perspectives of individuals with a past history of diagnosed AN or AAN, who were either directly or indirectly told by others they were "not sick enough" at some point during the course of their illness. Individuals with either diagnosis were included due to　diagnostic fluctuation or progression which may occur between AAN and AN over time [29], and to allow for possible inconsistency in diagnostic practices between providers, as AAN and AN diagnostic criteria are not always uniformly applied in clinical settings [30]. Qualitative research is particularly well-suited to gather in-depth insights from persons with lived experiences to concretize important directions for future research and to inform clinical practice [31, 32], To date, no study has specifically investigated the experience, and perceived impact, of being viewed by others as "not sick enough" with an ED. This is despite indications that some individuals delay help-seeking due to worries about the legitimacy of their eating problems, or some may deliberately—and dangerously—intensify efforts to lose weight to "prove" their ED or access treatment [28]. Understanding the views of persons with lived experiences informs hypotheses and outlines priorities for future studies, and may guide policy that reduces the overall suffering attributable to eating disorders by facilitating earlier or appropriate intervention.

Method
Sample
The participants were non-randomly selected using purposive, non-probability sampling via online adverts on social media (Facebook, Twitter) of Norway's two largest non-profit ED organizations (SPISFO, ROS) and the Regional Department of Eating Disorders (RASP) at Oslo University Hospital, which offers tertiary, specialized ED treatment to a catchment area of approximately 2.9 million people. Individuals aged 18 years and older who had previously received a diagnosis of AN or AAN and had at least one prior experience of being perceived as "not

sick enough" by others (e.g., family, friends, peers, teachers, healthcare professionals) were eligible for inclusion. Individuals who self-reported a *current* ED diagnosis were not eligible for inclusion. Being perceived as "not sick enough" was not formally operationalized, but based upon the participant's self-reported subjective experiences. Participants were instructed to reflect only upon experiences in which *others* perceived them as not sick enough, not the times when they personally didn't consider themselves ill, as denial or lack of recognition of the seriousness of the illness is diagnostic [4]. Respondents to the study advertisement were contacted by email and screened by phone. Recruitment was terminated with theoretical saturation [33, 34]. Participation was voluntary, with no financial compensation. Seven females participated, ranging age from 21 to 47 years, with a mean age of 28 years and median 25 years. Written consent was obtained from all participants. The study was conducted in accordance with the Helsinki convention and ethical approval was obtained from the Regional Ethics Committee (REK) and the Internal Review Board at Oslo University Hospital.

Procedure
Semi-structured interviews for this study were conducted in-person or over the phone (n = 2) on a one-to-one basis by KE. Qualitative interviews were considered well-suited to address the research aim by allowing the interviewer to gain insight into the subjective experience of the participant and provides a comprehensive set of data [35]. Care was taken to establish rapport and promote open discussion. Interviews were semi-structured around a topic guide that covered two main points: narration of the journey with an ED and experiences and reflections specific to the research question (e.g., "Can you describe your experience(s) of being viewed by others as "not sick enough"? I wondered if you could describe any specific instances when this occurred. Again, we're interested in your experiences when *others* perceived you as "not sick enough"––not the times when you *personally* didn't consider yourself ill with an eating disorder."). The topic guide (available upon request) was iteratively developed based on feedback from user representatives from SPISFO, ROS, and treatment providers at RASP, and was piloted with a volunteer who had lived experience with an ED. The average length of the interview was 45–60 min. All interviews were audio recorded and transcribed verbatim. Identifying information was removed at the point of transcription and pseudonyms were used hereafter.

Data analysis
Interpretive phenomenological analysis (IPA) is a useful methodological framework in qualitative psychology that

draws upon the epistemological foundation of phenomenology, hermeneutics, and idiography. The primary goal of IPA is to investigate how individuals make sense of their experiences, assuming people are 'self-interpreting beings'. The richness of the data produced by the semi-structured qualitative interview and the flexibility of interpretation in IPA was considered suitable for exploring individuals' experiences, particularly complex and difficult ones [35]. Following steps outlined by Smith [34], transcripts were read and re-read multiple times, reflections and observations noted, notes were transformed into emergent themes, and clustered based on conceptual similarities. To improve validity of the themes which emerged from the transcripts, both KE and TWH reviewed the material. Illustrative quotes were selected to exemplify less self-explanatory themes and to substantiate the findings. Quotes from the transcripts have been translated from Norwegian to English and edited for legibility, with explanations added in square brackets if required and are identified by initials to protect anonymity.

Results

As shown in Table 1, three main themes emerged from the material: (1) dealing with the focus upon physical appearance while battling a mental illness, (2) "project perfect": feeling pressure to prove oneself, and (3) the importance of being seen and understood.

Dealing with the focus upon one's physical appearance while battling a mental illness

This main theme revolved around the excessive, and untoward, attention that others place upon one´s physical appearance and weight while psychological aspects of the illness are neglected. The first subtheme captures being overlooked or under-recognized by others, including friends, family, school or health professionals, etc. largely due to not being considered "thin enough" to have an ED. The second subtheme is specific to treatment

settings, and captures the viewpoint that access to treatment, admission and discharge, is often reliant on the physical measure of body weight.

Not skinny enough to have an ED

Several of the participants shared that friends and family never believed they struggled with an eating disorder. This negatively affected participants, resulting in feelings of humiliation, shock, confusion, shame and feeling invisible. One participant shared,

"I have friends from high school, that are still my friends today that [they] don't believe I ever struggled with eating disorders. And that's friends who are supposed to be close friends, and it hurts a lot. I was skinny when I was actively struggling with the eating disorder, but when I started to recover and reached normal weight.... yeah, they point blank don't believe that I've ever had an ED because they didn't see me as being skinny enough." -Thea

Participants reported that these incidents caused self-doubt, and created a feeling of uncertainty over whether they actually were sick and deserved treatment. When one participant disclosed she had an eating disorder to a group of peers, she recalled,

"...It was very shameful, I felt, yeah, it was embarrassing to talk about it, and stuff like that. But, I thought, let's see if I am brave enough to do this. And then afterwards, almost everyone came up to me surprised and said "God, if you have an eating disorder...I know people [with EDs], but they are super-skinny, and you are not that skinny!" -Hege

These incidences illustrate some of the effects external comments had on the participant, as well as revealed the tendency to be concerned with how one was perceived by the surroundings. Several participants reacted to the fact that people would comment on their appearance but not ask how they were doing emotionally, and several were bothered by comments on the physical aspects. Several

Table 1 Overview of main themes and subthemes

Themes and subthemes	Number of participants
1. Dealing with the focus upon *physical* appearance while battling a *mental* illness	
(a) You are not skinny enough to have an ED!	5 of 7
(b) Weight-based access to treatment	7 of 7 (clearly in 5)
2. Project perfect: Feeling pressure to prove oneself	7 of 7 (clearly in 5)
3. The importance of being seen and understood	
(a) The lack of congruence between the internal experience and the response from the external environment	7 of 7
(b) Having someone to fight for you	7 of 7 (clearly in 5)

participants also described troubling incidents following recovery after weight restoration, in which others made weight-based comments seemingly without knowledge of the seriousness of an eating disorder:

> *"What I found maybe most difficult about it [weight gain] was that my fellow students who didn't know me very well, we were a pretty large class, right, and the ones that saw me every day and didn't know that I had been very sick, suddenly I'd gained a lot, (...) I was a little bit ashamed of having gained that much weight because I was thinking that now, they don't know... that I was life threateningly ill, sort of, so it is important that I gain weight." -Marie*

Weight-based threshold to access treatment

The need to become thinner, or "worse," to access treatment, or before being taken seriously by health care professionals, was a major theme for all participants. When one participant recognized a spike in ED symptoms following a break-up, she reached out for professional help to avoid a relapse,

> ... *"But they told me "no", they sort of just blew me off and said they just needed to monitor this, but there's nothing now that indicates that we need to take action because your weight is relatively stable, and your blood samples are fine". - Stine*

She further explained that her difficulties increased, she was eventually referred for treatment a second time, yet she was stunned at the intensity her illness needed to reach before she was taken seriously.

> *"After multiple rejections then, why, what's the point then? Why should I fight for something that nobody cares to fight for with me? Like three months went by until the doctor realized that this [the relapse] was serious, but by then my weight had gone drastically down. And that still annoys me today..."*

Project "perfect": under pressure to prove oneself

The second main theme that emerged from the data reflected the self-ascribed importance of being successful at the ED, to "prove" oneself to be "sick" enough, and for some, this had occurred within a context of perfectionistic and competitive traits. Several participants tied the onset of the illness to gaining control. The illness was described as an "area of expertise" and many participants were motivated to be "the best" at the ED. Being viewed as "not sick enough" dealt a blow to this endeavor, and in some instances, prompted additional weight loss and

a deterioration in symptoms. One participant recalled a visit to a school nurse,

> *"There I experienced... that I wasn't (...) sick enough. So, I remember that I, I had sessions with her once a week, or once a month, I don't remember exactly, anyways I remember that I made myself a goal that I would be f******* sick enough for her to tell me that "now you need help". - Tiril*

One participant described her ability to restrict made her feel special and unique, especially as most people tried yet failed to lose weight:

> *"Eh, and I got sort of an uncomfortable relationship with my weight, and then it was the summer before I started the second year of high school and I thought, "I'm gonna lose weight. But there are so many that lose weight and then they gain it again, but that's not me," I told myself. "I'm going to make it". - Thea*

The importance of being seen and heard

When looking at the material as a whole, the importance of being seen and understood was perhaps the most salient theme. Two subthemes emerged, the first of which captured experiences in dealing with an invalidating environment, where one's external surroundings directly or indirectly contradicted or minimized the internal feelings, beliefs, and experiences of the individual. The second subtheme reflected the importance of having someone available who is not only understanding and supportive, but who remains steadfast and persistent in encouraging and enabling, treatment motivation and access.

The lack of congruence between the internal experience of the individual and the response from the external environment

All of the participants described situations in which they felt misunderstood, or their symptoms were trivialized, leading to a sense of confusion and hurt. Failed attempts to acquire support and help left several participants feeling demotivated and uncertain.

> *"When I was admitted to the ER and was about to be discharged, I was told by a doctor there that I was supposed to just eat (...) three potatoes and two meatballs and then it will be OK. So just eat that, then everything will be fine, you'll see... And this is at the ER (...). So, comments from health professionals that I've gotten are completely out of touch, where I don't think they understand how sick you really are." -Tiril*

Most of the participants shared detailed accounts of aspects of their illness that were dramatic and scary, yet these experiences were often discounted or trivialized by others. This led to feelings of uncertainty and distrust, particularly towards the treatment system, and led to withdrawal and unwillingness to share additional information. One participant said this when describing her first meeting with her GP (general practitioner), after she disclosed that she had eating problems:

> "She started off by asking me questions, and they were really weird ones, like, "are you gay?", "have you (...) had a traumatizing childhood?", and all those things I answered "no" to...Then when she asked me how I ate on a normal day. I explained how I had eaten in January, when things were going well. Now things were much worse. But by that point in the assessment, I didn't dare to tell her...." - Maria

Having someone to "fight" for you

In contrast, the participants ardently recalled occasions during which they had felt seen and heard, naming specific encounters and individuals who "fought for them." One of the participants repeatedly mentioned her GP, and when asked what she would do if she felt at risk for a relapse, she said, without hesitation, that she would talk to her GP,

> "...because he is sort of the one who saved my life. If I lost some weight or like, hadn't managed what we had agreed on as my goals, then it was never like I was hopeless, but more like, "okay, we'll have to try again and then we'll have to see (...) where we went wrong and we'll try and see if we can find another way that works better for you..." Lise.

Another participant recalled feeling supported and validated by the sheer determination of a treatment provider, which was turning point in her recovery by boosting her motivation and lessening her ambivalence to engage in treatment.

> "... And then she said, "What did you just say? Oh my god, you can't leave here before we do something about this. Have you ever gotten help? After I replied no, she immediately called someone and I got an appointment right then and there, and she followed me to my appointment. So, I kind of realized that I wanted the help, you know." - Hege

One participant shared how she was first denied for local specialized treatment after being referred by her GP:

> "He [the GP] said, "that's not good enough, we can't

accept that. After that, I got an appointment quite fast, and I received the diagnosis of atypical anorexia." - Lise.

On the other hand, some participants recalled failed opportunities to be understood and taken care of by loved ones. One participant mentioned that her parents commented on her losing weight but they did not take action, and although it was a *"good comment to get"* she left feeling unseen and unsupported:

> "I'm left feeling very betrayed, sort of. Very betrayed, very, not to be seen, but I thought after that, that in fact your own parents didn't do anything because they thought it would pass." - Hege

Another participant remarked,

> "Mom said lots of times, like, "oh, now your losing... just don't lose control", and I was like "no, no, no, it is just a couple of kilos". But I didn't have control whatsoever....it's very much like... "Okay, we can see that there is something wrong with her, but we won´t ask her about it." Tiril.

Discussion

To our knowledge, this is the first study to explore the perspectives of individuals with a history of AN or AAN who have experienced being viewed as "not sick enough" by others at some point during their course of illness. Semi-structured interviews were administered face-to-face, and interpretive phenomological analysis was used to explore the in-depth experiences and perceived effects on prognosis, course, symptom development and motivation for recovery. Three main themes emerged from the interviews, (1) dealing with the focus upon one's physical appearance while battling a mental illness, (2) "project perfect": feeling pressure to prove oneself, and (3) the importance of being seen and understood.

The first main theme centered on the tendency of others to focus on physical measure of illness, such as weight, while psychological aspects of the illness were overlooked or under-recognized. All of the study participants had experienced at least one episode during the course of illness in which they perceived their symptoms were disregarded or trivialized by others—based on physical measures––as not serious enough to warrant, access, or continue treatment. Participants recalled feeling a variety of negative emotions in reaction to this experience, from annoyance and confusion, to despair, lack of trust, and an increased ambivalence to treatment and unwillingness to disclose information. A few participants directly linked trivialization of symptoms to an intentional intensification of restrictive eating behavior in an effort to "prove" their illness or to gain access to treatment. These findings are consistent with prior research detailing deleterious consequences in which individuals deliberately attempted to lose more weight to access treatment [28].

Relating to the second theme, one aspect which surfaced during the interviews was the desire to "be successful or good" at having an ED. In many ways, having an ED made the individual feel special and unique, and control over eating and weight provided a sense of mastery. Other studies have reported similar findings, that the ED provides the individual a feeling of being special, and this is generally described as one of the positive things connected to the illness [36]. In response to being perceived as "not sick enough," several participants reported they needed to "prove" the seriousness of their illness. Other research has also highlighted the interplay between a competitive nature of eating disorders and a weight-based access to treatment, in which individuals feel successful and taken seriously at lower weights [27].

The final theme related to the importance of being "seen" and "heard". This was an overarching theme and consistent with recent findings suggesting that the interaction of individuals with AN and their social environment, and specifically, the recognition of illness by family and peers, often functions as a facilitator in seeking timely help [12]. Several studies have confirmed that unconditional support from significant others, family, friends and health care providers is an important resource for an individual in recovery from EDs [37], and is related to lower levels of emotional distress and improved well-being generally [38]. Family support, and being believed when disclosing difficulties, has also proven important for seeking help and completing treatment [39, 40]. Some of the participants recalled feeling unseen or unsupported by family members who clearly recognized a problem yet didn't take action or ask questions. Feeling supported by healthcare providers is also a particularly salient predictor of treatment engagement and satisfaction [41]. Several of the participants recalled the exact moment, or series of moments, during which healthcare providers advocated, sometimes relentlessly, for a referral or admission. Being "fought for," despite privately harboring some level of ambivalence or uncertainty about the need for treatment, was identified by several participants as a turning point in motivation for recovery.

Clinical implications

This study offers novel evidence that, from the perspective of service users, that relying upon BMI as a marker for the presence or severity of an eating disorder may have adverse consequences to well-being and treatment motivation, in addition to mischaracterization or misclassification of health status [42, 43]. As such, our findings support prior arguments that treatment must "move beyond skinniness" [44] by not solely focusing on weight restoration, and address psychological and psychosocial aspects "from an early stage" [27].

Another implication of this study is that a weight-based approach to treatment is insufficient across all stages of the illness and treatment, from prodromal to residual phases. Waiting until significant weight loss occurs counteracts efforts to intervene early, and as observed in the present study, leaves patients feeling frustrated, less motivated to engage in treatment, and unsupported. Our participants also shared experiences of being discharged based upon meeting a weight threshold, without sufficient regard to the level of ED psychopathology, or conversely, being denied readmission following a relapse regardless of spikes in ED-related behaviors and cognitions. Indeed, one participant recalled frustration during a relapse, as she was not offered treatment until after three months of rapid weight loss had ensued. A focus on weight restoration without accompanying improvements in psychological, cognitive, and psychosocial function, for instance, is reflected in high relapse rates for AN [45], and indeed, several have argued for a broader focus beyond weight to define recovery and determine health needs [46, 47].

Within this context, it is important to note that an extremely low body weight due to malnutrition or starvation indeed propels a cascade of medical sequelae with potentially detrimental effects [48]. Nevertheless, prior studies have shown that a lack of currently low weight does not preclude medical compromise [2, 49]. One study, for example, found that a 5% weight loss in combination with significant ED-related cognitive concerns (i.e., undue influence of weight on self-evaluation and fears of weight gain) was a marker for a clinically meaningful restrictive eating disorder [50]. This also concurs with increasing evidence suggesting the importance of assessing relative weight status and weight history, not simply the current weight of the individual, when determining health status and treatment needs [51] [3].

Study limitations and future directions

Limitations of this study are important to mention. This study used a purposive sampling strategy to explore individual range of perspectives and experiences, and did not aim to generalize findings. Participants were self-selected and recruited via social media on user organization websites, and had previously sought treatment, and may have differed markedly from cases in the general community. Few individuals in the community with a diagnosable eating disorder seek treatment, and individuals with atypical symptoms seek treatment less often than the ones with more stereotypical presentations [23]. The present sample included recovered individuals willing to share their retrospective experiences, and data may be subject to recall or memory biases. The reflections of persons with lived experiences are valuable, and provide insight spanning the course of illness, including recovery and relapses; however, interviewing a current clinical sample, however, might have yielded different results.

Participants were screened by phone for eligibility based upon self-reported diagnostic status, but no diagnostic interview was administered to confirm current or past medical or psychiatric status or weight history. Additional information regarding diagnostic history, along with demographic and illness-related variables such as length of illness and time since recovery would be useful for the contextualization of findings, and future quantitative studies are encouraged to examine these variables in relation to participants' subjective experiences. In the current study, weight history, including current and past level of underweight, was not specifically related to the experiences of not feeling "sick enough", although this would also be an interesting area of future research. Additionally, further relevant aspects, such as insight into the disorder (self-evaluation of being sick enough, readiness to change), or age of onset, would be similarly interesting to explore in future investigations. We opted to include individuals with either a past diagnosis of AN or atypical AN in an effort to allow for diagnostic progression and inconsistency between providers in diagnostic practices, and a stricter approach to the inclusion criteria may have yielded different results.

Although both genders were eligible for participation, no males were identified via the recruitment process. Future research is needed to explore the views and experiences of ethnically and culturally diverse groups, as well as males, across the lifespan whose illness may be overlooked or trivialized due to a non-stereotypical presentation. It would also be interesting to broaden the scope to examine other types of eating disorders, for example, binge eating disorder, bulimia nervosa, avoidant-restrictive food intake disorder. A review of studies investigating public and healthcare professionals' knowledge and attitudes toward binge eating disorder, for instance, revealed limited public awareness that BED constitutes a diagnosable eating disorder [52].

Future research is also recommended to explore the experiences of carers. One study has found that carers of persons with mental illness experienced difficulties accessing services for their loved ones, being denied access due to their relative's illness being classified as "not in crisis" which had created feelings of frustration, distress and anxiety for families [53].

Conclusions
In conclusion, findings may help provide a framework for further investigation of the experience of being "not sick enough" from a restrictive eating disorder. Qualitative research can facilitate an improved understanding of the perspectives and priorities of persons with lived experience and provide the groundwork for additional research. Increased awareness of diverse, non-stereotypical presentations of restrictive eating disorders is needed to challenge beliefs among healthcare providers and the public-at-large that body weight is the primary indicator of the presence or severity of illness. Results underscore the importance of social support and being "seen" and understood, and the potentially deleterious consequences of disclosing symptoms which are then trivialized or disregarded by others. Assertively advocating, or being "fought for," by healthcare providers was viewed as especially powerful in motivating willingness to engage in treatment when battling a restrictive eating disorder.

Acknowledgements
The authors would like to thank the participants whose willingness to share their experiences made this study possible. Thank you to ROS, SPISFO and RASP for graciously providing feedback on the study design and for allowing us to advertise and recruit via your social media platforms.

Authors' contributions
KE conceived of the study, conducted and transcribed the interviews, performed the analyses, and prepared the first draft of the manuscript. DLR sought and received ethical approval for the project. TWG supervised the interviews and assisted with the analyses. DLR and TWH were involved in the study design, recruitment, interpretation of results, and preparation of the manuscript. All authors read and approved the final manuscript.

Competing interests
The authors declare that they have no competing interests.

Author details
[1] Institute of Psychology, Faculty of Social Sciences, University of Oslo, Oslo, Norway. [2] Regional Department of Eating Disorders, Division of Mental Health and Addiction, Oslo University Hospital-Ullevål, P.O. Box 4956, 0424 Nydalen Oslo, Norway.

References

1. Zipfel S, Giel KE, Bulik CM, Hay P, Schmidt U. Anorexia nervosa: aetiology, assessment, and treatment. Lancet Psychiatry. 2015;2(12):1099–111.
2. Rastogi R, Rome Md ES. Restrictive eating disorders in previously overweight adolescents and young adults. Cleve Clin J Med. 2020;87(3):165–71.
3. Whitelaw M, Gilbertson H, Lee KJ, Sawyer SM. Restrictive eating disorders among adolescent inpatients. Pediatrics. 2014;134(3):e758-764.
4. APA. Diagnostic and Statistical Manual of Mental Disorders. 5th ed. Washington, DC: American Psychiatric Publishing; 2013.
5. APA. Diagnostic and Statistical Manual of Mental Disorders. 4th ed. Arlington: American Psychiatric Publishing; 1994.
6. Sawyer SM, Whitelaw M, Le Grange D, Yeo M, Hughes EK. Physical and psychological morbidity in adolescents with atypical anorexia nervosa. Pediatrics. 2016;137(4):e20154080.
7. Le Grange D, Crosby RD, Engel SG, et al. DSM-IV-defined anorexia nervosa versus subthreshold anorexia nervosa (EDNOS-AN). Eur Eat Disord Rev. 2013;21(1):1–7.
8. Olivo G, Solstrand Dahlberg L, Wiemerslage L, et al. Atypical anorexia nervosa is not related to brain structural changes in newly diagnosed adolescent patients. Int J Eat Disord. 2018;51(1):39–45.
9. Forney KJ, Brown TA, Holland-Carter LA, Kennedy GA, Keel PK. Defining "significant weight loss" in atypical anorexia nervosa. Int J Eat Disord. 2017;50(8):952–62.
10. Moskowitz L, Weiselberg E. Anorexia nervosa/atypical anorexia nervosa. Curr Probl Pediatr Adolesc Health Care. 2017;47(4):70–84.
11. Ali K, Farrer L, Fassnacht DB, Gulliver A, Bauer S, Griffiths KM. Perceived barriers and facilitators towards help-seeking for eating disorders: a systematic review. Int J Eat Disord. 2017;50(1):9–21.
12. Kastner D, Weigel A, Buchholz I, Voderholzer U, Lowe B, Gumz A. Facilitators and barriers in anorexia nervosa treatment initiation: a qualitative study on the perspectives of patients, carers and professionals. J Eat Disord. 2021;9(1):28.
13. Treasure J, Russell G. The case for early intervention in anorexia nervosa: theoretical exploration of maintaining factors. Br J Psychiatry. 2011;199(1):5–7.
14. Von Holle A, Poyastro Pinheiro A, Thornton LM, et al. Temporal patterns of recovery across eating disorder subtypes. Aust N Z J Psychiatry. 2008;42(2):108–17.
15. Hughes EK, Le Grange D, Court A, Sawyer SM. A case series of family-based treatment for adolescents with atypical anorexia nervosa. Int J Eat Disord. 2017;50(4):424–32.
16. Lebow J, Sim LA, Kransdorf LN. Prevalence of a history of overweight and obesity in adolescents with restrictive eating disorders. J Adolesc Health. 2015;56(1):19–24.
17. Rockert W, Kaplan AS, Olmsted MP. Eating disorder not otherwise specified: the view from a tertiary care treatment center. Int J Eat Disord. 2007;40(Suppl):S99–103.
18. Kennedy GA, Forman SF, Woods ER, et al. History of overweight/obesity as predictor of care received at 1-year follow-up in adolescents with anorexia nervosa or atypical anorexia nervosa. J Adolesc Health. 2017;60(6):674–9.
19. Striegel-Moore RH, Silberstein LR, Rodin J. Toward an understanding of risk factors for bulimia. Am Psychol. 1986;41(3):246–63.
20. Puhl RM, Lessard LM. Weight stigma in youth: Prevalence, consequences, and considerations for clinical practice. Curr Obes Rep. 2020;9(4):402–11.
21. Hart LM, Granillo MT, Jorm AF, Paxton SJ. Unmet need for treatment in the eating disorders: a systematic review of eating disorder specific treatment seeking among community cases. Clin Psychol Rev. 2011;31(5):727–35.
22. Harrop EN, Mensinger JL, Moore M, Lindhorst T. Restrictive eating disorders in higher weight persons: a systematic review of atypical anorexia nervosa prevalence and consecutive admission literature. Int J Eat Disord. 2021. https://doi.org/10.1002/eat.23519.
23. Forrest LN, Smith AR, Swanson SA. Characteristics of seeking treatment among US adolescents with eating disorders. Int J Eat Disord. 2017;50(7):826–33.
24. Hay P, Mitchison D, Collado AEL, Gonzalez-Chica DA, Stocks N, Touyz S. Burden and health-related quality of life of eating disorders, including avoidant/restrictive food intake disorder (ARFID), in the Australian population. J Eat Disord. 2017;5:21.

25. Masheb RM, Ramsey CM, Marsh AG, Snow JL, Brandt CA, Haskell SG. Atypical Anorexia Nervosa, not so atypical after all: Prevalence, correlates, and clinical severity among United States military Veterans. Eat Behav. 2021;41:101496.
26. Thomas JJ, Schaefer J. Almost anorexic: is my (or my loved one's) relationship with food a problem? The almost effect series, harvard health publications, Harvard university. Center City: Hazelden Publishing; 2013.
27. Mitrofan O, Petkova H, Janssens A, et al. Care experiences of young people with eating disorders and their parents: qualitative study. BJPsych Open. 2019;5(1):e6.
28. Escobar-Koch T, Banker JD, Crow S, et al. Service users' views of eating disorder services: an international comparison. Int J Eat Disord. 2010;43(6):549–59.
29. Castellini G, Lo Sauro C, Mannucci E, et al. Diagnostic crossover and outcome predictors in eating disorders according to DSM-IV and DSM-V proposed criteria: a 6-year follow-up study. Psychosom Med. 2011;73(3):270–9.
30. Strand M, Zvrskovec J, Hubel C, Peat CM, Bulik CM, Birgegard A. Identifying research priorities for the study of atypical anorexia nervosa: A Delphi study. Int J Eat Disord. 2020;53(10):1729–38.
31. Bezance J, Holliday J. Adolescents with anorexia nervosa have their say: a review of qualitative studies on treatment and recovery from anorexia nervosa. Eur Eat Disord Rev. 2013;21(5):352–60.
32. Jansen YJ, Foets MM, de Bont AA. The contribution of qualitative research to the development of tailor-made community-based interventions in primary care: a review. Eur J Public Health. 2010;20(2):220–6.
33. Fossey E, Harvey C, McDermott F, Davidson L. Understanding and evaluating qualitative research. Aust N Z J Psychiatry. 2002;36(6):717–32.
34. Smith J, Flowers P, Larkin M. Interpretative phenomenological analysis: theory, method and research. London: Sage; 2009.
35. Smith J. Qualitative psychology—A practical guide to research methods. 2nd ed. London: Sage; 2008.
36. Serpell L, Treasure J, Teasdale J, Sullivan V. Anorexia nervosa: Friend or foe? Int J Eat Disord. 1999;25(2):177–86.
37. Marcos YQ, Cantero MCT. Assesment of social support dimensions in patients with eating disorders. Span J Psychol. 2009;12(1):226.
38. Fernandez-Aranda F, Poyastro Pinheiro A, Tozzi F, et al. Symptom profile of major depressive disorder in women with eating disorders. Aust N Z J Psychiatry. 2007;41(1):24–31.
39. Akey JE, Rintamaki LS, Kane TL. Health Belief Model deterrents of social support seeking among people coping with eating disorders. J Affect Disord. 2013;145(2):246–52.
40. Becker AE, Franko DL, Nussbaum K, Herzog DB. Secondary prevention for eating disorders: the impact of education, screening, and referral in a college-based screening program. Int J Eat Disord. 2004;36(2):157–62.
41. Clinton D, Button E, Norring C, Palmer R. Cluster analysis of key diagnostic variables from two independent samples of eating-disorder patients: evidence for a consistent pattern. Psychol Med. 2004;34(6):1035–45.
42. Shah NR, Braverman ER. Measuring adiposity in patients: the utility of body mass index (BMI), percent body fat, and leptin. PLoS ONE. 2012;7(4):e33308.
43. Tomiyama AJ, Hunger JM, Nguyen-Cuu J, Wells C. Misclassification of cardiometabolic health when using body mass index categories in NHANES 2005–2012. Int J Obes (Lond). 2016;40(5):883–6.
44. Garber AK. Moving beyond "skinniness": Presentation weight is not sufficient to assess malnutrition in patients with restrictive eating disorders across a range of body weights. J Adolesc Health. 2018;63(6):669–70.
45. Berends T, Boonstra N, van Elburg A. Relapse in anorexia nervosa: a systematic review and meta-analysis. Curr Opin Psychiatry. 2018;31(6):445–55.
46. Bardone-Cone AM, Hunt RA, Watson HJ. An overview of conceptualizations of eating disorder recovery, recent findings, and future directions. Curr Psychiatry Rep. 2018;20(9):79.
47. Phillipou A, Beilharz F. Should we shed the weight criterion for anorexia nervosa? Aust N Z J Psychiatry. 2019;53(6):501–2.
48. Mehler PS, Brown C. Anorexia nervosa - medical complications. J Eat Disord. 2015;3:11.

49. Bachmann KN, Schorr M, Bruno AG, et al. Vertebral volumetric bone density and strength are impaired in women with low-weight and atypical anorexia nervosa. J Clin Endocrinol Metab. 2017;102(1):57–68.

50. Forney KJ, Brown TA, Holland-Carter LA, Kennedy GA, Keel PK. Defining "significant weight loss" in atypical anorexia nervosa. Int J Eat Disord. 2017;50(8):952–62.

51. Berner LA, Feig EH, Witt AA, Lowe MR. Menstrual cycle loss and resumption among patients with anorexia nervosa spectrum eating disorders: Is relative or absolute weight more influential? Int J Eat Disord. 2017;50(4):442–6.

52. Reas DL. Public and healthcare professionals' knowledge and attitudes toward binge eating disorder: A narrative review. Nutrients. 2017;9(11):1267.

53. Olasoji M, Maude P, McCauley K. Not sick enough: Experiences of carers of people with mental illness negotiating care for their relatives with mental health services. J Psychiatr Ment Health Nurs. 2017;24(6):403–11.

9

A Standard Enteral Formula Versus an iso-caloric Lower Carbohydrate/High Fat Enteral Formula in the Hospital Management of Adolescent and Young Adults Admitted with Anorexia Nervosa

Elizabeth Kumiko Parker[1,2]* ●, Victoria Flood[2,3] ●, Mark Halaki[2], Christine Wearne[4], Gail Anderson[5], Linette Gomes[5], Simon Clarke[5,6,7], Frances Wilson[8], Janice Russell[7,9], Elizabeth Frig[10] and Michael Kohn[5,6,7]

Abstract

Background: The nutritional rehabilitation of malnourished patients hospitalised with anorexia nervosa is essential. The provision of adequate nutrition must occur, while simultaneously, minimising the risk of refeeding complications, such as electrolyte, metabolic, and organ dysfunction. The aim of this study was to compare the efficacy and safety of an iso-caloric lower carbohydrate/high fat enteral formula (28% carbohydrate, 56% fat) against a standard enteral formula (54% carbohydrate, 29% fat).

Methods: Patients (aged 15–25 years) hospitalised with anorexia nervosa were recruited into this double blinded randomised controlled trial. An interim analysis was completed at midpoint, when 24 participants, mean age 17.5 years ($\pm$1.1), had been randomly allocated to lower carbohydrate/high fat (n = 14) or standard (n = 10) feeds.

Results: At baseline, there was no significant difference in degree of malnutrition, medical instability, history of purging or serum phosphate levels between the two treatment arms. A significantly lower rate of hypophosphatemia developed in patients who received the lower carbohydrate/high fat formula compared to standard formula (5/14 vs 9/10, $p = 0.013$). The serum phosphate level decreased in both feeds, however it decreased to a larger extent in the standard feed compared to the lower carbohydrate/high fat feed (standard feed 1.11 $\pm$ 0.13 mmol/L at baseline vs 0.88 $\pm$ 0.12 mmol/L at week 1; lower carbohydrate/high fat feed 1.18 $\pm$ 0.19 mmol/L at baseline vs 1.06 $\pm$ 0.15 mmol/L at week 1). Overall, serum phosphate levels were significantly higher in the lower carbohydrate/high fat feed compared with standard feed treatment arm at Week 1 (1.06 $\pm$ 0.15 mmol/L vs 0.88 $\pm$ 0.12 mmol/L, $p < 0.001$). There was no significant difference in weight gain, number of days to reach medical stability, incidence of hypoglycaemia, or hospital length of stay.

*Correspondence: Elizabeth.Parker@health.nsw.gov.au
[1] Department of Dietetics and Nutrition, Westmead Hospital, PO Box 533, Wentworthville, NSW 2145, Australia
Full list of author information is available at the end of the article

Conclusions: The results of this study indicate that enteral nutrition provided to hospitalised malnourished young people with anorexia nervosa using a lower carbohydrate/high fat formula (28% carbohydrate, 56% fat) seems to provide protection from hypophosphatemia in the first week compared to when using a standard enteral formula. Further research may be required to confirm this finding in other malnourished populations.

Keywords: Anorexia nervosa, Enteral nutrition, Refeeding syndrome, Hypophosphatemia, Carbohydrate

Plain English Summary

Patients hospitalised with anorexia nervosa require nutrition support as part of their treatment, whilst refeeding complications are prevented. Of particular concern, is the reintroduction of carbohydrate to malnourished patients, which has been proposed to cause a surge in insulin levels and disturbance in electrolytes, particularly a decrease in blood phosphate levels. This double-blinded randomised controlled trial measured the occurrence of low phosphate blood levels and other refeeding complications, in adolescent and young adult patients hospitalised with anorexia nervosa. These patients were provided either a lower carbohydrate/high fat feed (28% carbohydrate, 56% fat) or a standard enteral feed (54% carbohydrate, 29% fat). Fewer patients in the lower carbohydrate/high fat feed group (5/14) than standard feed group (9/10) developed a low phosphate level. There was no significant difference in weight gain, number of days to reach medical stability, occurrence of hypoglycaemia, or hospital length of stay.

Introduction

Patients hospitalised with anorexia nervosa (AN) require nutritional rehabilitation to (1) achieve medical stability, (2) restore positive energy balance (3) commence weight restoration, and (4) reverse the medical complications associated with malnutrition [1, 2]. Malnourished patients, such as those with AN, are considered at increased risk of developing refeeding complications, such as the refeeding syndrome. While consensus is lacking on a definition of refeeding syndrome, it is generally described as the occurrence of electrolyte and fluid shifts which can occur when a person in a state of starvation undergoes nutrition repletion, leading to organ dysfunction and possible sudden death [1, 3].

A range of international refeeding guidelines provide consensus-based recommendations for initial energy intakes in malnourished patients at risk of developing refeeding complications. The United Kingdom based National Institute for Health and Care Excellence (NICE) guidelines initially published in 2006 and updated in 2017, recommend providing low energy intakes (5–10 kcal/kg/day) to prevent refeeding complications, and aim to increase slowly to meet nutrition needs by 4–7 days [4]. In the USA, the American Society for Parenteral and Enteral Nutrition (ASPEN) guidelines recommend initiating patients on 10–20 kcal/kg for the first 24 h and increasing by 33% of goal energy intake every 1–2 days [5]. These guidelines also suggest delaying increases in energy intakes in the presence of electrolyte derangement. The caloric prescription from these guidelines has been identified

as leading to an 'underfeeding syndrome' [6], whereby patients are provided with energy intakes below basal energy requirements, resulting in poor weight gain and even weight loss in an already malnourished patient group.

A growing body of evidence supports higher energy intakes in adolescent patients hospitalised with AN, ranging from 1200 to 2400 kcal/day commencing at admission [7]. However, evidence for the adult population is less robust; the fewer studies that exist suggest starting malnourished adults on energy intakes of 1200–1500 kcal/day [8–10].

Concern for the development of refeeding complications is increased when nutrition is commenced at a high caloric rate, the patient is severely malnourished (BMI < 14 kg/m^2) or when the carbohydrate intake is high [4, 11, 12]. During starvation the body is in a catabolic state. An "adaptive" shift from carbohydrate to fat and protein utilization occurs, which alters the body's insulin response [13]. Once adequate nutrition is reintroduced, the body returns to an anabolic state, and switches back from fat and protein utilisation to carbohydrate utilisation as the primary energy macronutrient. A sudden reintroduction of carbohydrate during this time is postulated to lead to a surge in insulin levels, which drives electrolytes such as phosphate into the cells, resulting in electrolyte derangements [14]. Hypophosphatemia, is considered a marker for refeeding complications, and serum phosphate levels are recommended to be maintained above 1.0 mmol/L during nutritional rehabilitation [15–18].

Strategies to avoid refeeding complications have been suggested, such as continuous delivery of nutrients (e.g. nasogastric feeding) with less than 40% of energy from carbohydrate [13]. Standard enteral formula usually contain > 50% energy from carbohydrate. A recent study published by Yamazaki T et al. [19], retrospectively reviewed 188 patients hospitalised with AN (mean age 28.77 ± 12.22 years) and found a diet high in carbohydrate (> 58.4%) was significantly associated with the occurrence of refeeding hypophosphatemia (Adjusted OR 5.37, 95% CI 1.60,18.1, $p = 0.007$)[19].

Not all studies of higher energy intakes (initiating ≥ 1200 kcal/day) have specified the macronutrient composition provided to patients during treatment [8, 17, 20, 21]. Studies which have specified the macronutrient content and utilised nasogastric feeding have ranged from starting calorie levels of 1500–2400 kcal/day and 44 to $\leq 50\%$ carbohydrate [10, 18, 22], whereas oral meal based programs have ranged from 1200 to 2000 kcal/day and 35–60% carbohydrate [15, 23–28].

This study compares refeeding treatment outcomes of a lower carbohydrate enteral formula (less than 40% energy from carbohydrate) against a standard enteral formula (54% energy from carbohydrate), in adolescent and young adult patients (aged 15–25 years), hospitalised with AN. In addition, the lower carbohydrate formula is also higher in fat compared to the standard enteral formula (56% energy from fat vs 29% energy from fat, respectively).

Our hypothesis is that compared with malnourished patients with AN provided with a standard higher carbohydrate enteral formula, malnourished patients with AN who are provided with a lower carbohydrate/high fat enteral formula will (1) have lower rates of hypophosphatemia, and (2) have less electrolyte disturbance, and thus safely reach the initial goal rate of feeding (1890 kcal Day 1) sooner. This will affect initial total energy intake, rate of weight gain, number of days to reach medical stability and length of hospital stay.

Methods
Study design
This double blinded randomised controlled trial was conducted in Sydney, Australia, from November 2017 to December 2018. A detailed research protocol has been published elsewhere [29]. This study received ethics approval from the Western Sydney Local Health District Human Research Ethics Committee (HREC/16/WMEAD/390) and site specific approvals from the Research Governance Offices of Western Sydney Local Health District (SSA/16/WMEAD/433) and Sydney Local Health District (SSA/17/RPAH/435). This study followed the Consolidated Standards of Reporting Trials (CONSORT) reporting guideline.

Participants and recruitment
Recruitment of participants was open at two public hospitals in New South Wales, Australia, with specialised inpatient eating disorder treatment services. Inclusion criteria specified adolescent and young adult patients (aged 15–25 years) hospitalised with AN (assessed by the treating medical officer using DSM-5 criteria [30]) who received nasogastric tube feeding. Exclusion criteria included patients transferred from another treatment facility, where they had already received nasogastric feeding and/or prophylactic phosphate replacement. Figure 1 describes the enrolment of participants into the trial.

Participants were invited to participate shortly after admission to hospital, and were approached after the treating team had made the decision the patient required nasogastric feeding, independent to the study. Written informed consent was obtained from all participants, and from guardians for participants aged less than 18 years.

Sample size
The sample size calculation of 48 participants (24 in each arm) was based on the primary outcome measure, incidence of hypophosphatemia, using a dichotomous endpoint two independent study sample, incidence of 45% hypophosphatemia [26] in the standard feed arm and 10% hypophosphatemia in the trial feed arm, 80% power, alpha 0.05.

An interim analysis was planned and completed at midpoint of recruitment, with the plan to cease recruitment early if a significant finding in the primary outcome measure of incidence of hypophosphatemia was found.

Randomisation
Random allocation was concealed by sequentially numbered, sealed opaque envelopes containing the feed allocation (Feed A vs Feed B), which was determined by a computer generated random number, stratified by gender. An external investigator (MH) generated the allocation sequence, and ward staff enrolled participants.

Blinding
The Department of Dietetics & Nutrition at the study hospital assisted in assigning participants to the randomised interventions and facilitated the blinding of participants and treating team during the intervention. The standard formula and lower carbohydrate/high fat formula were both decanted into generic containers and labelled either FEED A or FEED B. A record logbook of each participant and the enteral feed provided and the allocation to FEED A or FEED B was maintained

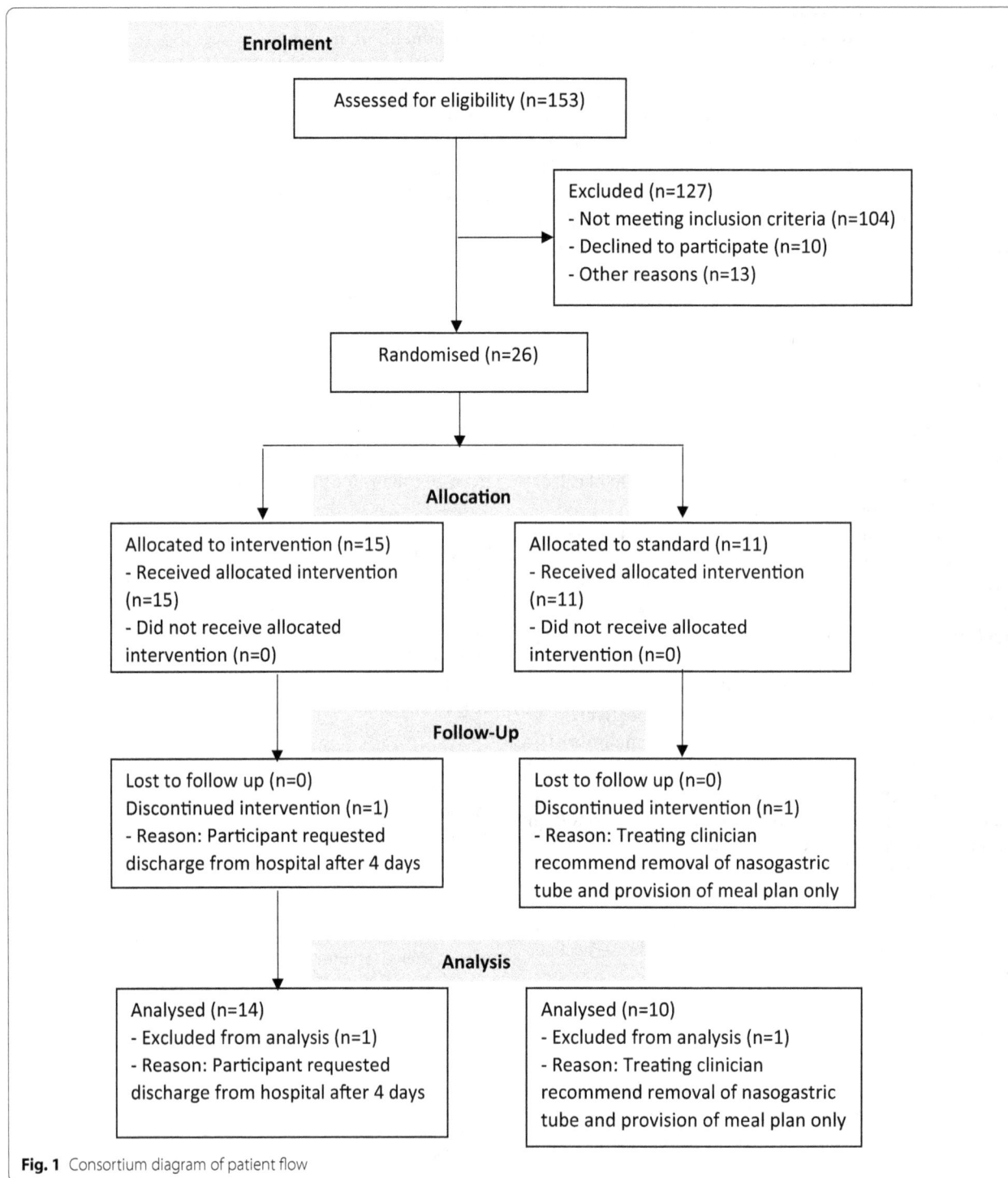

Fig. 1 Consortium diagram of patient flow

and stored in a locked cabinet for quality assurance and auditing purposes.

Intervention group
The trial enteral feed was a lower carbohydrate/high fat formula (Abbott Nutrition™), providing 1.5 kcal/mL

and 28% energy from carbohydrate, 56% energy from fat, 17% energy from protein.

Control group
Participants randomised to the standard enteral feed received an isocaloric formula (Abbott Nutrition™),

providing 1.5 kcal/mL, and 54% energy from carbohydrate, 29% energy from fat, 17% energy from protein.

Both groups were provided nutrition in a standardised and similar manner. Initially nasogastric tube feeds were commenced at 35 mL/h for 12 h. After 12 h, feeds were increased to goal rate 70 mL/h continuous infusion (total 1260 mL = 1890 kcal on Day 1), if electrolytes potassium and magnesium were within the normal reference range and serum phosphate was > 1.0 mmol/L, otherwise feed remained at 35 mL/h (total 840 mL = 1260 kcal on Day 1) until electrolytes had normalised.

Once patients were assessed as medically stable, defined as heart rate > 50 bpm, temperature > 35.5 °C, blood pressure > 80/50 mm Hg, postural hypotension < 20 mm Hg, nasogastric feeds were reduced to cyclic nocturnal at a rate of 70 mL/h over 10 h (2000–0600 h) and oral intake was introduced using standardised meal plans (energy content: 1800 kcal, 2300 kcal, 2800 kcal, 3300 kcal, 3800 kcal; macronutrient content: 47–57% carbohydrate, 30–38% fat, 13–15% protein) (Additional file 1: Table S1). Changes to the feeding regime were adjusted as per standard care, following a multidisciplinary team review three times/week, which aimed to support the development of anabolism and weight gain of at least 1 kg per week. Oral intake (main meals and mid meals) was supervised by a ward nurse and recorded on a daily food chart, and participants unable to finish the prescribed meal plan were provided with a nutrition supplement drink as a meal replacement.

Participants received a daily oral multivitamin. Participants did not receive prophylactic phosphate supplementation if baseline serum phosphate was > 1.0 mmol/L. Participants did receive 1 g oral phosphate supplementation prior to commencing nasogastric feeds if baseline serum phosphate levels were ≤ 1.0 mmol/L, and were provided with phosphate supplementation if serum phosphate levels were ≤ 1.0 mmol/L during nutritional rehabilitation. Participants did not receive prophylactic magnesium or potassium supplementation prior to commencing nasogastric feeds, however oral supplementation was provided if clinically indicated.

Primary and secondary outcomes

The primary outcome measure was incidence of hypophosphatemia. Secondary outcome measures were change in weight, total energy intake and macronutrient content, length of hospital stay, hypokalaemia, hypomagnesemia, hypoglycaemia, development of peripheral oedema, clinical refeeding syndrome, thiamine (Vitamin B1), admission to ICU, days required to reach medical stability.

Measurements of primary and secondary outcomes occurred during the first 3 weeks of hospital admission.

Nutrition assessment

Nutrition assessment was completed by an accredited practising dietitian, using a validated nutrition assessment tool the Subjective Global Assessment (SGA) [31], to assess change in weight, change in oral intake, nutrition impact symptoms, change in functional capacity, and the presence of muscle wasting, loss of subcutaneous fat stores and oedema. The nutritional status of participants was scored using an SGA rating of A (well nourished), B (mildly / moderately malnourished), or C (severely malnourished). In addition, degree of malnutrition was also assessed in participants using criteria defined in the Position Paper of the Society for Adolescent Health and Medicine [32], using percentage median Body Mass Index (%mBMI), calculated from the 50th percentile for age and sex [33]. Degree of malnutrition using %mBMI was categorised as mild malnutrition (80–90%mBMI), moderate malnutrition (70–79%mBMI), or severe malnutrition (< 70%mBMI) [32].

Nutritional intake of participants was assessed using recorded food charts and recorded administered enteral feed volumes.

Change in body weight was assessed at routine weight checks, minimum 3 days/week, using the ward scales recorded to the nearest 0.1 kg. These were early morning weights taken after voiding. Body mass index was calculated using the height recorded on admission using a wall mounted stadiometer.

Change in body composition was assessed by skinfold measurements using callipers (Holtain Ltd, Crymych, UK) and non-dominant hand-grip strength using a dynamometer (Jamar, Sammons Preston Roylan, Bolingbrook, IL, USA), with technique recommend in practice.

Blood tests

Blood tests monitoring electrolytes (potassium, magnesium, and phosphate), blood glucose level and thiamine were taken at baseline prior to initiating the nutrition intervention. Electrolyte levels were repeated 4–6 h after initiating enteral nutrition, and at least daily for the first week, and twice weekly in week 2 and week 3. Hypokalaemia was defined as a potassium level < 3.2 mmol/L, and hypomagnesemia was defined as a magnesium level < 0.70 mmol/L, as per the hospital reference range. Hypophosphatemia was defined as a phosphate level ≤ 1.0 mmol/L [16, 34]. Blood glucose levels were measured two times per day during the first week and at least weekly in week 2 and week 3. Hypoglycaemia was defined as a blood glucose level < 3.0 mmol/L [35]. The lowest serum potassium, magnesium, phosphate and blood glucose level was recorded for week 1, 2 and 3 and used in the analysis. Thiamine was repeated at week 1, 2 and 3. The hospital normal reference range for thiamine was 67–200 nmol/L.

Refeeding syndrome

For this study, refeeding syndrome was identified as the occurrence of life threatening complications (delirium, cardiac arrest, and coma) [6], as well as patients who exhibited all three diagnostic criteria involving electrolyte disturbance, acute circulatory fluid overload and organ dysfunction defined by Rio et al. [36].

Medical records

Electronic medical records were reviewed at least 3 times/week to review nursing observations (e.g. heart rate, blood pressure, temperature) and weekly physical assessment by the treating medical officer (e.g. monitoring for presence of peripheral oedema). The length of hospital stay, admission to ICU, and number of days to reach medical stability, was also reviewed.

Analysis

Data was collected and analysed using SPSS for Windows Version 26, IBM Corporation. Continuous outcomes were assessed for normality using the Shapiro–Wilk test. Mean, standard deviation, 95% CI, and effect size reported as d_{Cohen} or Partial Eta squared where appropriate, were reported for parametric data. Normally distributed variables were compared between the two treatment groups using independent t-tests for single measures, (e.g. hospital length of stay, age, white cell count on admission, heart rate on admission, % weight loss prior to admission, weight gain at weeks 1, 2 and 3) and two factor (between subject factor: group; within subject factor: time) repeated measures analysis of variance (ANOVA) for variables with multiple time point measures (e.g. weight, BMI, %mBMI, energy (kcal/kg/day), phosphate, magnesium, potassium, glucose, thiamine, handgrip strength, triceps skinfold, bicep skinfold, suprailiac skinfold). Change in phosphate levels between the two treatment groups was further analysed using analysis of covariance (ANCOVA) with %mBMI as a covariate as the literature has reported degree of malnutrition influencing development of refeeding complications such as hypophosphatemia [15].

Median, interquartile range, and effect size reported as d_{Cohen} were reported for variables not normally distributed (e.g. number of days to reach medical stability; energy intake (kcal/day) for oral, nasogastric feed and total; total and oral intake % macronutrient intake (carbohydrate, protein fat); subscapular skinfold), and between group differences were analysed using a Mann Whitney

U test, Wilcox matched pair test, and Friedman ANOVA. Binary outcomes (development of hypophosphatemia with degree of malnutrition as a covariate, medical stability on admission, degree of malnutrition, history of purging, electrolyte replacement, and incidence of hypoglycaemia), were compared using a chi-squared test, with odds ratio (OR) and 95% CI reported. A p value < 0.05 was required for statistical significance.

Results

A total of 26 participants were recruited between 01/11/2017 and 31/12/2018, with 2 patients excluded from analysis due to early discharge from treatment within the first week. Twenty-four participants were included in the analysis, all of whom were female with a diagnosis of AN (DSM 5). There was no significant difference at baseline between the lower carbohydrate/high fat feed (n = 14) and standard feed (n = 10) treatment arms in age (17.5 ± 1.3 vs 17.5 ± 0.9 years, $p = 0.979$), history of purging (3/14 vs 4/10, $p = 0.393$), degree of malnutrition using SGA (12/14 vs 6/10 mild-moderately malnourished; 2/14 vs 4/10 severely malnourished, $p = 0.192$) or %mBMI category (6/14 vs 3/10 mild malnutrition; 3/14 vs 6/10 moderate malnutrition; 4/14 vs 0/10 severe malnutrition, $p = 0.139$), % weight loss prior to admission (17.1% ± 7.8 vs 19.7% ± 8.5, $p = 0.443$), medical instability (10/14 vs 8/10, $p = 1.000$), heart rate (57.7 bpm ± 21.5 vs 59.1 bpm ± 16.2, $p = 0.865$), and white cell count (4.9 × 10^9/L ± 1.5 vs 5.1 × 10^9/L ± 1.6, $p = 0.798$).

During treatment, there was no significant difference between the lower carbohydrate/high fat feed (n = 14) and standard feed (n = 10) treatment arms in the number of days to reach medical stability [median (LQ,UQ) 2.0 (0.0, 3.3) vs 2.0 (0.8, 5.0) days, $p = 0.512$, d_{Cohen} effect size 2.982], phosphate replacement (5/14 vs 6/10, $p = 0.408$, OR 2.70, 95% CI 0.51, 14.37), magnesium replacement (2/14 vs 2/10, $p = 1.000$, OR 1.50, 95% CI 0.17, 12.94), potassium replacement (1/14 vs 2/10, $p = 0.550$, OR 3.25, 95% CI 0.25, 41.91), and hospital length of stay (24.3 ± 11.3 vs 24.4 ± 6.5 days, $p = 0.975$, d_{Cohen} effect size 0.01, 95% CI -0.80, 0.82). A significantly lower rate of hypophosphatemia developed in patients in the lower carbohydrate/high fat feed compared with standard feed treatment arm (5/14 vs 9/10, $p = 0.013$, OR 16.20, 95% CI 1.57, 167.74) during week 1 (Fig. 2). Although degree of malnutrition, defined by %mBMI, is a significant covariate ($p = 0.018$) in the development of hypophosphatemia, it did not affect the outcome as there was no significant association between development of hypophosphatemia and degree of malnutrition ($\chi^2 = 1.486$, $p = 0.686$). In all 14 patients that developed hypophosphatemia during week 1, this occurred between days 1–5 (mean day 2.9 ± 1.2). There was no significant difference in

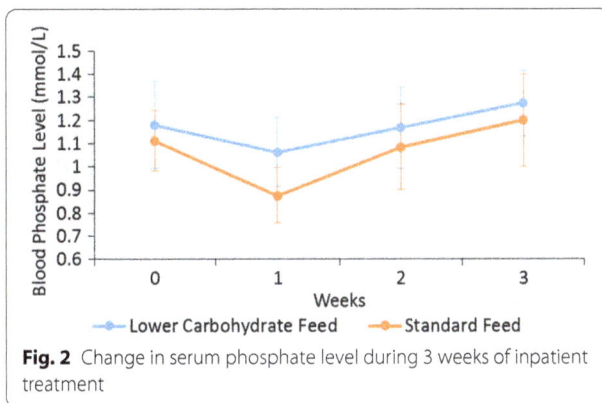

Fig. 2 Change in serum phosphate level during 3 weeks of inpatient treatment

incidence of hypoglycaemia between the lower carbohydrate/high fat feed and standard feed treatments arms at baseline (1/14 vs 0/10, $p = 1.000$) and at Week 1 (0/14 vs 1/10, $p = 1.000$). No patients developed oedema, clinical refeeding syndrome, or required admission to ICU.

Thiamine levels were measured in only 16 participants at baseline, 11 participants at week 1, and 10 participants at week 2 and 3. There was no significant difference between the lower carbohydrate/high fat feed (n = 9) compared with the standard feed (n = 7) treatment arm at baseline (130.9 nmol/L ± 19.1 vs 147.4 ± 21.0 nmol/L, $p = 0.122$). No significant differences in thiamine levels were found between the two treatment arms during the admission, and all thiamine levels measured at baseline and during treatment were within the normal reference range 67–200 nmol/L.

Additional patient characteristics and changes from baseline to week 1 are presented in Table 1 and Fig. 3. There was no significant difference in weight gain in the lower carbohydrate/high fat feed group compared to the standard feed group at Week 1 (2.7 kg ± 1.9 vs 2.7 kg ± 1.6, $p = 0.998$), Week 2 (4.9 kg ± 1.9 vs 4.6 kg ± 1.5, $p = 0.669$), and Week 3 (6.5 kg ± 2.3 vs 6.4 kg ± 2.0, $p = 0.959$).

At an interim point review, the trial was ceased, based on the significant finding of the primary outcome measure of development of hypophosphatemia reduced in the lower carbohydrate/high fat feed compared with the standard feed treatment arm at the interim analysis. No other significant differences were found after Week 1 in any of the variables analysed (Additional file 2: Table S2). There were no adverse or unintended outcomes reported in either treatment group.

Discussion

This is the first study to compare refeeding outcomes for malnourished adolescent and young adult patients given isocaloric nutritional therapy which was either

high (54%) or low (28%) carbohydrate enteral feeds. Our results show a lower carbohydrate/high fat enteral feed in adolescent and young adult patients hospitalised with AN resulted in lower levels of hypophosphatemia compared with those provided with a standard higher carbohydrate feed. No other significant differences were found between the two treatment arms during the first 3 weeks of admission.

Providing < 40% carbohydrate to refeed patients with eating disorders has been recommended [13]. Study outcomes of refeeding using nasogastric feeding tubes above current international recommendations (exceeding 1200 kcal/day), providing 44–46% [10, 22] or ≤ 50% carbohydrate [18] have been reported. Mathews et al. [10] reported no significant differences in rates of hypophosphatemia during the first 10 days of admission, in a retrospective pre-test-post-test study comparing a low-calorie (LC) protocol (1000 kcal, 45–55% carbohydrate, 20% protein, 30–35% fat) to a higher-calorie (HC) protocol (1500 kcal, 46% carbohydrate, 20% protein, 34% fat), in 119 medically compromised adult patients with eating disorders. The highest rate of hypophosphatemia (defined as below normal reference range 0.81–1.45 mmol/L) was on admission (23% LC vs 12% HC, $p = 0.196$), followed by Day 1 (19% LC vs 12% HC, $p = 0.307$). The LC group (n = 26) were provided with an oral based meal program, with nasogastric feeding provided only if oral feeding was deemed unsuccessful, whereas the HC group (n = 93) utilised nasogastric feeding within 24 h of admission. The authors did report a higher incidence of hypoglycaemia (defined as serum glucose level < 3.0 mmol/L or skin prick glucose level < 4.0 mmol/L) in the LC group compared to the HC group (31% vs 10%, $p = 0.012$), and suggested the use of continuous nasogastric feeding with constant supply of carbohydrate in the HC group may have contributed to the reduced incidence of hypoglycaemia. In the current study, both treatment arms reported a higher incidence of hypophosphatemia, compared with Mathews et al. [10], in the lower carbohydrate/high fat feed and the standard feed (35.7% vs 90%, $p = 0.013$). However, in addition to starting patients on a higher calorie intake (1890 kcal/day), hypophosphatemia was defined as $PO_4 \leq 1.0$ mmol/L in the current study rather than $PO_4 < 0.81$ mmol/L. Furthermore, there were no significant differences between treatment arms in blood glucose levels at baseline and week 1. The use of initial continuous nasogastric feeding in both treatment arms in the current study combined with the low rates of hypoglycaemia observed, further support the suggestion by Kohn et al. [13] and the results of Mathews et al. [10], that a constant supply of carbohydrate through the use of continuous NG feeds may reduce the rate of hypoglycaemia in this patient population.

Table 1 Baseline characteristics and changes after one week of nutritional rehabilitation

	Baseline						Week 1			
	Lower carbohydrate /high fat feed (n = 14)	95% CI	Standard feed (n = 10)	95% CI	Baseline comparison p value	Effect size	Lower carbohydrate /high fat feed (n = 14)	95% CI	Standard feed (n = 10)	95% CI
Anthropometry										
Body Mass, kg	43.7 ± 4.7	41.0, 46.4	45.1 ± 2.8	43.1, 47.1	0.37	0.35	46.4 ± 5.1	43.5, 49.3	47.9 ± 4.0	45.0, 50.8
BMI, kg/m^2	16.3 ± 1.7	15.3, 17.3	16.7 ± 0.9	16.1, 17.3	0.53	0.28	17.3 ± 1.8	16.3, 18.3	17.7 ± 1.1	16.9, 18.5
mBMI, %	77.8 ± 9.1	72.5, 83.1	79.3 ± 5.2	75.6, 83.0	0.63	0.19	82.7 ± 9.4	77.3, 88.1	84.0 ± 5.9	79.8, 88.2
Handgrip (L), kg	20.8 ± 3.3	18.9, 22.7	22.7 ± 3.7	20.1, 25.3	0.19	0.55	22.1 ± 4.4	19.6, 24.6	23.1 ± 3.5	20.6, 25.6
Handgrip (R), kg	24.2 ± 4.8	21.4, 27.0	23.2 ± 3.6	20.6, 25.8	0.58	-0.23	25.1 ± 5.0	22.2, 28.0	25.2 ± 3.6	22.6, 27.8
Tricep skinfold, mm	9.5 ± 2.9	7.8, 11.2	9.6 ± 2.7	7.7, 11.5	0.92	0.04	10.5 ± 3.5	8.5, 12.5	10.1 ± 2.5	8.3, 11.9
Bicep skinfold, mm	5.0 ± 1.7	4.0, 6.0	5.1 ± 1.4	4.1, 6.1	0.93	0.06	5.4 ± 2.0	4.2, 6.6	5.3 ± 1.3	4.4, 6.2
Suprailiac skinfold, mm	7.3 ± 2.6	5.8, 8.8	7.0 ± 1.9	5.6, 8.4	0.77	-0.13	8.3 ± 3.1	6.5, 10.1	8.2 ± 2.3	6.6, 9.8
Subscapular skinfold, mm	6.5 [5.6, 8.4]	N/A	6.7 [5.9, 8.4]	N/A	0.48^A	0.29	6.8 [6.0, 9.3]	N/A	7.5 [6.7, 8.9]	N/A
Nutrition										
Total kcal/day (Oral + NG feed)	1890 [1890, 1890]	N/A	1890 [1890, 1890]	N/A	1.00^A	0.00	3350 [3188, 3350]	N/A	3325 [2844, 3350]	N/A
Kcal/kg/day	43.7 ± 4.8	40.9, 46.5	42.0 ± 2.5	40.2, 43.8	0.28	-0.42	71.1 ± 9.9	65.4, 76.8	66.8 ± 7.5	61.4, 72.2
Energy from Carbohydrate, %	28.3 [28.3, 28.3]	N/A	54.4 [54.4, 54.4]	N/A	<0.001^A	3.06	44.8 [44.2, 45.3]	N/A	53.0 [52.9, 56.1]	N/A
Energy from Protein, %	16.8 [16.8, 16.8]	N/A	16.8 [16.8, 16.8]	N/A	1.00^A	0.00	14.5 [14.4, 14.5]	N/A	14.5 [14.1, 14.5]	N/A
Energy from Fat, %	55.8 [55.8, 55.8]	N/A	29.4 [29.4, 29.4]	N/A	<0.001^A	3.06	40.4 [39.8, 40.4]	N/A	32.2 [28.4, 32.3]	N/A
kcal/day from oral intake	0 [0,0]	N/A	0 [0,0]	N/A	1.00^A	0.00	2300 [1800, 2300]	N/A	2300 [1800, 2300]	N/A
Energy from Carbohydrate, %	0 [0,0]	N/A	0 [0,0]	N/A	1.00^A	0.00	52.3 [52.3, 57.4]	N/A	52.3 [52.3, 57.4]	N/A
Energy from Protein, %	0 [0,0]	N/A	0 [0,0]	N/A	1.00^A	0.00	13.4 [12.6, 13.4]	N/A	13.4 [12.6, 13.4]	N/A
Energy from Fat, %	0 [0,0]	N/A	0 [0,0]	N/A	1.00^A	0.00	33.4 [27.6, 33.4]	N/A	33.4 [27.6, 33.4]	N/A
Biochemical parameters										
Phosphate, mmol/L	1.18 ± 0.19	1.07, 1.29	1.11 ± 0.13	1.02, 1.20	0.35	-0.42	1.06 ± 0.15 *	0.97, 1.15	0.88 ± 0.12 *†	0.79, 0.97
Magnesium, mmol/L	0.94 ± 0.09	0.89, 0.99	0.94 ± 0.05	0.90, 0.98	0.85	0.00	0.86 ± 0.08	0.81, 0.91	0.85 ± 0.05	0.81, 0.89
Potassium, mmol/L	3.75 ± 0.44	3.50, 4.00	3.72 ± 0.32	3.49, 3.95	0.84	-0.08	3.67 ± 0.23	3.54, 3.80	3.59 ± 0.10	3.52, 3.66
Glucose, mmol/L	4.8 ± 0.9	4.3, 5.3	5.5 ± 1.2	4.6, 6.4	0.22	0.68	4.4 ± 0.7	4.0, 4.8	4.5 ± 0.8	3.9, 5.1

Table 1 (continued)

| | ANOVA Results | | | | | |
| | Time | | Feed | | Interaction | |
	p value	Effect size	p value	Effect size	p value	Effect size
Anthropometry						
Body Mass, kg	<0.001	0.71	0.428	0.03	0.998	0.00
BMI, kg/m²	<0.001	0.72	0.566	0.02	0.978	0.00
mBMI, %	<0.001	0.72	0.670	0.01	0.931	0.00
Handgrip (L), kg	0.059	0.15	0.346	0.04	0.289	0.05
Handgrip (R), kg	0.006	0.30	0.790	0.00	0.274	0.05
Tricep skinfold, mm	0.001	0.43	0.935	0.00	0.241	0.06
Bicep skinfold, mm	0.001	0.41	0.954	0.00	0.214	0.07
Suprailiac skinfold, mm	<0.001	0.60	0.857	0.00	0.616	0.01
Subscapular skinfold, mm	0.395[B]	0.35	0.002[C]	2.87	0.005[D]	3.96
Nutrition						
Total kcal/day (Oral + NG feed)	0.599[B]	0.20	0.001[C]	4.00	0.005[D]	2.30
Kcal/kg/day	<0.001	0.94	0.248	0.06	0.365	0.04
Energy from Carbohydrate, %	<0.001[B]	3.06	0.001[C]	4.00	0.797[D]	0.16
Energy from Protein, %	0.478[B]	0.25	0.001[C]	4.67	0.004[D]	4.11
Energy from Fat, %	<0.001[B]	3.06	0.001[C]	4.67	0.027[D]	1.95
kcal/day from oral intake	0.841[B]	0.07	0.001[C]	4.08	0.004[D]	2.49
Energy from Carbohydrate, %	0.841[B]	0.07	0.001[C]	4.08	0.004[D]	2.49
Energy from Protein, %	0.841[B]	0.07	0.001[C]	4.08	0.004[D]	2.49
Energy from Fat, %	0.841[B]	0.07	0.001[C]	4.08	0.004[D]	2.49
Biochemical parameters						
Phosphate, mmol/L	0.086	0.13	0.013	0.26	0.035	0.20
Magnesium, mmol/L	<0.001	0.71	0.853	0.00	0.396	0.03
Potassium, mmol/L	0.193	0.08	0.584	0.01	0.779	0.00
Glucose, mmol/L	0.058	0.21	0.141	0.13	0.994	0.00

Data are presented as means ± standard deviations when normally distributed and medians [interquartile range] when not normally distributed

*Significant difference to baseline based on ANCOVA Bonferonni post hoc results and using percent median BMI on admission as a covariate

† Significant difference to Lower carbohydrate/high fat feed at same time point on ANCOVA Bonferonni post hoc results and using percent median BMI on admission as a covariate

A Mann Whitney U test for lower carbohydrate/high fat feed versus standard feed at Baseline

B Mann Whitney U test for lower carbohydrate/high fat feed versus standard feed at Week 1

C Wilcoxon matched paired test for lower carbohydrate/high fat feed Baseline versus Week 1

D Wilcoxon matched paired test for standard feed Baseline versus Week 1

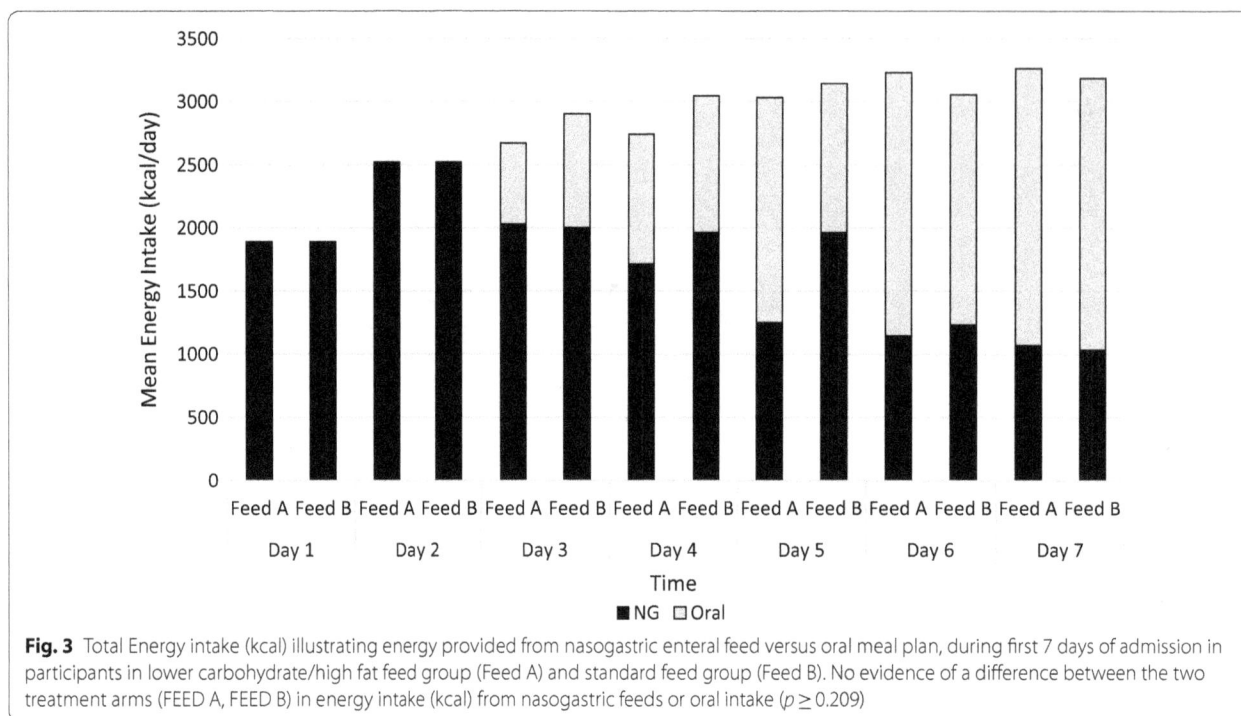

Fig. 3 Total Energy intake (kcal) illustrating energy provided from nasogastric enteral feed versus oral meal plan, during first 7 days of admission in participants in lower carbohydrate/high fat feed group (Feed A) and standard feed group (Feed B). No evidence of a difference between the two treatment arms (FEED A, FEED B) in energy intake (kcal) from nasogastric feeds or oral intake ($p \geq 0.209$)

Other studies that reported outcomes on patients hospitalised with AN provided with enteral feeds, include Madden et al. [18] providing 2400 kcal/day, limiting carbohydrate to $\leq 50\%$ energy; and Agostino et al. [22] providing 1617 kcal/day, 44% carbohydrate to adolescent patients. However, while both studies report 0% hypophosphatemia in patients receiving NG feeds, these results are not comparable to the current study as both studies prescribed prophylactic phosphate supplementation prior to nutrition intervention which would mask the development of hypophosphatemia.

Our results suggest the use of an enteral feed providing only 28% energy from carbohydrate reduced the incidence of hypophosphatemia observed compared with a standard feed. Both treatment arms in this study received a higher calorie protocol providing patients with 1890 kcal on admission. Electrolyte disturbances were treated with oral supplementation, and no cases of clinical refeeding syndrome or admissions to ICU occurred. These results support higher caloric prescription than recommendations in current guidelines. The use of a lower carbohydrate/high fat enteral feed provides a further option for clinicians to consider when treating patients hospitalised with AN, rather than providing low energy intakes and risking an underfeeding syndrome and even weight loss in this already malnourished and often medically compromised patient population. There were no significant differences in any variables observed between the two treatment arms after week 1, and this

may be explained by the increase in oral intake and reduction of calories provided through nasogastric tube feeding after week 1, thereby reducing the difference in macronutrient composition received by the two treatment arms in Week 2 and 3.

Several limitations affect the generalisability and interpretation of results. The sample size of this study and the effect size observed were both small. The small sample size was attributed to the trial being ceased early following the interim analysis identifying a significant difference between the two treatment arms in the primary outcome measure of incidence of hypophosphatemia. The age range in the inclusion criteria prohibits the findings of this study being applicable to older patients who may also have a more severe and enduring course of illness. Furthermore, while all patients were diagnosed as malnourished using a validated nutrition assessment tool, the admission BMI or %mBMI categorised the majority of patients as mild to moderately malnourished therefore limiting the validity of results in severely malnourished patients who are at the highest risk of developing refeeding complications.

The strengths of the study are that it is the first of its kind to compare two different feeding formulas with different macronutrient compositions, in patients hospitalised with AN using a double-blinded randomised controlled trial design with controls for bias, thereby enhancing reliability of study findings. Furthermore, by focusing on the adolescent and young adult population hospitalised with AN, the study addresses the urgent need to identify effective treatments to reduce length of hospital stay and associated costs, with the hope of preventing severe and enduring course of illness in the longer term.

Further research is required to assess the safety and efficacy of the use of a lower carbohydrate/high fat enteral feed in more severely malnourished and older patients with AN, as well as other patient groups considered at risk of developing refeeding complications, specifically patients with a history of prolonged fasting or low energy intake [37]. A comparison of patient outcomes in higher energy oral based feeding protocols versus enteral feeding protocols manipulating macronutrient content is also warranted to examine the safety, feasibility and discomfort that may be experienced by patients in either treatment model.

Furthermore, while the current study did not report a significant difference in weight gain between the two treatment arms, future studies incorporating indirect calorimetry measurements into the study design are recommended. This will help confirm if patients fed a high carbohydrate/low fat diet have a higher basal metabolic rate due to increased diet-induced thermogenesis, compared to patients fed a low carbohydrate/high fat diet, as reported by Russell et al. [38].

Conclusion

The results of this study indicate that enteral nutrition provided to hospitalised malnourished young people with AN using a lower carbohydrate/high fat formula (28% carbohydrate, 56% fat) seems to provide protection from hypophosphatemia in the first week compared to when using a standard enteral formula. Further research is required to confirm this finding in more severely malnourished and older patients with AN, as well as other malnourished populations with a history of prolonged fasting or low energy intake.

Abbreviations

AN: Anorexia nervosa; ANCOVA: Repeated measures analysis of covariance; ANOVA: Repeated measures analysis of variance; APA: American Psychiatric Association; ASPEN: American Society for Parenteral and Enteral Nutrition; BMI: Body mass index; %mBMI: Percent median body mass index; HC: High-calorie; LC: Lower-calorie; MARSIPAN: Management of really sick patients with anorexia nervosa; NICE: National Institute for Health and Care Excellence; OR: Odds ratio.

Acknowledgements
The authors would like to thank the Department of Dietetics & Nutrition, Westmead Hospital, Australia, for facilitating the blinding of enteral feeds during the study. We would also like to thank the young people who participated in this research.

Authors' contributions
The study was designed by EP, VF, MK and FW and further refined by LG, GA, SC, MH, EF and JR; EP conducted the research; EP analysed the data with assis-

tance from MH; EP wrote the paper with major contributions from VF, MH and MK; EP has primary responsibility for final content. All authors critically revised the manuscript and approved the final version of the manuscript.

Competing interests
The authors declare that they have no competing interests.

Author details
[1]Department of Dietetics and Nutrition, Westmead Hospital, PO Box 533, Wentworthville, NSW 2145, Australia. [2]Sydney School of Health Sciences, Faculty of Medicine and Health, The University of Sydney, Sydney, NSW 2006, Australia. [3]Western Sydney Local Health District, Westmead, NSW 2145, Australia. [4]Department of Medical Psychology, Westmead Hospital, Westmead, NSW 2145, Australia. [5]Department of Adolescent and Young Adult Medicine, Westmead Hospital, Westmead, NSW 2145, Australia. [6]Centre for Research Into Adolescents' Health (CRASH), Westmead Hospital, Westmead, NSW 2145, Australia. [7]Sydney School of Medicine, Faculty of Medicine and Health, The University of Sydney, Sydney, NSW 2006, Australia. [8]Department of Psychiatry, Westmead Hospital, Westmead, NSW 2145, Australia. [9]NSW Statewide Eating Disorder Service, Peter Beumont Unit, Professor Marie Bashir Centre, Royal Prince Alfred Hospital, Camperdown, NSW 2050, Australia. [10]Department of Nutrition and Dietetics, Royal Prince Alfred Hospital, Camperdown, NSW 2050, Australia.

References
1. Cuerda C, Vasiloglou MF, Arhip L. Nutritional management and outcomes in malnourished medical inpatients: anorexia nervosa. J Clin Med. 2019;8:1042. https://doi.org/10.3390/jcm8071042.
2. Brown C, Mehler PS. Medical complications of anorexia nervosa and their treatments: an update on some critical aspects. Eat Weight Disord. 2015;20:419–25.
3. Friedli N, Stanga Z, Sobotka L, et al. Revisiting the refeeding syndrome: results of a systematic review. Nutrition. 2017;35:151–60.
4. National Institute for Clinical Excellence (NICE). Nutrition support in adults: oral nutrition support, enteral tube feeding and parenteral nutrition. NICE clinical guideline 32, National Institute for health and clinical excellence. London, UK, 2006.
5. Da Silva JSV, Seres DS, Sabino K, et al. ASPEN consensus recommendations for refeeding syndrome. Nutr Clin Pract. 2020;35:178–95.
6. Garber AK, Kohn MK. Newer approaches to acute nutritional rehabilitation for patients with anorexia nervosa. Adolesc Med. 2018;29:344–58.
7. Garber AK, Sawyer SM, Golden NH, et al. A systematic review of approaches to refeeding in patients with anorexia nervosa. Int J Eat Disord. 2016;49:293–310.
8. Redgrave GW, Coughlin JW, Schreyer CC, et al. Refeeding and weight restoration outcomes in anorexia nervosa: challenging current guidelines. Int J Eat Disord. 2015;48:866–73.
9. Gentile MG, Pastorelli P, Ciceri R, et al. Specialized refeeding treatment for anorexia nervosa patients suffering from extreme undernutrition. Clin Nutr. 2010;29:627–32.
10. Matthews K, Hill J, Jeffrey S, et al. A higher-calorie refeeding protocol does not increase adverse outcomes in adult patients with eating disorders. J Acad Nutr Diet. 2018;118:1450–63.
11. Hay P, Chinn D, Forbes D, et al. Royal Australian and New Zealand College of Psychiatrists clinical practice guidelines for the treatment of eating disorders. Aust N Z J Psychiatry. 2014;48:977–1008.
12. Royal College of Psychiatrists, Royal College of Physicians. MARSIPAN: management of really sick patients with anorexia nervosa (College report CR189). 2nd edn. Royal College of Psychiatrists, 2014.
13. Kohn MR, Madden S, Clarke SD. Refeeding in anorexia nervosa: increased safety and efficiency through understanding the pathophysiology of protein calorie malnutrition. Curr Opin Pediatr. 2011;23:390–4.
14. O'Connor G, Goldin J. The refeeding syndrome and glucose load. Int J Eat Disord. 2011;44:182–5.

15. Golden NH, Keane-Miller C, Sainani KL, et al. Higher caloric intake in hospitalized adolescents with anorexia nervosa is associated with reduced length of stay and no increased rate of refeeding syndrome. J Adolesc Health. 2013;53:573–8.

16. O'Connor G, Dasha N. Refeeding hypophosphatemia in adolescents with anorexia nervosa: a systematic review. Nutr Clin Pract. 2013;28:358–64.

17. Ornstein RM, Golden NH, Jacobson MS, et al. Hypophosphatemia during nutritional rehabilitation in anorexia nervosa: implications for refeeding and monitoring. J Adolesc Health. 2003;32:83–8.

18. Madden S, Miskovic-Wheatley J, Clarke S, et al. Outcomes of a rapid refeeding protocol in adolescent anorexia nervosa. J Eat Disord. 2015;3:8.

19. Yamazaki T, Inada S, Sawada M, et al. Diets with high carbohydrate contents were associated with refeeding hypophosphatemia: a retrospective study in Japanese inpatients with anorexia nervosa. Int J Eat Disord. 2020. https://doi.org/10.1002/eat.23416.

20. Whitelaw M, Gilbertson H, Lam P-Y, et al. Does aggressive refeeding in hospitalized adolescents with anorexia nervosa result in increased hypophosphatemia? J Adolesc Health. 2010;46:577–82.

21. Parker EK, Faruquie SS, Anderson G, et al. High caloric refeeding is safe in hospitalised adolescent patients with restrictive eating disorders. J Nutr Metab. 2016;2016:1–9.

22. Agostino H, Erdstein J, Di Meglio G. Shifting paradigms: continuous nasogastric feeding with high caloric intakes in anorexia nervosa. J Adolesc Health. 2013;53:590–4.

23. O'Connor G, Nicholls D, Hudson L, et al. Refeeding low weight hospitalized adolescents with anorexia nervosa: a multicenter randomized controlled trial. Nutr Clin Pract. 2016;31:681–9.

24. Garber AK, Mauldin K, Michihata N, et al. Higher calorie diets increase weight gain and shorten hospital stay in hospitalized adolescents with anorexia nervosa. J Adolesc Health. 2013;53:579–84.

25. Maginot TR, Kumar MM, Shiels J, et al. Outcomes of an inpatient refeeding protocol in youth with anorexia nervosa: Rady children's Hospital San Diego/University of California, San Diego. J Eat Disord. 2017;5:1.

26. Smith K, Lesser J, Brandenburg B, et al. Outcomes of an inpatient refeeding protocol in youth with anorexia nervosa and atypical anorexia nervosa at children's hospitals and clinics of Minnesota. J Eat Disord. 2016;4:35.

27. Davis C, Hong WJN, Zhang SL, et al. Outcomes of a higher calorie inpatient refeeding protocol in Asian adolescents with anorexia nervosa. Int J Eat Disord. 2021;54:95–101.

28. Garber AK, Cheng J, Accurso EC, et al. Short-term outcomes of the study of refeeding to optimize inpatient gains for patients with anorexia nervosa. JAMA Pediatr. 2021;175:19–27.

29. Parker E, Flood V, Halaki M, et al. Study protocol for a randomised controlled trial investigating two different refeeding formulations to improve safety and efficacy of hospital management of adolescent and young adults admitted with anorexia nervosa. BMJ Open. 2020;10: e038242. https://doi.org/10.1136/bmjopen-2020-038242.

30. American Psychiatric Association. Diagnostic and statistical manual of mental disorders. 5th ed. Arlington, VA: American Psychiatric Publishing; 2013.

31. Detsky AS, McLaughlin JR, Baker JP, et al. What is subjective global assessment of nutritional status? J Parenter Enteral Nutr. 1987;11:8–13.

32. Golden NH, Katzman DK, Sawyer SM, et al. Society for Adolescent Health and Medicine. Position paper of the Society for adolescent health and medicine: medical management of restrictive eating disorders in adolescents and young adults. J Adolesc Health. 2015;56:121–5.

33. Centres for Disease Control and Prevention, "CDC 2000 data sets," 2000, http://www.cdc.gov/nchs/nhanes.htm

34. Katzman DK, Garber AK, Kohn M, Golden NH. Refeeding hypophosphatemia in hospitalized adolescents with anorexia nervosa. J Adolesc Health. 2014;55:455–7.

35. World Health Organization. Management of severe malnutrition : a manual for physicians and other seniorhealth workers. World Health Organization, 1999.

36. Rio A, Whelan K, Goff L, et al. Occurrence of refeeding syndrome in adults started on artificial nutrition support: prospective cohort study. BMJ Open. 2013;3:e002173.

37. Mehanna HM, Moledina J, Travis J. Refeeding syndrome: what it is, and how to prevent and treat it. BMJ. 2008;336:1495–8.

38. Russell J, Baur L, Beumont P, Byrnes S, Zipfel S. Refeeding of anorexics: wasteful not wilful. The Lancet. 1998;352:1445–6.

10

Understanding Implicit and Explicit Learning in Adolescents with and without Anorexia Nervosa

Lot C. Sternheim[1,2]* ⓘ, Miriam I. Wickham[3], Unna N. Danner[1,4], Todd W. Maddox[5], Vincent J. Filoteo[6], Megan E. Shott[6,7] and Guido K. W. Frank[6,7]

Abstract

Background: Cognitive disturbances such as impairments in learning are thought to play a role in adult Anorexia Nervosa (AN). It is remains unclear to what extent these disturbances result from starvation of the brain, or relate to an abnormal premorbid cognitive profile. This study investigates learning processes in adolescents with AN, hypothesizing that implicit learning is intact, as found previously in explicit learning tasks. Secondly, we hypothesized that anxiety and depression symptoms, inherent to AN, are associated to learning processes in AN.

Methods: In total 46 adolescents diagnosed with AN and 44 control participants were administered an implicit category learning task in which they were asked to categorize simple perceptual stimuli (Gabor patches) based on a linear integration (i.e., an implicit task) of orientation and spatial frequency of the stimulus. A subgroup of adolescents ($n = 38$) also completed a task assessing explicit learning.

Results: Model-based analyses indicated that adolescents with AN performed significantly more accurately compared to their healthy peers regardless of whether they used the optimal strategy or not. Depression and anxiety did not relate to learning performance in the AN group.

Conclusions: Overall, our findings of augmented implicit and explicit learning in adolescents with AN corroborate recent studies that suggested higher stimulus-response learning during prediction error paradigms. Learning disturbances in adult AN may then be at least partly due to long-term malnourishment, highlighting the importance of early recognition and refeeding in treatments for AN.

* Correspondence: l.c.sternheim@uu.nl
[1]Department of Clinical Psychology, Universiteit Utrecht, Heidelberglaan 1, 3508, TC, Utrecht, The Netherlands
[2]Utrecht, The Netherlands
Full list of author information is available at the end of the article

Plain English summary

We know that some adults with anorexia nervosa (AN) experience difficulties in learning processes. It is remains unclear to what extent these difficulties result from long-term starvation of the brain. This study looked at learning processes in adolescents with AN who have a relatively short duration of illness. We also investigated whether anxiety and depression affected learning. Forty-six adolescents diagnosed with AN and 44 control participants completed tasks that assessed learning and questionnaires assessing depression and anxiety. We found that adolescents with AN performed more accurately compared to their healthy peers. However, depression and anxiety did not relate to learning performance. Overall, our findings suggest that individuals with AN, relative to their healthy peers, may be quicker in forming automatic responses and behaviors to cues. Learning disturbances in adult AN may then be at least partly due to long-term malnourishment, which highlights the importance of early recognition of AN and refeeding in treatments for AN.

Keywords: Anorexia nervosa, Adolescents, Implicit learning, Explicit learning

Background

Anorexia nervosa (AN) is a severe psychiatric disorder with the highest mortality rates across mental disorders [1]. AN is characterized by extreme restriction of intake or purging of food, fear of gaining weight and disturbed experience of body weight or shape (DSM-5, [2]). The lifetime prevalence of AN among women is up to 4% [3] with a crude mortality rate of approximately 5% per decade [1, 2]. This debilitating disorder most typically develops during adolescence or young adulthood [4] and research suggests that prepubertal and early adolescent onset of AN may be on the rise [5].

Whilst available treatments for adolescents, in particular family-based interventions, are associated with good rates of remission (approximately 70% [6];) there is still a subgroup of young people who do not benefit from this treatment. lLittle is known about factors contributing to a more chronic prognosis [6, 7].

Recently it has been suggested that the focus for AN treatment should shift from mainly treating physical symptoms (i.e weight loss), and psychiatric symptoms (i.e., depression), to potentially underlying pathologies, such as disturbed cognitive processes, which have been described in adults with AN [8]. To further advance this direction, we investigated specific learning processes and whether these are comparable in younger AN patients to their peers without AN. Findings will contribute to unravelling whether impairments in cognitive processes such as learning are implicated in the development of AN, or whether these impairments are related to chronic starvation of AN. Subsequently, this knowledge will inform treatment directions.

Over the last few years studies have shown that some individuals with AN experience impairments in cognitive functioning. Studies in adults with AN show problems across a wide range of cognitive domains, such as, motor inhibition, visual processing speed, central coherence, visual–spatial ability, attention, learning and memory as well as decision making and cognitive flexibility [9, 10]. Currently it remains unknown however to what extent these difficulties are contributing to the development and maintenance of AN, or in turn, to what extent the chronic underweight of AN causes these cognitive impairments. Although longitudinal studies are the desirable method for answering these questions, these types of studies are costly and hindered by high levels of attrition in AN [11]. An alternative approach to gaining insight into the relation between cognitive functioning and AN is to study patients with a relative short duration of illness (i.e., adolescents) to compare with results in older samples. Seeing that the common age of onset of AN is early to mid-adolescents, studying young people with AN may provide important information about cognitive disturbances in AN at younger age [5].

Interestingly, published data on cognitive functioning in adolescent patients with AN posit a more mixed picture compared to the adult literature. Many studies, commonly including neuropsychological instruments, report no deficits at all or only subtle impairments in e.g. nonverbal intelligence functions and cognitive flexibility impairments such as audiomotor responses, and set-shifting abilities (e.g. [12–18]). In terms of general cognitive functioning, Schilder et al. [19] found that IQ was in fact higher in adolescent AN patients then the norm which suggests a superior cognitive functioning compared to peers.

Looking specifically at learning in AN there is less literature available. One increasingly popular hypothesis, based on recent advances in cognitive neuroscience, posits that persistent AN behaviors may be understood as maladaptive habits, which are driven by abnormal learning processes [20, 21]. This neurobiological "habit model of AN" [22, 23] suggests that for AN patients, eating behaviors become automatic responses very quickly and that little effort is needed to maintain these behaviors. On the other hand, *discontinuing* these dysfunctional habits becomes very difficult, as expressed in the often unsuccessful treatment of AN. In other words, *stimulus-response learning* may be augmented in individuals with AN.

Another important type of learning is category learning, which refers to the ability to make adaptive responses across a wide variety of situations and as such is a fundamental decision making process. Two separate but overlapping learning systems that contribute to category learning are the explicit and implicit learning systems. Explicit learning involves conscious learning, including (sets of) rules and feedback processes (rule-based learning) [24].

On the other hand, implicit learning refers to extracting predictive relationships in the form of statistical regularities or sequence of events from the environment without putting conscious effort into the process or even realizing the learning process at all (procedural-based learning [24]. The two types of learning are related to different brain areas and neural pathways, whereby explicit learning involves the hippocampal and medial temporal areas, whilst implicit learning engages frontal cortico-striatal circuits [25].

Explicit category learning involves both initial acquisition learning and updating explicitly-learned associations. This latter learning aspect is partly determined by a cognitive process called set-shifting, i.e. being able to shift attention between one task and another, whereby poor set-shifting interferes with being able to successfully update these explicitly-learned associations. In recent years set-shifting has gained a lot of attention in AN. While the literature suggests impaired set shifting in adults with AN [26], findings related to set-shifting in adolescent AN samples are mixed and whilst some studies show set-shifting impairments, other studies find that adolescents with AN perform on equal measure to HC groups (for a review see [15]). Mixed findings may be attributable to the complexity of different paradigms assessing different components of set-shifting. One task that has been previously used in studies investigating set-shifting and, more broadly, the ability to update explicitly-learned associations is the Houses and Castle task [27]. Set shifting deficits have been found in individuals with AN and individuals weight restored from AN [18, 28]. Individuals weight restored from AN also displayed hyper-learning, defined as a steeper learning curve, and learned the rules of the task faster than their healthy counterparts. This learning slope, however, was not significantly associated with the shift cost [28]. As far as we know, there are no studies explicitly examining hyper-learning in adolescents with AN. Following the theory that an amplification in learning processes, for example habit learning, is characteristic of AN, arguably then we may expect to find altered learning processes in

adolescents with AN. Research on implicit category learning on the other hand is scarce. In fact, to our knowledge only one study looked at implicit learning in adolescents with AN [29]. Firk and colleagues [29] studied an adolescent sample before and after weight gain and found implicit sequence learning, which refers to learning the order of a sequence of stimuli, which is thought to be random, to be impaired, and that this was related to lower BMI. Looking at the adult literature, Shott et al. [30] found that in adults with AN, implicit category learning, which refers to learning how to categorize stimuli according to an unknown and non-verbalizable rule, was impaired. Other studies in adults showed (implicit) attention interferences for food-related words in individuals with patients with AN, but no implicit memory bias [31].

Furthermore, Shott et al. [30] found that implicit category learning was related to heightened novelty-seeking and lower sensitivity to punishment in adults with AN, which hints at the potential association with reward processes. Studies in adults show that the reward-related dopamine system is indeed implicated in cognitive functioning (e.g., reinforcement learning) [32]. Moreover, alterations in dopamine system activity has been associated with depression [33] and anxiety traits [34], both of which are pertinent to AN [34–36]. All of the studies above include adult samples; studies including adolescent samples are scarce. There is some evidence from cerebrospinal fluid and neuroimaging studies that the dopaminergic (DA) system is abnormal in adults ánd adolescents with AN, studies are lacking that directly linked DA function to behavior in AN [37–39]. The DA system is involved in Pavlovian model free learning, as well as habit and goal directed learning [40]. Elevated brain response during reward prediction error tasks may indicate altered Pavlovian stimulus-response learning in AN [38]. However, the interactions between the DA system and learning in AN needs further study. Nevertheless, it has been speculated that plasticity of brain DA function in adolescents is higher than in adults, and that this more flexible DA response may protect from DA-related learning inefficiencies [18]. It is therefore possible that whilst adults with AN display impaired learning, adolescents with AN will have *intact* learning due to age-dependent greater flexibility of their learning circuitry. Alongside the possible influence of the reward system, other potentially important effects on attention-dependents tasks include age-related, motivational and mood-related effects. For example, it has been suggested that those with a relatively short duration of AN (either adult or adolescent) may have ways to compensate poor cognitive functioning by activating more neural activity, or different neural circuits, or both [41]. High levels of perfectionism and fear for making mistakes, often reported by both adults and adolescents with AN [42] may also serve as a compensatory feature contributing to a performance comparable to healthy peers despite perhaps poorer cognitive functioning. With regards to mood disturbances there is evidence suggesting that both depressive and anxious symptomatology contribute to poorer performance on cognitive tasks in adults with AN [43, 44]. Whether depressive and anxious symptomatology contribute to implicit learning in adolescents with AN is another unexplored area. Recent studies have, for instance, indicated that individuals who score high on intolerance of uncertainty perform poorly on threat extinction (as assesses with responses to uncertain auditory stimuli that varied in threat level), which may contribute to suboptimal learning [45]. Intolerance of uncertainty is an important anxiety-related factor and refers to approach and avoidance responses to uncertainty whereby those with higher intolerance levels, are more likely to interpret ambiguous stimuli as more threatening, and have less confidence in their decisions in ambiguous situations [46]. Intolerance of uncertainty has been associated with the reward system [47] and may be an important factor for understanding learning processes in AN seeing that it is pertinent to both adults with AN [48–50] and adolescents [51, 52].

Depression has also been associated with altered learning and specifically in reward related context [53]. Our understanding of what brain regions and neurotransmitter systems are involved is still limited and again studies including adolescent samples are lacking However, several factors could play a role. Anxiety and depression as well as AN are associated with elevated cortisol levels as a sign of high stress, which could interfere with cognitive flexibility and learning [54]. Stress has been found to alter dopamine and noradrenaline circuitry and thereby altering working memory function and learning [55]. In sum, whilst there is some evidence for altered learning processes in adults with AN, and associations with affective states, studies investigating learning processes in adolescents with AN are scarce. Building on the theory that altered learning processes are characteristic of AN, we expect to find these alterations in adolescents as well.

Aims & hypotheses
The aims of this study were twofold. We wanted to test the hypothesis that implicit learning is intact in adolescent AN, similarly to explicit learning studies, as this may provide insight into the development of cognitive functioning from childhood years to adulthood and may shed some light onto the relation between learning abnormalities and the (long-term) neurobiological starvation effects in AN. Second, we wanted to test whether

depressive and anxiety symptoms are related to worse learning performance in adolescents with AN.

Method
Participants
A total of 90 adolescent participants (11–17 years old) were recruited from two different sites (the Netherlands - NL, United States of America - USA), which will be described here separately. No participants were excluded in the USA groups; 3 participants were excluded in the NL groups.

NL sample
Twenty adolescents with a current diagnosis of AN according to DSM 5 criteria were recruited from a Dutch specialized Eating Disorders center (AN-NL group). Diagnoses were established by psychiatrists or clinical psychologists and confirmed with the Eating Disorder Examination (EDE [56];). Participants were excluded in the case of alcohol and drug abuse, history of or current diagnoses of other psychiatric disorders such as dementia, schizophrenia or mental retardation, and current diagnoses of diabetes, or a neurological disorder. Of these 20, 6 were taking anti-psychotics and 1 was taking mood-stabilizers. None were taking anti-depressants or sedatives. Eighteen healthy control adolescents were recruited in the Utrecht (NL) area through local advertisement flyers posted in a number of high schools, sports clubs and community centers (HC-NL group). They were included if they had no history of neurological medical diagnoses that may affect cognitive functioning, and no first-line relatives with a diagnosis of an eating disorder. Before participation, the experimenter completed the Mini International Neuropsychiatric Interview (M.I.N.I.: [57]; Dutch version: [58]), in order to screen for any possible (undiagnosed) psychiatric disorders. If there was any indication of an (undiagnosed) disorder (as seen from any of the subsections of the M.I.N.I.) participants were excluded from the study ($n = 3$).

USA sample
Twenty-six adolescents with a diagnosis of AN (AN-USA group) were recruited through an Eating Disorders program at a children's hospital and a specialized Eating Disorder center (USA). All participants met DSM 5 criteria for AN ($n = 24$) or broadly defined AN (restricting atypical AN, $n = 2$) at the time of enrolment of the study. All individuals with AN completed the Clinical Diagnostic Interview Schedule for Children 4.0, to assess all major psychiatric diagnoses [59]. Participants were excluded if there was any indication of current substance use or other psychiatric disorders including dementia, mental retardation, schizophrenia or any neurological disorder. Those with diagnoses of anxiety and depression

were included. Of these 26, 10 were taking anti-depressants and 4 were taking anti-psychotics. None were taking mood-stabilizers or sedatives. Twenty-six adolescent non-AN controls (HC-USA group) were recruited through local advertisements in the Denver metropolitan areas (USA). They completed the Clinical Diagnostic Interview Schedule for Children 4.0, to rule out any current or previous psychiatric disorders [59]. Non-AN controls had a lifetime history of body weight between 90 and 110% of ideal body weight since menarche.

Clinical measures

The NL-AN group's BMI was assessed before participation, by measuring weight on a digital Tanita scale (Tanita Cooperation of America, Inc., Arlington Heights, IL) and height with a stadiometer. The NL-HC group's BMI was assessed by asking participants to state their height and weight. All BMI were then calculated as kg/m^2.

The USA-AN group's BMI (kg/m^2) was obtained from their hospital chart (weight was measured on a digital scale daily). The weight date was on the day of the testing session, which was between 1 and 2 weeks into treatment. The USA-HC group's BMI (kg/m^2) was assessed immediately before the testing session by weighing them on a digital Detecto scale (Detecto, Webb City, Missouri) and measuring their height with a Seca stadiometer.

All four groups of participants (NL-AN, NL-HC, USA-AN and USA-HC) were asked to fill out two questionnaires; the Children's Depression Inventory to measure possible depressive symptoms (CDI: [60], α = 0.92; Dutch version: [61], α = 0.88 and a scale measuring intolerance of uncertainty (IUS: [62], α = 0.96; Dutch version: [63], α = 0.93). We used the Intolerance of Uncertainty Scale (IUS) to assess symptoms of anxious pathology. Intolerance of uncertainty is a key component of anxiety, and a wealth of evidence shows the contribution of intolerance of uncertainty to anxiety across a wide range of anxiety disorders and other psychological disorders (see a recent review by [64]).

Implicit category learning task

All 908 participants were asked to do an implicit category learning task, as previously used in Shott et al. [30]. In this task, participants were presented with Gabor patches (see Fig. 1 for examples), which they were asked to categorize into one of two categories (A and B). Each Gabor patch was presented until the participant's response was made ("z" and "/" keys for categories A and B, respectively). After this, the participant received feedback for 1 s: the screen displayed the words "correct" or "wrong" respectively. Immediately after 1 s of feedback, a mask was displayed for 5 s in order to prevent participants from responding to the after-image of the previous stimulus. Then, the next trial began. The rule, unknown to participants, by which the Gabor patches had to be categorized, required a linear integration of two stimulus dimensions (spatial frequency and orientation of the lines in the stimulus). In each testing session, each of the presented stimuli was unique in its combined spatial frequency and orientation dimensions. For each testing session there were 80 trials, for which an equal number of Gabor patches from category A and B were generated randomly by sampling from two bivariate normal distributions (as originally done by [65]). Each Gabor patch was generated using MATLAB routines from Brainard's [66] Psychophysics Toolbox.

The NL groups performed this task on a computer with a 15.4" screen with a 1680 × 1050 resolution. The Gabor patches were thereby approximately 5 cm in height and at an approximate viewing distance of 45 cm, they subtended a visual angle of about 6.4°. The USA groups performed this task on a computer with a 21" screen with a 1360 × 1024 resolution. Each Gabor patch was thereby 7 cm in diameter, which subtended a visual angle of about 8.9° from an approximate viewing distance of 45 cm.

This paradigm has been used extensively to gain a better understanding of the underlying processes in category learning in both normal and patient populations [67, 68].

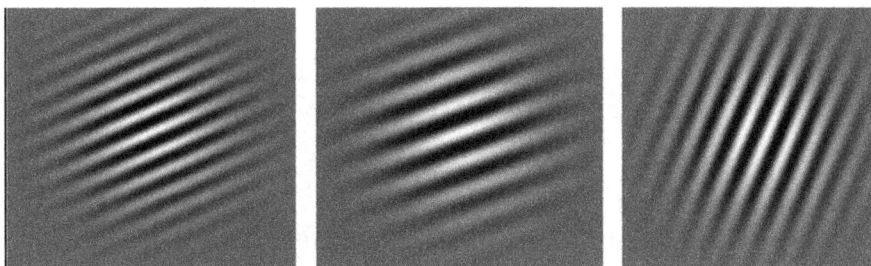

Fig. 1 Examples of Gabor patch stimuli, image taken from Shott et al. [30]

Explicit category learning task

A selection of our sample (AN-NL and HC-NL; total $n = 38$) additionally completed an explicit category learning task, in addition to the implicit category learning task, i.e. the Houses & Castles task [18]. In this task, participants were randomly categorized into two groups: Houses group and Castles group. In each trial, participants were presented with either a cartoon image of a house or a castle (see Fig. 2 for examples), depending on their group, which was presented until the participant made a response. Each stimulus belonged to a category ("A" or "B") based on an unknown rule. Participants were asked to categorize the stimuli by pressing a key ("z" key and "/" key for categories "A" and "B" respectively). Immediately after the participant's response, feedback was shown for 0.75 s: displaying either the word "correct" or "wrong" beneath the image of the stimulus. This was followed by 1 s of blank screen, after which the next trial began. There was a total of 160 trials. Four dimensions with binary values could differ per stimulus per trial: castle stimuli – shape of foundation (diamond or square), location of ramparts (above or sunken into walls), number of rings around castle (one or two), color of drawbridge (yellow or green); house stimuli – color of door (red or blue), lighting inside window (light on or off), shape of roof (flat or triangular), type of plant (shrub or tree). During the first 80 trials, the rules for categorization were as follows: castle stimuli – shape of foundation (category "A": square, category "B": diamond); house stimuli – shape of roof (category "A": flat, category "B": triangular). During the last 80 trials, the rules for categorization were as follows: castle stimuli – number of rings (category "A": one, category "B": two), house stimuli – type of plant (category "A": tree, category "B": shrub). Participants were never informed of the rule shift and had to infer all rules from the provided feedback. Participants were given feedback on every trial and the contingencies were the same in each trial.

This task has been used many times before to reliably test set shifting/explicit and implicit category learning across normal and patient populations [18, 27].

Participants performed this task on a computer with a 15.4″ screen with a 1680 × 1050 resolution. Stimuli were approximately 6.5 cm in height and at an approximate viewing distance of 45 cm, they subtended a visual angle of about 8.3°. The stimuli were generated using MATLAB routines from Brainard's [66] Psychophysics Toolbox.

Procedure

This study was approved by both appropriate USA and Dutch (medical) ethical committees. All participants and their parents or legal guardians gave consent for participation in this study. USA data was collected between February 2012–February 2014. An additional Dutch sample was included between October 2014 and August 2016 in order to 1) increase power for the implicit learning task; and 2) build on the [18] study by analyzing associations between the explicit learning processes and intolerance of uncertainty.

Primary analyses included a between-subjects design, where all participants were asked to do an implicit category learning task, and a sub-group of participants (NL-AN and NL-HC groups only) were asked to additionally do an explicit learning task.

In the case of participants who were not administered the additional explicit learning task (USA-AN and USA-HC groups), they were asked to complete the implicit category learning task at the beginning of the testing session. In the case of the other sub-group of participants (NL-AN and NL-HC groups), they were asked to first perform the explicit learning task, followed by the implicit learning task after a small break. This order was chosen as the explicit learning task is the easier one of the two so we expected that participants would thereby stay motivated enough after the first task to complete the second task.

All participants were asked to fill out all questionnaires at the end of the testing session. The experimenter stayed with the participant at all times during the testing session in case of fatigue, questions about the tasks or questionnaires, or in case of early termination of the experiment. Participants were not given compensation for their participation.

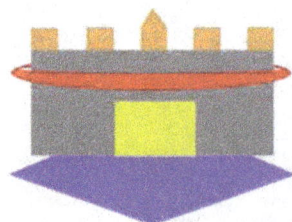

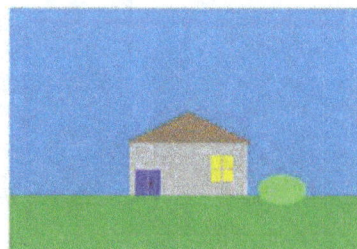

Fig. 2 Examples of castle and house stimuli, image taken from Shott et al. [18]

Statistical analyses

Statistical Package for the Social Sciences version 26 was used for the analyses. In order to see whether there were any significant differences in age or BMI between the AN adolescents and the non-AN controls, and between the USA and NL groups, independent samples t-tests were run with Bonferroni corrections for multiple testing. Sphericity as well as homogeneity of variances were checked and corrected for accordingly at all times. Where sphericity could not be assumed within an ANOVA, the Greenhouse-Geisser results are reported. Estimates of effect size are calculated using partial eta squares or Cohen's D [69], where .2 = small effect, .5 = medium effect and .8 = large effect.

Learning outcomes

Model-based analyses implicit learning task

Using mathematical models, this task allows for insight into the specific approach participant use when learning the task [67, 70, 71]. As explained by Shott et al. [30], these models can identify AN patients who adopted a procedural-based approach to learning compared to healthy controls, in order to assess impairments in procedural-based learning in patients. Two classes of models will be compared, namely the *procedural-based* (PB) approach, and the *hypothesis-testing* (HT) approach. The optimal PB model assumes that participant used the rule displayed in Fig. 1 as the solid line. The second PB model was the general linear classifier (GLC), which also assumes that the participant's decision on each trial is based on a linear integration. HT models assume that the participant set a criterion and that there were four response regions: low frequency/ shallow angle, low frequency/steep angle, high frequency/shallow angle and high frequency/ steep angle (for a detailed explanation of these models see Shott et al. [30].

Statistical analyses

Following procedures as described by Shott et al. [30], to explore differences in implicit learning performance, a 2 (group) × 4 (block) mixed-design ANOVA (to compare AN to HC) was run with the following measures: 1) accuracy (number of correct responses divided by number of trials), 2) reaction time (RT, in seconds) and 3) reaction time variability (standard deviation of reaction time). Moreover, 4) a learning curve (accuracy in block 4 – accuracy in block 1) was computed and 4-way ANOVA'S were used to examine group differences. Post-hoc tests were examined to ensure no country group differences (NL versus USA AN groups).

Following procedures from Shott et al. [30], for the explicit learning task, to explore differences in accuracy (number of correct responses divided by the number of trials) in the explicit learning task, a 2 (group) × 8 (block) mixed-design ANOVA was run (in the Dutch samples only).

Learning outcomes and anxious and depressive symptomatology

To explore associations between implicit learning outcomes and anxious and depressive symptoms Pearson's correlation analyses were run in all four groups including, depression, BMI age, and learning curve (implicit learning) variables (for an elaborate explanation on the using the learning curve within the correlation analyses, rather than the other outcomes we refer to procedures described by Shott & colleagues [18].

To explore associations between implicit learning outcomes, explicit learning, anxious and depressive symptoms, Pearson's correlation analyses were run in AN (NL-AN only) and in HC (NL-HC only) separately including learning curve (implicit learning outcome), accuracy block 5 (explicit learning), intolerance of uncertainty, depression, BMI and age.

Results

Age and BMI

There were no significant difference in age between AN patients (NL versus USA (NL: mean = 15.60, SD =1.23; USA: mean = 14.73, SD = 1.56)) and non-AN controls (NL versus USA (NL: mean = 15.22, SD = 1.47; USA: mean 14.19, SD: 1.86)). There was a significant difference in age between the two USA and the NL groups whereby the USA groups were slightly younger than the AN-NL group ($t(86.34) = -3.73$, $p < 0.01$, Cohen's $d = 0.79$), but including age as a covariate did not change the results.

As expected a significant difference in BMI between ANs and HCs was found (see Table 1). Low BMI is inherent to AN diagnosis and was therefore not added into the analyses as covariate. No significant differences in BMI between the two AN groups or between the two HC groups were found.

Implicit learning task

Due to the mixed design ANOVA on implicit learning data showing heterogeneity of variance on all measures (i.e. non-normal distribution), all data was logarithmically transformed to normalize the data and reduce heterogeneity of variances (according to [72]). A skewness analysis of the untransformed data showed that implicit learning data was indeed skewed (max skewness value = 4.78, *SES* = 0.25). The skewness observed in the logarithmically transformed data was improved as compared to the untransformed data, with all skewness values lying between – 0.54 and 0.36 (*SES* = 0.25), which is within the acceptable range of skewness (e.g. [73]). We therefore deemed the logarithmic transformation adequate to

Table 1 Age, BMI, depression, intolerance of uncertainty, implicit leaning (means, standard deviations and ranges; $N = 90$)

Measure	AN-USA N = 26	AN-NL N = 20	HC-USA N = 26	HC-NL N = 18	Test statistic ANOVA
Age ** [a]	$M = 14.73$ $SD = 1.56$ Range = 12–17	$M = 15.60$ $SD = 1.23$ Range = 13–17	$M = 14.19$ $SD = 1.86$ Range = 11–17	$M = 15.22$ $SD = 1.47$ Range = 12–17	$F(3,85) = 5.61$ $p < 0.01$ $\eta^2 = 0.17$
BMI ** [b] [c]	$M = 16.14$ $SD = 1.53$ Range = 12.49–18.34	$M = 17.28$ $SD = 1.82$ Range = 13.30–20.07	$M = 20.21$ $SD = 2.45$ Range = 16.41–25.88	$M = 20.37$ $SD = 2.53$ Range = 15.82–24.40	$F(3,85) = 23.56$ $p < 0.01$ $\eta^2 = 0.45$
CDI ** [a] [b] [c]	$M = 12.31$ $SD = 9.00$ Range = 0–28	$M = 23.89$ $SD = 2.23$ Range = 20–27	$M = 3.04$ $SD = 2.72$ Range = 0–9	$M = 7.56$ $SD = 5.44$ Range = 2–22	$F(3,85) = 51.23$ $p < 0.01$ $\eta^2 = 0.64$
IUS ** [b] [d]	$M = 71.31$ $SD = 20.55$ Range = 35–107	$M = 80.53$ $SD = 14.55$ Range = 41–107	$M = 48.27$ $SD = 18.09$ Range = 27–104	$M = 64.83$ $SD = 15.69$ Range = 28–92	$F(3,85) = 13.66$ $p < 0.01$ $\eta^2 = 0.33$
Implicit learning accuracy (log) * [c]	$M = -.21$ $SD = .07$ Range = -.33 - -.08	$M = -.18$ $SD = .07$ Range = -.33 - -.07	$M = -.21$ $SD = .06$ Range = -.34 - -.14	$M = -.27$ $SD = .05$ Range = -.34 - -.14	$F(3,85) = 3.28$ $p = 0.02$ $\eta_p^2 = 0.10$
Implicit learning reaction time (log)	$M = .09$ $SD = .15$ Range = -.18–.49	$M = .04$ $SD = .11$ Range = -.15–.29	$M = .14$ $SD = .14$ Range = -.11 - -.42	$M = .06$ $SD = .17$ Range = -.28–.30	$F(3,85) = 2.18$ $p = 0.10$
Implicit learning reaction time variability (log)	$M = -.15$ $SD = .24$ Range = -.63–0.31	$M = -.18$ $SD = .19$ Range = -.60–.15	$M = -.03$ $SD = .31$ Range = -.57–.58	$M = -.05$ $SD = .24$ Range = -.51–.45	$F(3,85) = 1.74$ $p = 0.16$
Implicit learning curve (accuracy in last block minus accuracy in first block)	$M = .10$ $SD = .12$ Range = -.11–.31	$M = .03$ $SD = .10$ Range = -.13–.2	$M = .09$ $SD = .12$ Range = -.11–.31	$M = .04$ $SD = .10$ Range = -.13–.20	$F(3,85) = 1.92$ $p = 0.13$

CDI Children's Depression Inventory, *IUS* Intolerance of Uncertainty

* = $p < 0.05$; ** = $p < 0.01$

[a] AN-USA and AN-NL differ significantly

[b] AN-USA and HC-USA differ significantly

[c] AN-NL and HC-NL differ significantly

[d] HC-USA and HC-NL differ significantly

normalize the data. Another 2 (group) × 4 (block) mixed-design ANOVA was then run on the log10 transformations of accuracy, reaction time and reaction time variability. For a summary of all implicit learning task results, see Table 1.

Implicit learning task: accuracy

The ANOVA revealed a main effect of group, $F(1,88) = 7.77$, $p = 0.01$, $\eta_p^2 = 0.08$, where the AN groups were overall more accurate than the HC groups (small effect). A main effect of block was found, $F(2.30,201.92[1]) = 20.59$, $p < 0.01$, $\eta_p^2 = 0.19$, where all groups improved across blocks. No significant interaction of block x group was found. For an illustration of the accuracy results, see Fig. 3. The NL and USA AN groups did not differ significantly from each other.

Implicit learning task: reaction time

No significant main effect of group on reaction time was found. There was a significant main effect of block on

reaction time, $F(2.58,227.17) = 28.54$, $p < 0.01$, $\eta_p^2 = 0.25$, where participants' reaction times decreased across blocks. No significant group x block interaction was found. The NL and USA AN groups did not differ significantly from each other.

Implicit learning task: reaction time variability

For the reaction time variability, a significant main effect of group was found, $F(1,88) = 5.51$, $p = 0.02$, $\eta_p^2 = 0.06$, where the AN group showed less variability in reaction times than the HC group. A significant main effect of block was found, $F(2.31,203.22) = 25.32$, $p < 0.01$, $\eta_p^2 = 0.22$, where all participants' variability decreased over time. No significant block x group interaction was found. The reaction time variability results are displayed in Fig. 4. The NL and USA AN groups did not differ significantly from each other.

Implicit learning task: learning curve

No significant differences in learning curve (accuracy in last block minus accuracy in first block) between the AN and HC groups were found. The NL and USA AN groups also did not differ significantly from each other.

[1] As Mauchly's test of sphericity was violated Greenhouse-Geisser corrected values are reported

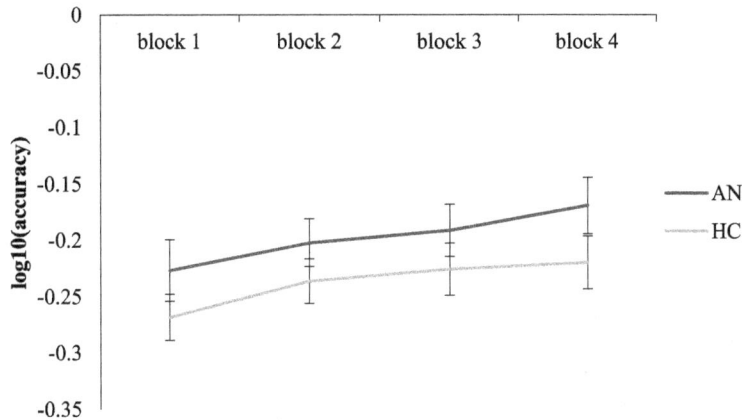

Fig. 3 Changes in accuracy (number of correct responses divided by the number of trials, log transformed) in implicit learning task across blocks, differentially between AN HC groups. Error bars show standard error

Implicit learning task: model results

In line with Shott et al. [30], to determine whether the model-based subgroups differed, accuracy rates in the final block for the AN and HC participants who used either *procedural-based* (PB) or *hypothesis-testing* (HT) approach were contrasted (see Fig. 5). T-tests showed that for both the AN and HC participants accuracy for the PB approach was significantly better compared to the HT approach (AN: $p < .01$; HC: $p < .05$). Moreover, for both the PB and HT approach, the AN participants performed more accurately than the HC participants ($p < .01$, when controlling for depression, anxiety or medication $p < .05$).

Explicit learning task

No heterogeneity of variance was found for the planned ANOVA, therefore no transformation had to be

performed on the set-shifting data. For a summary of explicit learning task results, see Table 2.

Explicit learning: accuracy

The ANOVA revealed a significant main effect of group, $F(1,36) = 11.35$, $p = 0.01$, $\eta_p^2 = 0.24$, where the AN group was consistently more accurate than the HC group (large effect). A significant main effect of block was found, $F(3.39,122.02) = 10.94$, $p < 0.01$, $\eta_p^2 = 0.23$. No significant block x group interaction was revealed. For a visualization of the explicit learning task accuracy results, see Fig. 6.

Explicit learning: shift costs

To explore whether there were any differences in shift cost (accuracy in block 5 minus accuracy in block 4) between the two groups, an independent samples t-test was run. To determine the impact of the actual shift, a

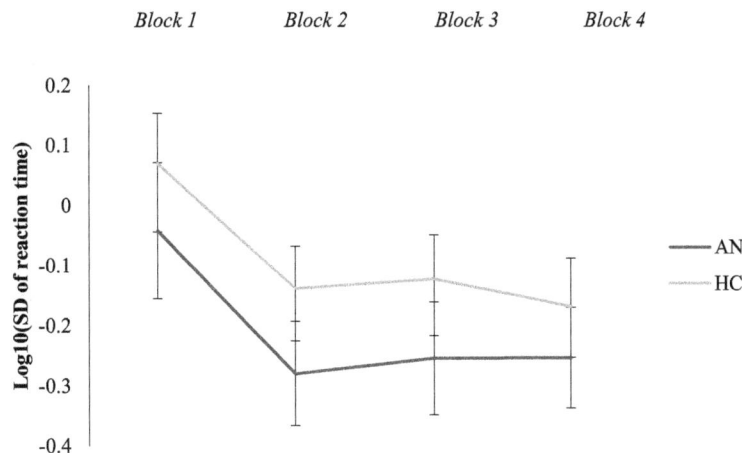

Fig. 4 Changes in reaction time variability (standard deviation of reaction time in seconds, log transformed) in implicit learning task across blocks, differentially for AN and HC group

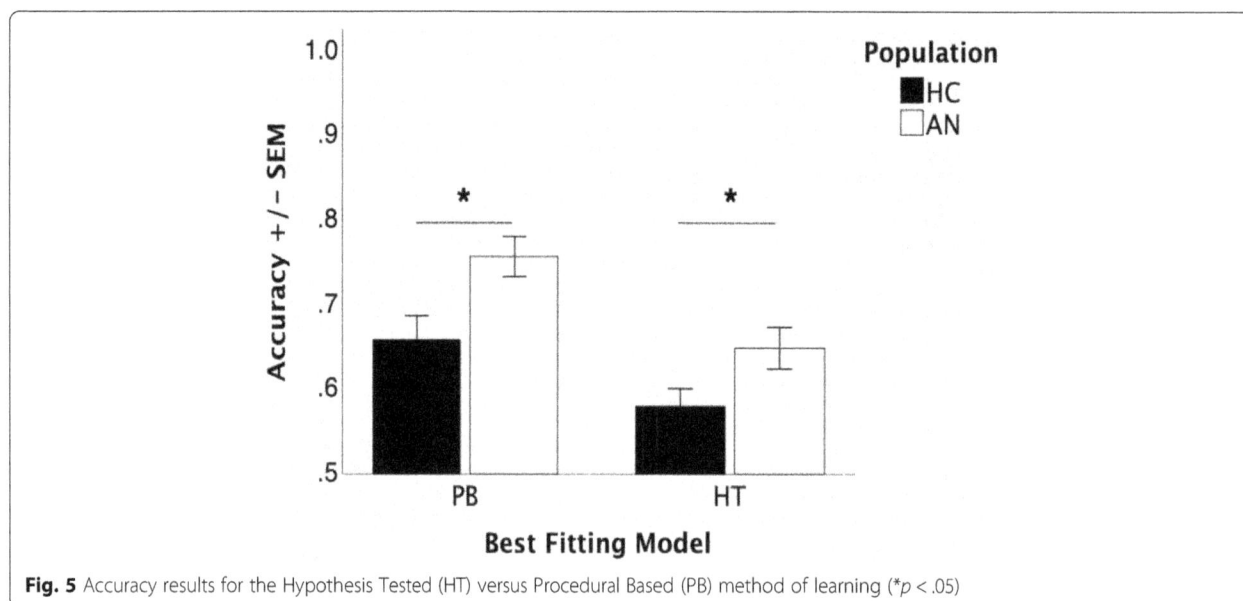

Fig. 5 Accuracy results for the Hypothesis Tested (HT) versus Procedural Based (PB) method of learning (*$p < .05$)

Shift-Cost score was computed by subtracting each participant's accuracy on block 5 from their accuracy on block 4 (higher scores equaled a greater shift-cost). Group differences indicate how well a particular group did, compared to the other, at coping with the rule change. No significant differences were found. To investigate this further, an independent samples t-test was run on accuracy in block 5, as well as accuracy in block 4, between groups. After Bonferroni corrections, it was found that accuracy in block 5 differed between groups, $t(36) = 2.76$, $p = 0.02$, Cohen's d = 0.90, but not accuracy in block 4 (this only yielded a significant result before Bonferroni corrections, $t(36) = 2.13$, $p = 0.04$, Cohen's d = 0.69). This suggests that participants were nearly as good as each other at the end of block 4, *but dealt with the set change after the rule shift differently, yielding different accuracies in block 5.*

Relationships between implicit learning, intolerance of uncertainty, depression, BMI and age

As there were significant differences between the USA and NL groups regarding the Intolerance of Uncertainty Scale and Children's Depression Inventory in both the HC and AN groups 4 different analyses were run including learning curve, intolerance of uncertainty, depression age and BMI. In the USA-AN, NL-AN and NL-HC groups no significant correlations were found between any of the implicit learning outcomes and the clinical variables. In the USA-HC group a smaller learning curve was associated to a higher BMI ($r = -.47$, $p = 0.02$) and to a higher age ($r = -.43$, $p = 0.03$).

Relationships between implicit learning, intolerance of uncertainty, depression, BMI, age and explicit learning (NL groups only).

Table 2 Means, standard deviations and ranges of explicit learning task results in the NL groups ($N = 38$)

Statistic	AN N = 20	HC N = 18	Test statistic t-test
Set-shifting overall accuracy**	M = 0.86 SD = 0.21 Range = 0.25–1.00	M = 0.80 SD = 0.15 Range = 0.46–0.99	$t(36) = -3.37$ $p < 0.01$ d = 1.10
Set-shifting accuracy block 4*	M = 0.90 SD = 0.21 Range = 0.25–1.00	M = 0.83 SD = 0.24 Range = 0.25–1.00	$t(36) = -2.13$ $p = 0.04$ d = 0.69
Set-shifting accuracy block 5*	M = 0.73 SD = 0.15 Range = 0.25–0.95	M = 0.67 SD = 0.17 Range = 0.25–0.95	$t(36) = -2.76$ $p < 0.01$ d = 0.90
Shift cost (accuracy block 5 minus accuracy block 4)	M = 0.18 SD = 0.24 Range = −0.45-0.75	M = 0.18 SD = 0.25 Range = −0.45-0.75	$t(36) = 0.23$ $p = 0.82$ d = 0.07

* = $p < 0.05$; ** = $p < 0.01$

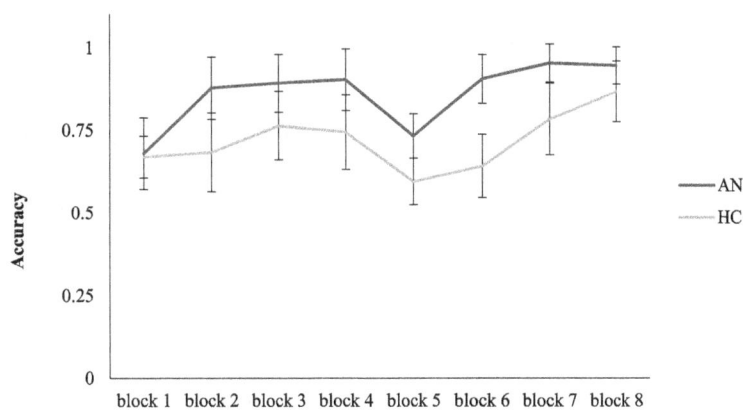

Fig. 6 Changes in accuracy (number of correct responses divided by number of trials) in the explicit learning task across blocks, differentially for both groups. Error bars show standard error

In the NL-AN group, IUS scores were significantly associated to explicit learning outcomes (Accuracy: $r = .49$, $p = 0.03$; Costs: $r = -.46$, $p = 0.05$), whereby higher intolerance of uncertainty was associated to higher SS accuracy and lower SS costs (i.e. more/stronger intolerance of uncertainty was related to better learning).

Discussion

In this study we aimed to understand implicit and explicit learning in adolescents with AN, and to explore associations between learning outcomes and anxious and depressive symptomatology. Interestingly, in terms of implicit learning, accuracy performance of AN participants was superior to that of the HC, and this was true for both the *procedural-based* (PB) and the *hypothesis-testing* (HT) model types. As expected, performance on the other implicit learning outcomes, reaction time and variability in these times, were comparable between the AN and HC participants. Similarly, for explicit learning, AN participants had higher accuracy rates compared to HCs. In both the combined AN and HC groups there were no associations between the implicit learning outcomes and clinical variables such as age, BMI, intolerance of uncertainty and depression. In the USA-HC group poorer implicit learning was associated to lower BMI and lower age, which may be due to developmental processes.

The finding of superior accuracy outcomes in AN on both tasks applied in this study is particularly interesting, seeing that a recent systematic review by Olivo et al. [74] concludes that on most cognitive domains, adolescents with AN are *comparable* to their peers in term of behavioral performance. Our finding of better performance compared to non-AN controls on a specific type of learning task adds new important information regarding cognitive functioning in adolescents with AN. Looking at learning more broadly, findings fit with the theory

that individuals with AN may have augmented *stimulus-response learning*. As posited by the "habit model of AN" ([20]; Walsh, 2013), for individuals with AN, behaviors become automatic responses quickly and are then also maintained without much effort. Discontinuing these habits however is much harder, which may explain why some AN symptoms remain difficult to treat.

Furthermore, an earlier study showed that patients with AN had higher IQs than the population norm, which may also contribute to better performance [19]. Another possible explanation for more optimal behavioral performance may lie with high levels of perfectionism that may partly drive this overperformance [75]. That is, adolescents who develop AN put in more effort to "get it right", which would reflect the high perfectionism commonly present in individuals with AN [42]. A limitation of the study however is that it did not include IQ or perfectionism measures so this remains speculation. Future studies on learning in AN should apply perfectionism scales and test this hypothesis.

It is also possible that adolescents with AN, with a (usually) shorter duration of illness are in a state of cognitive and perfectionistic overdrive, driven by a brain pathophysiology that is in a state of overexcitability and associated with high intellectual capacity. Interestingly, such an "overexcitable cognitive ability" has been associated with hyper-reactivity of the central nervous system [76], which is associated to a risk for psychopathology [77]. An important neural system implicated in cognitive functioning and perhaps explanatory for our results of better learning performance in adolescent AN is the dopamine system. Striatal dopamine pathways are involved in major cognitive domains such as feedback sensitivity, which in turn affects learning processes. Indeed, previous literature highlights alterations in feedback sensitivity, especially punishment sensitivity, in adults and adolescents with AN [37, 78] which may affect learning strategies [32]. Furthermore, brain dopamine circuitry is a major contributor to model free and model based learning, namely Pavlovian prediction error learning, habit learning and goal directed instrumental learning [40]. This study was not designed to test dopamine circuit function and thus does not allow testing for these hypotheses. We are currently planning future studies that will include biological markers of the dopamine system when investigating learning in AN.

Our results are in line with previous literature showing that cognitive processes that may be disturbed in adults with AN are intact in adolescents with AN [12, 13, 15, 16, 18, 30]. It is therefore possible that cognitive deficits in adults are at least partly contributable to the illness itself, which may be explained by the neurobiological effects of long-term starvation [79]. The initial hyper-drive in adolescent AN during the continuing duration of illness (and associated long-term malnourishment) then transfers into a state of burn-out (and associated cognitive problems) in adults with long-term AN (as theorized by [74, 80]). Indeed, Shott et al. [30] found that adults with AN still performed poorly on the same implicit learning task used in this study, even if they applied the correct model or strategy. Whether these suspected illness-related changes are permanent is an important question for further research to examine, yet the relation between cognitive functioning and malnourishment in AN is complex, and study findings aiming to entangle this relationship are mixed. For example, as highlighted by a recent review [81], whilst some literature suggests that cognitive difficulties in AN are related to low weight, other studies find that cognitive deficits were not or only partly associated with malnourishment in AN (see also [82]). Also data on the reversibility of these potential malnourishment-related cognitive deficits is mixed; some studies find that AN-related cognitive difficulties are reversable after weight gain [83], whilst others find that even short-term malnourishment can lead to irreversible brain changes in adolescents with AN (for a review see [84]). The lack of associations between learning outcomes and clinical variables in the AN group was unexpected, in particular seeing that some recent studies demonstrated negative effects of anxious and depressive symptoms on cognitive functioning in AN (i.e. social problem solving; [85]) and central coherence [86]. Due to group differences in scores on the clinical instruments analyses were run in the separate smaller groups. This may have resulted in a power issue which in turn may have resulted in non-significant associations that in fact could be significant with a larger sample. On the other hand, a recent meta-analysis concluded that depression is not associated to set-shifting in adults [10]. In line with this finding, a recent study including adolescents showed that despite higher levels of depression in the

AN group, set-shifting ability did not differ between AN and healthy controls [16]. Of note, results of the current study show that intolerance of uncertainty was significantly higher in the AN adolescents than in the non-AN controls, and that stronger intolerance of uncertainty was related to better explicit learning confirming that intolerance of uncertainty may be an important clinical factor in adolescents with AN [52]. How and to what extent intolerance of uncertainty fits into AN pathology requires further examination in future studies. Whilst no differences between the NL and USA groups on learning outcomes were found, interestingly, the NL and USA groups did differ in terms of anxious and depressive symptomology, with the NL-AN group reporting more severe depression and intolerance of uncertainty. Whether this is indeed a cultural difference in terms of severity, or can be explained by other cultural differences (i.e. interpretation of questions) we can't conclude from this study.

Whilst these results are promising, it is important to keep in mind that the observed effects are small and that due to relatively small groups, interpretation should be done with caution and replication studies are warranted, in particular the findings for the explicit learning task seeing that only the NL groups completed these (18 HC versus 20 AN = total $n = 38$). However, for the associations between learning outcomes and clinical variables, some correlation coefficients were in fact quite high, suggesting that in larger groups significant correlations may be detected. Further studies should include larger samples and it is recommendable to record (clinical characteristics of) those who were invited but refused to take part in order to avoid any participation biases. Future studies may also want to ensure matching the HC group to the patient groups to optimize comparability.

Although we did include age in this study, we did not include illness duration, which may well be an important factor seeing the effects of more chronic and long-term AN on the brain, and cognitive processes. Lastly, due to a technical error we had to rely on self-report weight data for some participants, future studies should ensure objective weight information. Moreover, studies aiming to understand the complex relation between BMI and cognitive processes in adolescents may benefit from using the WHO values (% median BMI).

Conclusions
Taken together these findings shed light on learning processes in adolescents with AN, in that learning appears intact, or even enhanced, compared to their peers. This may be an indication that cognitive difficulties such as impaired implicit and explicit learning in adults with AN may result from (enduring) starvation or other illness related factors. Future research should aim

to examine the effects of acute and long-term malnourishment and weight gain on learning processes.. The better performance in the adolescent AN group is in line with other research examining cognitive functions in adolescents, and the opposite compared to research in adults. It is therefore possible that the brain activation in AN when young is in a form of hyper-learning, i.e. showing steeper learning curves then their peers without AN, and that this hyper-learning is in turn potentially driven by anxiety and perfectionism to result in excellent task performance [76, 77]. However, this state is not sustainable, food restriction may also take its toll on the brain, and this may eventually lead to poor performance in adults.

Taking into account studies that do find learning impairments in adolescents with AN, further research should focus on unravelling different learning processes and their underlying neurocircuits. This may have direct clinical implications in that identifying the underlying pathophysiology of altered category learning in AN may allow us to identify interventions that maintain normal cognitive flexibility from young to adult age, which could improve outcome when treating adults with AN.

Abbreviations
AN: Anorexia nervosa; APA: American Psychology Association; BMI: Body mass index; CDI: Children's Depression Inventory; DA system: Dopaminergic system; DSM-IV: Diagnostic statistical manual-IV; EDE: Eating Disorder Examination; HC: Healthy control; HT approach: Hypothesis-testing approach; IQ: Intelligence quotient; NL: Netherlands; IUS: Intolerance of Uncertainty Scale; PB approach: Procedural-based approach

Acknowledgements
Not applicable.

Authors' contributions
LS coordinated the study, obtained ethical approval, analyzed and interpreted the data and was a major contributor in writing the manuscript. MW collected the data for the Dutch samples, analyzed the data and contributed to writing the manuscript. UD coordinated the data collection for the AN Dutch sample and contributed to writing the manuscript.TM analyzed the data. VF analyzed the data. MS coordinated the data collection for the USA samples and helped interpreting the data. GF supervised LS, contributed to analyzing and interpreting the data and contributed to writing the manuscript. All authors read and approved the final manuscript.

Declarations

Ethics approval and consent to participate
USA: The study was approved by the Colorado Multiple Institutional Review Board. We obtained written assent from the participant and consent from the legal guardian prior to conducting any of the study procedures.
NL: This study was approved by the Medische Ethische Toetsingscommisie Universitair Medisch Centrum Utrecht (13–139). All participants and their parents or legal guardians gave consent for participation in this study.

Competing interests
The authors declare that they have no competing interests.

Author details
[1]Department of Clinical Psychology, Universiteit Utrecht, Heidelberglaan 1, 3508, TC, Utrecht, The Netherlands. [2]Utrecht, The Netherlands. [3]Department of Social Health and Organisation Psychology, Universiteit Utrecht, Heidelberglaan 1, 3508, TC, Utrecht, The Netherlands. [4]Altrecht Eating Disorders Rintveld, Wenshoek 4, 3705, WE, Zeist, The Netherlands. [5]Department of Psychology, University of Texas, Austin, USA. [6]Department of Psychiatry, University of California San Diego, La Jolla, CA, USA. [7]Eating Disorders Center for Treatment and Research, University of California San Diego, San Diego, CA, USA.

References
1. Fichter MM, Quadflieg N. Mortality in eating disorders-results of a large prospective clinical longitudinal study. Int J Eat Disord. 2016;49(4):391–401. https://doi.org/10.1002/eat.22501.
2. American Psychiatric Association. Diagnostic and statistical manual of mental disorders (DSM-5®). American Psychiatric Pub; 2013.
3. Smink FR, Van Hoeken D, Hoek HW. Epidemiology of eating disorders: incidence, prevalence and mortality rates. Curr Psychiatry Rep. 2012;14(4): 406–14. https://doi.org/10.1007/s11920-012-0282-y.
4. Campbell K, Peebles R. Eating disorders in children and adolescents: state of the art review. Pediatrics. 2014;134(3):582–92.
5. Petkova H, Simic M, Nicholls D, Ford T, Prina AM, Stuart R, et al. Incidence of anorexia nervosa in young people in the UK and Ireland: a national surveillance study. BMJ Open. 2019;9(10):e027339. https://doi.org/10.1136/bmjopen-2018-027339.
6. Couturier J, Kimber M, Szatmari P. Efficacy of family-based treatment for adolescents with eating disorders: a systematic review and meta-analysis. Int J Eat Disord. 2013;46(1):3–11. https://doi.org/10.1002/eat.22042.
7. Marucci S, Ragione LD, De Iaco G, Mococci T, Vicini M, Guastamacchia E, et al. Anorexia nervosa and comorbid psychopathology. Endocr Metab Immune Disord Drug Targets (Formerly Curr Drug Targets Immune Endocr Metabol Disord). 2018;18(4):316–24.
8. Zipfel S, Giel KE, Bulik CM, Hay P, Schmidt U. Anorexia nervosa: aetiology, assessment, and treatment. Lancet Psychiatry. 2015;2(12):1099–111.
9. Lena SM, Fiocco AJ, Leyenaar JK. The role of cognitive deficits in the development of eating disorders. Neuropsychol Rev. 2004;14(2):99–113. https://doi.org/10.1023/B:NERV.0000028081.40907.de.
10. Smith KE, Mason TB, Johnson JS, Lavender JM, Wonderlich SA. A systematic review of reviews of neurocognitive functioning in eating disorders: the state-of-the-literature and future directions. Int J Eat Disord. 2018;51(8):798–821. https://doi.org/10.1002/eat.22929.
11. Abdelbaky G, Hay P, Touyz S. Factors associated with treatment attrition in anorexia nervosa: a systematic review. OA Evid Based Med. 2013;1:1–3.
12. Bühren K, Mainz V, Herpertz-Dahlmann B, Schäfer K, Kahraman-Lanzerath B, Lente C, et al. Cognitive flexibility in juvenile anorexia nervosa patients before and after weight recovery. J Neural Transm. 2012;119(9):1047–57. https://doi.org/10.1007/s00702-012-0821-z.
13. Calderoni S, Muratori F, Leggero C, Narzisi A, Apicella F, Balottin U, et al. Neuropsychological functioning in children and adolescents with restrictive-type anorexia nervosa: an in-depth investigation with NEPSY–II. J Clin Exp Neuropsychol. 2013;5(2):167–79.
14. Kjaersdam Telléus G, Jepsen JR, Bentz M, Christiansen E, Jensen SO, Fagerlund B, et al. Cognitive profile of children and adolescents with anorexia nervosa. Eur Eat Disord Rev. 2015;23(1):34–42. https://doi.org/10.1002/erv.2337.
15. Lang K, Stahl D, Espie J, Treasure J, Tchanturia K. Set shifting in children and adolescents with anorexia nervosa: an exploratory systematic review and meta-analysis. Int J Eat Disord. 2014;47(4):394–9. https://doi.org/10.1002/eat.22235.

16. Rößner A, Juniak I, van Noort BM, Pfeiffer E, Lehmkuhl U, Kappel V. Cognitive flexibility in juvenile anorexia nervosain relation to comorbid symptoms of depression, obsessive compulsive symptoms and duration of illness. Z Kinder Jugendpsychiatr Psychother. 2016; Dec 12.

17. Sarrar L, Ehrlich S, Merle JV, Pfeiffer E, Lehmkuhl U, Schneider N. Cognitive flexibility and agouti-related protein in adolescent patients with anorexia nervosa. Psychoneuroendocrinology. 2011;36(9):1396–406. https://doi.org/10.1016/j.psyneuen.2011.03.014.

18. Shott ME, Filoteo JV, Bhatnagar KA, Peak NJ, Hagman JO, Rockwell R, et al. Cognitive set-shifting in anorexia nervosa. Eur Eat Disord Rev. 2012b;20(5):343–9. https://doi.org/10.1002/erv.2172.

19. Schilder CM, van Elburg AA, Snellen WM, Sternheim LC, Hoek HW, Danner UN. Intellectual functioning of adolescent and adult patients with eating disorders. Int J Eat Disord. 2017;50(5):481–9.

20. Davis L, Walsh BT, Schebendach J, Glasofer DR, Steinglass JE. Habits are stronger with longer duration of illness and greater severity in anorexia nervosa. Int J Eat Disord. 2020;53(5):683–9. https://doi.org/10.1002/eat.23265.

21. Walsh BT. The enigmatic persistence of anorexia nervosa. Am J Psychiatry. 2013;170(5):477–84.

22. Haynos AF, Hall LM, Lavender JM, Peterson CB, Crow SJ, Klimes-Dougan B, et al. Resting state functional connectivity of networks associated with reward and habit in anorexia nervosa. Hum Brain Mapp. 2019;40(2):652–62. https://doi.org/10.1002/hbm.24402.

23. Steinglass JE, Walsh BT. Neurobiological model of the persistence of anorexia nervosa. J Eat Disord. 2016;4(1):1–7.

24. Reber AS. Implicit learning and tacit knowledge: essay on the cognitive unconscious (Oxford Psychology Series). Oxford: Oxford University Press Inc; 1993.

25. Yang J, Li P. Brain networks of explicit and implicit learning. PLoS One. 2012;7(8):e42993. https://doi.org/10.1371/journal.pone.0042993.

26. Fuglset TS. Set-shifting, central coherence and decision-making in individuals recovered from anorexia nervosa: a systematic review. J Eat Disord. 2019;7(1):1–4.

27. Filoteo JV, Maddox WT, Ing AD, Zizak V, Song DD. The impact of irrelevant dimensional variation on rule-based category learning in patients with Parkinson's disease. J Int Neuropsychol Soc. 2005;11(5):503.

28. Filoteo JV, Paul EJ, Ashby FG, Frank GK, Helie S, Rockwell R, et al. Simulating category learning and set shifting deficits in patients weight-restored from anorexia nervosa. Neuropsychol. 2014;28(5):741–51. https://doi.org/10.1037/neu0000055.

29. Firk C, Mainz V, Schulte-Ruether M, Fink G, Herpertz-Dahlmann B, Konrad K. Implicit sequence learning in juvenile anorexia nervosa: neural mechanisms and the impact of starvation. J Child Psychol Psychiatry. 2015;56(11):1168–76. https://doi.org/10.1111/jcpp.12384.

30. Shott ME, Filoteo JV, Jappe LM, Pryor T, Maddox WT, Rollin MD, et al. Altered implicit category learning in anorexia nervosa. Neuropsychol. 2012a;26(2):191–201. https://doi.org/10.1037/a0026771.

31. Hermans D, Pieters G, Eelen P. Implicit and explicit memory for shape, body weight, and food-related words in patients with anorexia nervosa and nondieting controls. J Abnorm Psychol. 1998;107(2):193–202. https://doi.org/10.1037/0021-843X.107.2.193.

32. Cavanagh JF, Frank MJ, Allen JJ. Social stress reactivity alters reward and punishment learning. Soc Cogn Affect Neurosci. 2011;6(3):311–20. https://doi.org/10.1093/scan/nsq041.

33. Ayano GJ. Dopamine: receptors, functions, synthesis, pathways, locations and mental disorders: review of literatures. J Ment Disord Treat. 2016;2(120):2.

34. Lawford BR, Young R, Noble EP, Kann B, Ritchie T. The D 2 dopamine receptor (DRD2) gene is associated with co-morbid depression, anxiety and social dysfunction in untreated veterans with post-traumatic stress disorder. Eur Psychiatry. 2006;21(3):180–5.

35. Allen KL, Byrne SM, Oddy WH, Crosby RD. DSM–IV–TR and DSM-5 eating disorders in adolescents: prevalence, stability, and psychosocial correlates in a population-based sample of male and female adolescents. J Abnorm Psychol 2013;122(3):720, 732, https://doi.org/10.1037/a0034004.

36. Lloyd EC, Haase AM, Verplanken B. Anxiety and the development and maintenance of anorexia nervosa: protocol for a systematic review. Syst Rev. 2018;7(1):1–5.

37. DeGuzman M, Shott ME, Yang TT, Riederer J, Frank GK. Association of elevated reward prediction error response with weight gain in adolescent anorexia nervosa. Am J Psychiatry. 2017;174(6):557–65. https://doi.org/10.1176/appi.ajp.2016.16060671.

38. Frank GK, DeGuzman MC, Shott ME, Laudenslager ML, Rossi B, Pryor T. Association of brain reward learning response with harm avoidance, weight gain, and hypothalamic effective connectivity in adolescent anorexia nervosa. JAMA Psychiatry. 2018;75(10):1071–80.

39. Kaye WH, Ebert MH, Raleigh M, Lake CR. Abnormalities in CNS monoamine metabolism in anorexia nervosa. Arch Gen Psychiatry. 1984;41(4):350–5. https://doi.org/10.1001/archpsyc.1984.01790150040007.

40. Daw ND, O'Doherty JP. Chapter 21: multiple systems for value learning. In: Glimcher PW, Fehrs E, editors. Neuroeconomics. 2nd ed. San Diago: Academic Press; 2014. p. 393–410.

41. Wildes JE, Forbes EE, Marcus MD. Advancing research on cognitive flexibility in eating disorders: the importance of distinguishing attentional set-shifting and reversal learning. Int J Eat Disord. 2014;47(3):227–30. https://doi.org/10.1002/eat.22243.

42. Lloyd S, Yiend J, Schmidt U, Tchanturia K. Perfectionism in anorexia nervosa: novel performance based evidence. PLoS One. 2014;9(10):e111697. https://doi.org/10.1371/journal.pone.0111697.

43. Andrés-Perpiña S, Lozano-Serra E, Puig O, Lera-Miguel S, Lázaro L, Castro-Fornieles J. Clinical and biological correlates of adolescent anorexia nervosa with impaired cognitive profile. Euro Child Adol Psych. 2011;20(11-12):541–9. https://doi.org/10.1007/s00787-011-0216-y.

44. Wilsdon A, Wade TD. Executive functioning in anorexia nervosa: exploration of the role of obsessionality, depression and starvation. J Psychiatr Res. 2006;40(8):746–54. https://doi.org/10.1016/j.jpsychires.2005.10.006.

45. Morriss J, Saldarini F, Van Reekum CM. The role of threat level and intolerance of uncertainty in extinction. Int J Psychophysiol. 2019;142:1–9. https://doi.org/10.1016/j.ijpsycho.2019.05.013.

46. Birrell J, Meares K, Wilkinson A, Freeston M. Toward a definition of intolerance of uncertainty: a review of factor analytical studies of the intolerance of uncertainty scale. Clin Psychol Rev. 2011;31(7):1198–208. https://doi.org/10.1016/j.cpr.2011.07.009.

47. Nelson BD, Shankman SA, Proudfit GH. Intolerance of uncertainty mediates reduced reward anticipation in major depressive disorder. J Affect Disord. 2014;158:108–13. https://doi.org/10.1016/j.jad.2014.02.014.

48. Frank GK, Roblek T, Shott ME, Jappe LM, Rollin MD, Hagman JO, et al. Heightened fear of uncertainty in anorexia and bulimia nervosa. Int J Eat Disord. 2012;45(2):227–32. https://doi.org/10.1002/eat.20929.

49. Kesby A, Maguire S, Brownlow R, Grisham JR. Intolerance of uncertainty in eating disorders: an update on the field. Clin Psychol Rev. 2017;56:94–105. https://doi.org/10.1016/j.cpr.2017.07.002.

50. Sternheim L, Konstantellou A, Startup H, Schmidt U. What does uncertainty mean to women with anorexia nervosa? An interpretative phenomenological analysis. Eur Eat Disord Rev. 2011;19(1):12–24. https://doi.org/10.1002/erv.1029.

51. Konstantellou A, Hale L, Sternheim L, Simic M, Eisler I. The experience of intolerance of uncertainty for young people with a restrictive eating disorder: a pilot study. Eat Weight Disord Stud Anorexia Bulimia Obesity. 2019;24(3):533–40.

52. Sternheim L, Harrison A. The acceptability, feasibility and possible benefits of a group-based intervention targeting intolerance of uncertainty in adolescent inpatients with anorexia nervosa. Cogn Psychol. 2018;5(1):1441594. https://doi.org/10.1080/23311908.2018.1441594.

53. Vrieze E, Pizzagalli DA, Demyttenaere K, Hompes T, Sienaert P, de Boer P, et al. Reduced reward learning predicts outcome in major depressive disorder. Biol Psychiatry. 2013;73(7):639–45. https://doi.org/10.1016/j.biopsych.2012.10.014.

54. Shields GS, Sazma MA, Yonelinas AP. The effects of acute stress on core executive functions: a meta-analysis and comparison with cortisol. Neurosci Biobehav Rev. 2016;68:651–68. https://doi.org/10.1016/j.neubiorev.2016.06.038.

55. Hernaus D, Quaedflieg CW, Offermann JS, Casales Santa MM, van Amelsvoort T. Neuroendocrine stress responses predict catecholamine-dependent working memory-related dorsolateral prefrontal cortex activity. Soc Cogn Affect Neurosci. 2018;13(1):114–23. https://doi.org/10.1093/scan/nsx122.

56. Fairburn CG. Cognitive behavior therapy and eating disorders. Guilford Press; 2008.

57. Sheehan DV, Lecrubier Y, Sheehan KH, Amorim P, Janavs J, Weiller E, et al. The Mini-International Neuropsychiatric Interview (MINI): the development

and validation of a structured diagnostic psychiatric interview for DSM-IV and ICD-10. J Clin Psychiatry. 1998;59(20):22–33.

58. Overbeek I, Schruers K, Griez E. Mini international neuropsychiatric interview: Nederlandse versie 5.0. 0. *DSM-IV [Dutch version]*. Maastricht: Universiteit Maastricht; 1999.

59. Shaffer D, Fisher P, Lucas CP, Dulcan MK, Schwab-Stone ME. NIMH Diagnostic Interview Schedule for Children Version IV (NIMH DISC-IV): description, differences from previous versions, and reliability of some common diagnoses. J Am Acad Child Adolesc Psychiatry. 2000;39(1):28–38. https://doi.org/10.1097/00004583-200001000-00014.

60. Kovacs M. Children's depression inventory. North Tonawanda: Multi-Health System; 1992.

61. Timbremont B, Braet C. Psychometrische evaluatie van de Nederlandstalige children's depression inventory. Gedragstherapie. 2001;34:229–42.

62. Buhr K, Dugas MJ. The intolerance of uncertainty scale: psychometric properties of the English version. Behav Res Ther. 2002;40(8):931–45. https://doi.org/10.1016/S0005-7967(01)00092-4.

63. de Bruin GO, Rassin E, van der Heiden C, Muris P. Psychometric properties of a Dutch version of the intolerance of uncertainty scale. Neth J Psychol. 2006;62(2):87–92. https://doi.org/10.1007/BF03061055.

64. Rosser BA. Intolerance of uncertainty as a transdiagnostic mechanism of psychological difficulties: a systematic review of evidence pertaining to causality and temporal precedence. Cog Ther Res. 2019;43(2):438–63. https://doi.org/10.1007/s10608-018-9964-z.

65. Ashby FG, Gott RE. Decision rules in the perception and categorization of multidimensional stimuli. J Exp Psychol Learn Mem Cogn. 1988;14:33.

66. Brainard DH. The psychophysics toolbox. Spat Vis. 1997;10(4):433–6. https://doi.org/10.1163/156856897X00357.

67. Maddox WT, Ashby FG. Dissociating explicit and procedural-learning based systems of perceptual category learning. Behav Process. 2004;66(3):309–32. https://doi.org/10.1016/j.beproc.2004.03.011.

68. Maddox WT, Filoteo JV. Striatal contributions to category learning: quantitative modeling of simple linear and complex nonlinear rule learning in patients with Parkinson's disease. J Int Neuropsychol Soc. 2001;7(6):710–27. https://doi.org/10.1017/S1355617701766076.

69. Cohen J. Statistical power analysis for the behavioral sciencies. UK: Routledge; 1977.

70. Maddox WT, Ashby FG, Bohil CJ. Delayed feedback effects on rule-based and information-integration category learning. J Exp Psychol Learn Mem Cogn. 2003;29(4):650.

71. Zeithamova D, Maddox WT. Dual-task interference in perceptual category learning. Memory Cog. 2006;34(2):387–98. https://doi.org/10.3758/BF03193416.

72. Bartlett MS, Kendall DG. The statistical analysis of variance-heterogeneity and the logarithmic transformation. Suppl J R Stat Soc. 1946;8(1):128–38. https://doi.org/10.2307/2983618.

73. Trafimow D, Wang T, Wang C, Myuz HA. Does slight skewness matter? Int J Aviation Res. 2019;11(1):11–24.

74. Olivo G, Gaudio S, Schiöth HB. Brain and cognitive development in adolescents with anorexia nervosa: a systematic review of FMRI studies. Nutrients. 2019;11(8):1907. https://doi.org/10.3390/nu11081907.

75. Schilder C, Sternheim LC, Aarts E, van Elburg AA & Danner UN. Do adolescents with eating disorders ask too much of themselves in school? Relationships between educational achievement, intelligence and perfectionism. n.d.. *under review* IJED-20-0296.

76. Chang HJ, Kuo CC. Overexcitabilities: empirical studies and application. Learn Individ Differ. 2013;23:53–63.

77. Karpinski RI, Kolb AM, Tetreault NA, Borowski TB. High intelligence: a risk factor for psychological and physiological overexcitabilities. Intel. 2018;66:8–23.

78. Jappe LM, Frank GK, Shott ME, Rollin MD, Pryor T, Hagman JO, et al. Heightened sensitivity to reward and punishment in anorexia nervosa. Int J Eat Disord. 2011;44(4):317–24.

79. Johnson JG, Cohen P, Kasen S, Brook JS. Eating disorders during adolescence and the risk for physical and mental disorders during early adulthood. Arch Gen Psychiatry. 2002;59(6):545–52. https://doi.org/10.1001/archpsyc.59.6.545.

80. Kingston K, Szmukler G, Andrewes D, Tress B, Desmond P. Neuropsychological and structural brain changes in anorexia nervosa before and after refeeding. Psychol Med. 1996;26(1):15–28. https://doi.org/10.1017/S0033291700033687.

81. Reville MC, O'Connor L, Frampton I. Literature review of cognitive neuroscience and anorexia nervosa. Curr Psychiatry Rep. 2016;18(2):18. https://doi.org/10.1007/s11920-015-0651-4.

82. Tchanturia K, Anderluh MB, Morris RG, Rabe-Hesketh S, Collier DA, Sanchez P, et al. Cognitive flexibility in anorexia nervosa and bulimia nervosa. J Int Neuropsychol Soc. 2004;10(4):513–20. https://doi.org/10.1017/S1355617704104086.

83. Lozano-Serra E, Andrés-Perpiña S, Lázaro-García L, Castro-Fornieles J. Adolescent anorexia nervosa: cognitive performance after weight recovery. J Psychosom Res. 2014;76(1):6–11. https://doi.org/10.1016/j.jpsychores.2013.10.009.

84. Katzman DK, Christensen B, Young AR, Zipursky RB. Starving the brain: structural abnormalities and cognitive impairment in adolescents with anorexia nervosa. In Sem Clin Neuropsychiatry. 2001;6(2):146–52. https://doi.org/10.1053/scnp.2001.22263.

85. Sternheim L, Danner U, van Elburg A, Harrison A. Do anxiety, depression, and intolerance of uncertainty contribute to social problem solving in adult women with anorexia nervosa?. Brain Behav. 2020;10(6):e01588.

86. Roberts ME, Tchanturia K, Treasure JL. Is attention to detail a similarly strong candidate endophenotype for anorexia nervosa and bulimia nervosa? World J Bio Psychiatry. 2013;14(6):452–63. https://doi.org/10.3109/15622975.2011.639804.

11

Early Weight Gain Trajectories in First Episode Anorexia: Predictors of Outcome for Emerging Adults in Outpatient Treatment

A. Austin[1]* [iD], M. Flynn[1], K. L. Richards[1], H. Sharpe[2], K. L. Allen[1,3], V. A. Mountford[1,3,4], D. Glennon[3], N. Grant[3], A. Brown[5], K. Mahoney[6], L. Serpell[6,7], G. Brady[8], N. Nunes[8], F. Connan[8], M. Franklin-Smith[9], M. Schelhase[9], W. R. Jones[9], G. Breen[10] and U. Schmidt[1,3]

Abstract

Background: Early response to treatment has been shown to be a predictor of later clinical outcomes in eating disorders (EDs). Specifically, early weight gain trajectories in anorexia nervosa (AN) have been shown to predict higher rates of later remission in inpatient treatment. However, no study has, as of yet, examined this phenomenon within outpatient treatment of first episode cases of AN or in emerging adults.

Methods: One hundred seven patients with AN, all between the ages of 16 and 25 and with an illness duration of < 3 years, received treatment via the first episode rapid early intervention in eating disorders (FREED) service pathway. Weight was recorded routinely across early treatment sessions and recovery outcomes (BMI $\geq$ 18.5 kg/m^2 and eating psychopathology) were assessed up to 1 year later. Early weight gain across the first 12 treatment sessions was investigated using latent growth mixture modelling to determine distinct classes of change. Follow-up clinical outcomes and remission rates were compared between classes, and individual and clinical characteristics at baseline (treatment start) were tested as potential predictors.

Results: Four classes of early treatment trajectory were identified. Three of these classes ($n = 95$), though differing in their early change trajectories, showed substantial improvement in clinical outcomes at final follow-up. One smaller class ($n = 12$), characterised by a 'higher' start BMI (> 17) and no early weight gain, showed negligible improvement 1 year later. Of the three treatment responding groups, levels of purging, depression, and patient reported carer expressed emotion (in the form of high expectations and low tolerance of the patient) determined class membership, although these findings were not significant after correcting for multiple testing. A higher BMI at treatment start was not sufficient to predict optimal clinical outcomes.

Conclusion: First episode cases of AN treated via FREED fit into four distinct early response trajectory classes. These may represent subtypes of first episode AN patients. Three of these four trajectories included patients with substantial improvements 1 year later. For those in the non-response trajectory class, treatment adjustments or augmentations could be considered earlier, i.e., at treatment session 12.

* Correspondence: amelia.1.austin@kcl.ac.uk
[1]Department of Psychological Medicine, King's College London, Institute of Psychiatry, Psychology, and Neuroscience, 16 De Crespigny Park, London, UK
Full list of author information is available at the end of the article

Plain English summary

A key feature of anorexia nervosa (AN) is an unhealthily low body weight. Previous studies show that more weight gained early in inpatient treatment leads to better outcomes. This study tried to see if this was also true for outpatients receiving treatment for the first time. All participants were emerging adults between the ages of 16 and 25 who had been ill for less than 3 years. Weight was recorded across the first 12 weekly treatment sessions. Statistics showed that the patients fit roughly into four different groups in early treatment, each with different starting weights and rates of weight gain in the first 12 treatment sessions. The group a patient belonged to could sometimes be predicted by vomiting behaviours, level of depression, and patients' perception of parental tolerance and expectations at the start of treatment. Out of the four groups, three did relatively well 1 year later, but one small group of patients did not. This small group had a higher starting weight than many of the other groups but did not gain any weight across the first 12 sessions. These patients could benefit from a change or increase in the amount or intensity of treatment after the first 12 treatment sessions

Keywords: Anorexia nervosa, Eating disorder, Early intervention, Outpatient, Treatment, Growth mixture modelling

Introduction

Outpatient psychological therapies for adults with anorexia nervosa (AN) are associated with modest improvement in body mass index (BMI) and other outcomes, and there is no evidence for superiority of any specific approach. Such findings highlight the need to further develop and improve treatments [1]. A better understanding of individual characteristics, moderators, and trajectories in treatment is crucial in order to tease apart what works best for whom (i.e., to develop a precision medicine approach), and also to reduce unsuccessful treatment attempts [2].

Early response to treatment has been identified as a possible predictor of later clinical outcomes in eating disorders (EDs) [3, 4], i.e., those who have early symptom reduction after starting treatment are likely to have better outcomes at end of treatment and at later follow-ups. Recent studies evaluating early treatment response in EDs have adopted a latent growth modelling approach [5–7]. The purpose of this approach is to identify meaningful subgroups of patients with distinct growth (recovery) trajectories within a larger heterogeneous patient group [8]. Specific to AN, weight gain during early treatment has been shown to predict later rates of remission [9]. Application of a latent growth modelling approach to the treatment of AN, with the identification of these early weight gain subgroups, and individual and clinical characteristics that predict membership to these groups, may allow clinicians to determine the prognosis of patients and consequently tailor treatment to their needs.

Previous studies looking at treatment response in AN using a latent growth modelling approach have largely focused on full and partial hospitalisation settings. In a study of 102 adolescents and young adults with AN who were partially hospitalised, Berona, Richmond, and Rienecke found three distinct early weight gain trajectories: a slow, a moderate, and a rapid class. The rapid weight gain class

membership was predicted by three characteristics at baseline (i.e., treatment start): the presence of compensatory behaviours, lower parental expressed emotion, and the absence of a comorbid mood disorder [10]. Similarly, in an inpatient sample, Makhzoumi et al. found that a rapid weight gain trajectory was associated with regular restriction, bingeing, and purging, and further determined that a faster weight gain trajectory was associated with greater weight restoration at follow-up [11].

Most recently, Wade et al. investigated the trajectories of early weight gain in AN during outpatient treatment [12]. Four distinct trajectories were found, and the class with the highest weight gain over the early treatment period had the greatest rates of later remission. Results also showed that a class with higher BMI at treatment start did not automatically have better clinical outcomes than a class with a low BMI at treatment start [12]. This supports the need for the consideration of growth patterns rather than only severity of BMI at baseline for appropriate treatment selection.

To date, no studies have specifically assessed early weight gain trajectories for outpatients experiencing their first episode of AN, i.e., in a treatment naïve state. This is important to assess as first episode AN patients tend to have a more favourable treatment response compared to those with a more established illness [13, 14]. Thus, previous trajectory analyses in outpatient AN may not generalise to a first episode population.

In the current study we attempt to address this gap, with the aim to:

1. Investigate typical weight gain trajectory classes in outpatient treatment for first episode AN.
2. Evaluate baseline variables to determine if any predict membership of trajectory classes.
3. Evaluate outcome (remission) variables of each class.

Methods

Design

This study involves an analysis of weekly BMI and ED behavioural symptom data, logged weekly by clinicians during the multi-centre FREED-Up study. This study had a quasi-experimental pre-post design comparing 278 First Episode Rapid Early Intervention for Eating Disorders (FREED) patients to 224 treatment-as-usual controls, who were similar patients seen in the 2 years before FREED was introduced. The study and its findings are described in detail elsewhere [15, 16].

Participants

Participants were consecutive referrals from four specialist ED centres in England. All were emerging adults who entered treatment for a first episode ED (illness duration < 3 years) between 2016 and 2018 and were between 16 and 25 years old at study enrolment. Patients were excluded if they needed an immediate inpatient admission, were pregnant, had a severe learning disability, or had a comorbid physical or mental disorder needing primary treatment (e.g., psychosis). One hundred and twenty-one met diagnostic criteria for DSM-5 AN or other specified feeding and eating disorder [17] at assessment and had a BMI ≤ 18.5 at the start of treatment. Of these, 107 patients (88.4%) had symptom log data available, which constituted our final sample.

Procedure

Details of the FREED service model and care pathway has been previously described [18–21]. In brief, FREED patients were given a phone call within 48 h of referral to screen for eligibility for the service, and to increase engagement. Patients potentially suitable for FREED were offered a clinical assessment adapted for FREED, taking a biopsychosocial, person-centred approach, with family involvement encouraged. The adapted assessment emphasised the importance of early intervention on ED-related changes to the brain and body. Patients were then allocated to treatment, with the aim of starting this within 2 weeks of assessment. Treatment was NICE-concordant [22], evidence based (e.g., ED focused cognitive behavioural [CBT-ED] or Maudsley Anorexia Nervosa Treatment for Adults [MANTRA]), tailored to the needs of emerging adults in early-stage illness, and typically lasting between 20 and 30 individual sessions. Developmentally informed adaptations included a focus on early dietetic involvement and nutritional change, reduction of any unhelpful/excessive social media and health-related app use, effective management of transitions (e.g., to university, in treatment), the developmental tasks of emerging adulthood and age-appropriate family involvement.

Measures

Clinician symptom log

Therapist-recorded BMI and ED behaviour frequency at weekly therapy sessions.

Eating disorder examination questionnaire (EDE-Q)

The EDE-Q [23] is a 28-item measure which captures the frequency and severity of ED behaviours over the past 28 days. It provides a score on four subscales (dietary restraint, eating concerns, shape concerns, and weight concerns) as well as a global score. A total global score ≥ 2.8 suggests a clinical ED. [24] The EDE-Q also measures the frequency of binge and compensatory behaviours over the last 28 days [23].

Depression anxiety stress scale-21 (DASS-21)

The DASS-21 [25] is a 21-item screener which captures mood over the past week. It contains subscales for depression, anxiety, and distress, as well as a global score.

Clinical impairment assessment (CIA)

The CIA [26] is a 16-item measure used to evaluate psychosocial impairment from an ED. It covers four domains: mood and self-perception, cognitive function, work performance, and interpersonal function.

Level of expressed emotion (LEE)

The LEE [27] is a 60-item true or false questionnaire used to evaluate the perception of expressed emotion of one's most influential relationship. It includes subscales for attitude toward illness, emotional response, intrusiveness, and low tolerance/high expectations.

Analysis

Derivation of latent classes

The rate of change in weekly BMI over the first 12 therapy sessions (the approximate halfway point) was used to determine latent class membership in the current study. Patients who took a break for more than 30 days between treatment sessions (e.g., for exams, holidays) during the first 12 weeks only had data included up to the point of absence. Latent growth mixture modelling (LGMM) was used, which categorises individuals with similar patterns of longitudinal change into subgroups while also allowing for individual variation [28]. The optimal number of subgroups was informed by fit statistics including the Akaike Information Criteria (AIC), the Bayesian Information Criteria (BIC), and the sample-size adjusted Bayesian Information Criteria (aBIC), with lower absolute values indicating a better model fit. Entropy, or the separateness of the classes, was also evaluated in each model, with a value above 0.8 suggesting good separation [29]. Finally, the Vuong-Lo-Mendell-Rubin likelihood ratio test (VLMR-LRT) and the adjusted Lo-Mendell-Rubin likelihood ratio test (adjusted LRT) were used to compare a model with X classes to a model with X-1 classes, with a *p* value < 0.05 indicating that a model with X classes fits better the model with X-1 classes. LGMM was first conducted with a one class model, increasing up to a five-class model. Analysis was performed in Mplus version 8.4 (Muthén & Muthén, 2019).

Latent classes and clinical characteristics

Latent classes were compared on baseline variables (predictors) and 12-month follow-up variables (outcomes) using a 3-step approach as recommended by Herle et al. [30]. One way analysis of variance (ANOVA) was used to compare trajectory classes on continuous variables (e.g., EDE-Q score) while chi-squared and Fisher's exact tests were used for categorical variables (e.g., ethnicity). Significant findings were then subject to post-hoc testing to determine which classes differed. Binge, purge, and laxative use frequencies were zero-inflated and so groups were compared on the presence or absence of these behaviours. Remission was defined as BMI $\geq 18.5\,\mathrm{kg/m^2}$ and an EDE-Q global score ≤ 2.8 as suggested by Mond et al. [24]. For participants with missing data at the 12-month follow-up, data from the 6-month timepoint were used. Analysis was done in SPSS version 26.

Results

Latent classes

Fit statistics from the latent class analyses are presented in Table 1. One to five class solutions were tested, with entropy (i.e., separateness of the classes) increasing with each subsequent analysis. As recommended, the best fitting solution was determined by both fit statistics and existing findings/previous theory. Following previous evidence, we anticipated a three to four class solution [10–12, 31]. Two of the three fit statistics (AIC and aBIC) were lowest for the four-class solution. Thus, a four-class solution best fit the data, as is presented in Fig. 1. This includes one class starting with a higher BMI, making little change across the first 12 therapy sessions (*higher, stable*). A second class also starts at a higher BMI but makes steady, moderate gains across this

same time period (*higher, moderate*). A third class starts treatment with a very low BMI but makes large gains in early treatment (*low, rapid*). Finally, a fourth class begins at a moderate BMI and makes little early change (*medium, stable*).

Baseline predictors

Baseline characteristics of each latent class can be seen in Table 2. Participants in Class 2 (*high, moderate*) were significantly more likely to report higher scores on depression than Class 3 (*low, rapid*) and higher patient reported carer expressed emotion (low tolerance/greater expectations) compared to participants in Class 4 (*medium, stable*). Class 2 also had the highest rates of binge, purge, and laxative use behaviours at baseline, although only the presence of purging significantly predicted membership into Class 2 compared to Class 3 (*low, rapid*). These baseline findings are non-significant after a Bonferroni correction.

Recovery outcomes

Outcome characteristics of each latent class are presented in Table 3.

Follow-up BMI at 12 months was higher for Class 2 (*high, moderate*) compared to Class 1 (*high, stable*), although this was no longer significant after a Bonferroni correction to account for multiple testing.

The trajectory with the lowest starting BMI (Class 3: *low, rapid*) had significantly greater BMI change between treatment start and 12-month follow-up than Class 1 (*high, stable*) and Class 2 (*high, moderate*).

No other significant differences between classes were found. Class 1 (*high, stable*) had the lowest proportion of weight restored participants (BMI $\geq 18.5\,\mathrm{kg/m^2}$) and the lowest rates of full remission (10%), although these finding were not statistically significant.

Discussion

Our first aim was to investigate the typical trajectory classes of early weight gain across outpatients with first episode AN. Fit statistics suggested that a four-class solution best fit the data. This consisted of 1) a class of patients with relatively high BMI ($> 17\,\mathrm{kg/m^2}$) at treatment

Table 1 Fit statistics for latent growth mixture modelling

Classes	# free parameters	AIC	BIC	aBIC	Entropy	[a]LRT P
1	19	1602.64	1653.60	1593.56	–	–
2	23	1593.16	1654.85	1582.17	0.76	0.32/0.34
3	27	1589.36	1661.78	1576.47	0.87	0.34/0.36
4	31	1584.38	1667.53	1569.58	0.88	0.48/0.49
5	35	1588.67	1682.55	1571.96	0.90	0.24/0.24

aBIC sample-size adjusted Bayesian information criteria, *AIC* Akaike information criteria, *BIC* Bayesian information criteria
[a]*LRT* likelihood ratio tests (Vuong-Lo-Mendell-Rubin likelihood ratio test; adjusted Lo-Mendell-Rubin adjusted LRT test) quantify specific comparisons between the model of interest and a model with one fewer class, C-1

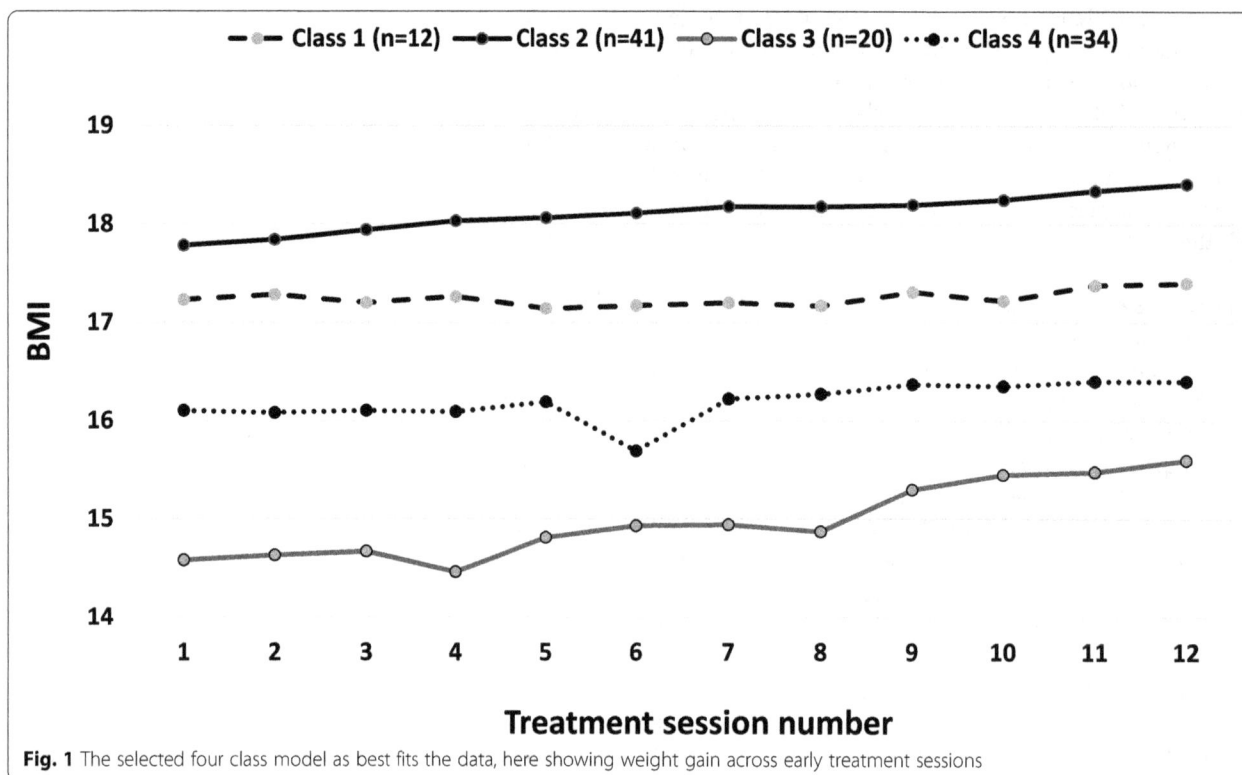

Fig. 1 The selected four class model as best fits the data, here showing weight gain across early treatment sessions

start and stable weight (i.e., no improvement) across early treatment (*high, stable*), 2) a class with relatively high BMI at treatment start but with moderate weight gains (about half a BMI point) across early treatment (*high, moderate*), 3) a class with a medium starting BMI relative to other classes but with little improvement over early treatment (*medium, stable*), and 4) a class with extremely low BMI ($< 15 \, \text{kg/m}^2$) and fast improvement across early treatment (*low, rapid*). This is similar to Wade et al., who found four classes with similar start BMIs (two with higher values, one medium, and one low) [12].

The second aim was to determine whether any characteristics may predict class membership. Those in Class 2 (*high, moderate*) were more likely to report higher levels of depression than Class 3 (*low, rapid*) and higher reported parental expressed emotion (greater expectations/lower levels of tolerance) compared to those in Class 4 (*medium, stable*). A previous study by Berona et al. found that the presence of a comorbid mood disorder and higher levels of parental expressed emotion were predictive of slower early weight gain [10]. However, it is still unclear exactly how depression/mood and parental expressed emotion contribute to trajectory change classes in first episode AN. For example, depression scores were more severe in a group (Class 2) with higher starting BMI and moderate trajectory improvements and lower in a group (Class 3) with poorer

starting BMI and rapid trajectory improvements. Future research will need to tease apart the relationship between these predictive variables and their relationship to intercept (start BMI) and slope (trajectory change).

Class 2 (*high, moderate*) also had the highest rates of binge, purge, and laxative use behaviours at baseline, although only the presence of purging predicted membership into Class 2 compared to Class 3 (*low, rapid*). Previous work has found compensatory behaviours to be predictors of more rapid weight gain trajectories in early inpatient treatment [10, 11]. However, it is difficult to directly compare our results to this previous work as these studies focused on the rate of weight gain irrespective of a patient's starting weight (i.e., all patients started at 'zero'). A transdiagnostic study by Espel-Huynh et al. found that the presence of vomiting at baseline was more common in patients with a rapid response trajectory in early treatment as measured by ED symptoms and emotional functioning [5]. As such, compensatory behaviour should be considered a specific variable of interest in any future treatment response trajectory studies. Overall, after correcting for multiple testing, there were no robust baseline predictors of later clinical outcomes.

Our third aim was to compare classes by later clinical outcomes. Three of the four classes achieve substantial improvements at 12-months. For the classes with a lower starting BMI, these improvements were 'propped

Table 2 Baseline characteristics (predictors) of each latent class, with mean and standard deviation

Variable	Class1, $n = 12$ (high, stable)	Class2, $n = 41$ (high, moderate)	Class3, $n = 20$ (low, rapid)	Class4, $n = 34$ (medium, stable)	Group comparison
Age (years)	19.50 (1.45)	19.22 (2.15)	20.10 (2.08)	20.15 (2.32)	$F_{(3,103)} = 1.46, p = 0.23$
DUED (months)	14.73 (9.19)	16.98 (12.17)	16.05 (9.01)	16.88 (10.83)	$F_{(3,101)} = 0.15, p = 0.93$
Baseline BMI	17.91 (0.66) [1]	17.66 (0.97) [1]	14.74 (0.65) [2]	16.23 (0.72) [3]	**$F_{(3,87)} = 3.44, p = 0.02$** [a]
Ethnicity, n (%)					$X^2 (3) = 4.57, p = 0.21$
White	9/11 (81.8%)	28/36 (77.8%)	17/19 (89.5%)	22/32 (68.8%)	
BAME	2/11 (18.2%)	8/36 (22.2%)	2/19 (10.5%)	10/32 (31.3%)	
Occupation, n (%)					$X^2 (6) = 3.64, p = 0.74$
Student	10/12 (83.3%)	28/41 (68.3%)	12/20 (60.0%)	21/34 (61.8%)	
Employed	1/12 (8.3%)	7/41 (17.1%)	6/20 (30.0%)	7/34 (20.6%)	
Unemployed	1/12 (8.3%)	6/41 (14.6%)	2/20 (10.0%)	6/34 (17.6%)	
Home, n (%)					$X^2 (3) = 6.84, p = 0.08$
With family	3/10 (30.0%)	29/40 (72.5%)	10/19 (52.6%)	21/34 (61.8%)	
Other	7/10 (70.0%)	11/40 (27.5%)	9/19 (47.4%)	13/34 (38.2%)	
EDE-Q	4.42 (1.21)	3.95 (1.25)	3.62 (1.28)	3.33 (1.57)	$F_{(3,103)} = 2.39, p = 0.07$
Binge	6/12 (50.0%)	21/41 (51.2%)	9/20 (45.0%)	9/34 (26.5%)	$X^2 (3) = 5.18, p = 0.16$
Purge	3/12 (25.0%)	15/41 (36.6%) [1]	1/20 (5.0%) [2]	5/34 (14.7%)	**Fisher's exact = 9.23, $p = 0.02$** [a]
Laxative	2/12 (16.7%)	9/41 (22.0%)	3/20 (15.0%)	1/34 (2.9%)	Fisher's exact = 6.26, $p = 0.08$
DASS - 21	32.83 (14.06)	35.17 (14.04)	27.45 (9.90)	33.50 (14.62)	$F_{(3, 103)} = 1.48, p = 0.23$
Depression	11.92 (4.98)	13.02 (5.61) [1]	8.80 (4.51) [2]	11.24 (5.56)	**$F_{(3, 103)} = 2.86, p = 0.04$** [a]
Anxiety	8.42 (4.70)	9.49 (5.71)	5.90 (4.04)	9.24 (5.38)	$F_{(3,103)} = 2.35, p = 0.08$
Stress	12.50 (5.90)	12.66 (4.54)	12.75 (4.46)	13.03 (5.18)	$F_{(3,103)} = 0.05, p = 0.99$
CIA	34.83 (8.6)	32.20 (10.86)	32.20 (9.68)	29.76 (11.03)	$F_{(3,103)} = 0.79, p = 0.50$
LEE	13.58 (13.91)	18.26 (11.99)	15.1 (11.52)	11.97 (8.45)	$F_{(3, 103)} = 2.08, p = 0.53$
Intrusiveness	4.92 (3.73)	5.80 (3.88)	4.95 (3.62)	4.64 (2.74)	$F_{(3, 102)} = 0.74, p = 0.53$
Emotional response	2.58 (4.14)	4.50 (3.60)	3.95 (3.89)	2.74 (3.51)	$F_{(3, 102)} = 1.77, p = 0.16$
Attitude toward illness	2.58 (2.61)	3.50 (2.72)	2.60 (2.52)	2.09 (1.48)	$F_{(3, 102)} = 2.32, p = 0.08$
Tolerance/expectations	3.50 (4.08)	4.93 (3.77) [1]	3.60 (3.56)	2.50 (2.54) [2]	**$F_{(3, 102)} = 3.12, p = 0.03$** [a]

BAME Black, Asian, and minority ethnic, *CIA* Clinical Impairment Assessment, *DASS-21* Depression, Anxiety, and Stress Scale, 21-item version, *DUED* duration of untreated eating disorder, *EDE-Q* Eating Disorder Examination Questionnaire, *LEE* Level of Expressed Emotion Scale
[1,2,3] Different superscripts indicate significant differences between the classes. For example, Class 2 and Class 3 have significantly different rates of depression. [a] Non-significant after Bonferroni correction

up' by higher use of additional intensive treatments, although the difference in use of intensive treatments was not significantly different between classes. While these three classes had differing early treatment trajectories, i.e., some classes responding rapidly and others taking longer, all three achieved substantial and similar clinical outcomes. Conversely, those in Class 1 (*high, stable*) had the lowest rate of remission (10%) compared to the other classes (31–43%). This demonstrates that, similar to Wade et al.'s findings [12], a higher BMI at treatment start is not sufficient to predict later remission or even weight restoration in AN, and this seems to be even more pronounced in first episode cases.

One clinical implication of these results is the consideration of adjunct or alternative treatments for those

with first episode AN. In our study, a small group ($n = 12$) of patients with a 'relatively' higher BMI (i.e., > 17) who do not gain weight over the first 12 sessions (Class 1: *high, stable*) had the poorest recovery rates at 12 months, at only 10%. It may be that a change or augmentation to therapy for a first episode patient is more suitable at the mid-point of treatment rather than simply carrying on 'as is.' This could include intensifying session frequency, increasing family involvement, or changing treatment setting (e.g., day treatment). Alternatively, adjunctive medications (e.g., antidepressants or olanzapine) focused on the ED or a comorbidity might be considered [32], or emerging treatments such as cognitive remediation therapy [33], or neuromodulation approaches [34].

Table 3 Outcome characteristics of each latent class

Variable	Class1, $n = 12$ (high, stable)	Class2, $n = 41$ (high, moderate)	Class3, $n = 20$ (low, rapid)	Class4, $n = 34$ (medium, stable)	Group comparison
Follow-Up BMI	17.56 (1.69) [1]	19.32 (1.73) [2]	18.03 (2.95)	18.17 (1.49)	**$F_{(3,87)} = 3.44$, $p = 0.02$** [a]
Follow-Up BMI $\geq$ 18.5	4 /11 (36.4%)	20/32 (62.3%)	7/16 (43.8%)	15/32 (46.9%)	$X^2 (3) = 3.18$, $p = 0.39$
BMI change	0.38 (1.68) [1]	1.57 (1.80) [1]	3.40 (2.95) [2]	1.95 (1.55)	**$F_{(3,87)} = 5.66$, $p < 0.001$**
Follow-Up EDE-Q	2.50 (1.48)	2.64 (1.88)	2.28 (1.80)	1.91 (1.41)	$F_{(3,77)} = 0.96$, $p = 0.42$
Follow-Up EDE-Q $\leq$ 2.8	6/10 (60.0%)	19/29 (65.5%)	9/14 (64.3%)	23/29 (79.3%)	$X^2 (3) = 2.14$, $p = 0.59$
EDE-Q change	−1.75 (1.31)	−1.51 (1.67)	− 1.30 (1.75)	−1.44 (1.24)	$F_{(3,69)} = 0.19$, $p = 0.90$
Completed treatment	11/12 (91.7%)	28/41 (68.3%)	13/20 (65.0%)	29/34 (85.3%)	Fisher's Exact = 5.61, $p = 0.14$
Intensive treatment [b]	–	2/41 (4.9%)	4/20 (20.0%)	3/34 (8.8%)	Fisher's Exact = 0.18, $p = 0.15$
Remission at Follow-up	1/10 (10.0%)	13/30 (43.3%)	5/16 (31.3%)	10/30 (33.3%)	Fisher's Exact = 3.84, $p = 0.28$

BMI Body mass index, in kg/m², *EDE-Q* Eating Disorder Examination Questionnaire
[1,2,3]Different superscripts indicate significant differences between the classes. For example, Class 1 and Class 2 have significantly different follow-up BMI
[a]Non-significant with Bonferroni correction; [b] Intensive treatment refers to stepped up care into day or inpatient during the 12-month follow-up period

A key limitation of this work is the relatively small sample size. This may impact the reliability of results, and as such, these findings should be considered exploratory. However, the sample size was above the minimum of 100 as recommend for LGMM [5, 35]. Additionally, while patients' weight for BMI calculations was measured at each weekly treatment session by a clinician, all other variables were assessed by self-report. Data gathered by self-report rely on patient memory and insight, which may reduce validity. Finally, clinical outcome data were analysed using complete case analysis with 6-month outcomes substituted when 12-month outcomes were unavailable, which poses a risk for bias. Future research would ideally have longer and more complete follow-up data.

In conclusions, patients with first episode AN fit into four distinct trajectory classes, three of which had substantial weight gain at 12-months. Depression scores, the presence of purging, and perceived levels of parental/carer expressed emotion in the form of high expectations/low levels of tolerance were predictive of class membership. A higher BMI at treatment start was not sufficient to produce better weight restoration at 12-month follow-up. These results are exploratory in nature and should be interpreted with caution until larger studies can clarify findings.

Abbreviations
CBT-ED: Eating disorder focused cognitive behavioural therapy;
DUED: Duration of untreated eating disorder; FREED: First episode rapid early intervention for eating disorders; LGMM: Latent growth mixture modelling; MANTRA: Maudsley model of anorexia nervosa treatment for adults; NICE: National Institute for Health and Care Excellence

Acknowledgements
AA and MF are funded by King's College London (KCL) International Postgraduate Research Scholarship. US receives salary support from the National Institute for Health Research (NIHR) Biomedical Research Centre for Mental Health, South London and Maudsley NHS Foundation Trust, and Institute of Psychiatry, Psychology and Neuroscience, KCL and is also supported by an NIHR Senior Investigator Award. The views expressed in this publication are those of the authors and not necessarily those of the National Health Service, the NIHR, or the UK Department of Health.

Authors' contributions
All authors made substantial contributions to this work, such as conception, design, data acquisition, interpretation, or substantive revision. AA performed the statistical analysis and prepared the first draft of the manuscript. All authors read and approved the final manuscript.

Competing interests
The authors declare that they have no competing interests.

Author details
[1]Department of Psychological Medicine, King's College London, Institute of Psychiatry, Psychology, and Neuroscience, 16 De Crespigny Park, London, UK. [2]School of Health in Social Sciences, University of Edinburgh, Edinburgh, UK. [3]South London and Maudsley NHS Foundation Trust, London, UK. [4]Maudsley Health, Abu Dhabi, UAE. [5]Sussex Partnership NHS Foundation Trust, Brighton, UK. [6]North East London NHS Foundation Trust, London, UK. [7]Division of Psychology and Language Sciences, University College London, London, UK. [8]Central and North West London NHS Foundation Trust, London, UK. [9]Leeds and York Partnership NHS Foundation Trust, Leeds, UK. [10]Department of Social, Genetic & Developmental Psychiatry, King's College London, London, UK.

References

1. Solmi M, Wade TD, Byrne S, Del Giovane C, Fairburn CG, Ostinelli EG, et al. Comparative efficacy and acceptability of psychological interventions for the treatment of adult outpatients with anorexia nervosa: a systematic review and network meta-analysis. Lancet Psychiatry. 2021;8(3):215–24. https://doi.org/10.1016/S2215-0366(20)30566-6.

2. Mirnezami R, Nicholson J, Darzi A. Preparing for precision medicine. N Engl J Med. 2012;366(6):489–91. https://doi.org/10.1056/NEJMp1114866.

3. Vall E, Wade TD. Predictors of treatment outcome in individuals with eating disorders: a systematic review and meta-analysis. Int J Eat Disord. 2015;48(7): 946–71. https://doi.org/10.1002/eat.22411.

4. Chang P, Delgadillo J, Waller G. Early response to psychological treatment for eating disorders: a systematic review and meta-analysis. Clin Psychol Rev. 2021;86:102032. https://doi.org/10.1016/j.cpr.2021.102032.

5. Espel-Huynh HM, Zhang F, Boswell JF, Thomas JG, Thompson-Brenner H, Juarascio AS, et al. Latent trajectories of eating disorder treatment response among female patients in residential care. Int J Eat Disord. 2020;53(10): 1647–56. https://doi.org/10.1002/eat.23369.

6. Hilbert A, Herpertz S, Zipfel S, Tuschen-Caffier B, Friederich HC, Mayr A, et al. Early change trajectories in cognitive-behavioral therapy for binge-eating disorder. Behav Ther. 2019;50(1):115–25. https://doi.org/10.1016/j.beth.2018.03.013.

7. Lebow J, Sim L, Crosby RD, Goldschmidt AB, Le Grange D, Accurso EC. Weight gain trajectories during outpatient family-based treatment for adolescents with anorexia nervosa. Int J Eat Disord. 2019;52(1):88–94. https://doi.org/10.1002/eat.23000.

8. Jung T, Wikrama KAS. An introduction to latent class growth analysis and growth mixture modeling. Soc Personal Psychol Compass. 2008;2(1):302–17. https://doi.org/10.1111/j.1751-9004.2007.00054.x.

9. Nazar BP, Gregor LK, Albano G, Marchica A, Coco GL, Cardi V, et al. Early response to treatment in eating disorders: a systematic review and a diagnostic test accuracy meta-analysis. Eur Eat Disord Rev. 2017;25(2):67–79. https://doi.org/10.1002/erv.2495.

10. Berona J, Richmond R, Rienecke RD. Heterogeneous weight restoration trajectories during partial hospitalization treatment for anorexia nervosa. Int J Eat Disord. 2018;51(8):914–20. https://doi.org/10.1002/eat.22922.

11. Makhzoumi SH, Coughlin JW, Schreyer CC, Redgrave GW, Pitts SC, Guarda AS. Weight gain trajectories in hospital-based treatment of anorexia nervosa. Int J Eat Disord. 2017;50(3):266–74. https://doi.org/10.1002/eat.22679.

12. Wade TD, Allen K, Crosby RD, Fursland A, Hay P, McIntosh V, et al. Outpatient therapy for adult anorexia nervosa: Early weight gain trajectories and outcome. Eur Eat Disord Rev. 2021;29(3):472–481. https://doi.org/10.1002/erv.2775.

13. Ambwani S, Cardi V, Albano G, Cao L, Crosby RD, Macdonald P, et al. A multicenter audit of outpatient care for adult anorexia nervosa: symptom trajectory, service use, and evidence in support of "early stage" versus "severe and enduring" classification. Int J Eat Disord. 2020;53(8):1337–48. https://doi.org/10.1002/eat.23246.

14. Fernández-Aranda F, Treasure J, Paslakis G, Agüera Z, Giménez M, Granero R, et al. The impact of duration of illness on treatment nonresponse and drop-out: exploring the relevance of enduring eating disorder concept. Eur Eat Disord Rev. 2021;29(3):499–513. https://doi.org/10.1002/erv.2822

15. Flynn M, Austin A, Lang K, Allen K, Bassi R, Brady G, et al. Assessing the impact of first episode rapid early intervention for eating disorders on duration of untreated eating disorder: a multi-centre quasi-experimental study. Eur Eat Disord Rev. 2021;29(3):458–71. https://doi.org/10.1002/erv.2797https://doi.org/10.1002/erv.2797.

16. Austin A, Flynn M, Shearer J, Long M, Allen K, Mountford V, et al. The first episode rapid early intervention for eating disorders – upscaled (FREED-Up) study: clinical outcomes. Early Interv Psychiatry. 2021;1–9. https://doi.org/10.1111/eip.13139.

17. American Psychiatric Association. Diagnostic and statistical manual of mental disorders. 5th ed. Arlington: American Psychiatric Association; 2013.

18. Allen KL, Mountford V, Brown A, Richards K, Grant N, Austin A, et al. First episode rapid early intervention for eating disorders (FREED): from research to routine clinical practice. Early Interv Psychiatry. 2020;14(5):625–30. https://doi.org/10.1111/eip.12941.

19. Schmidt U, Brown A, McClelland J, Glennon D, Mountford VA. Will a comprehensive, person-centered, team-based early intervention approach to first episode illness improve outcomes in eating disorders? Int J Eat Disord. 2016;49(4):374–7. https://doi.org/10.1002/eat.22519.

20. Brown A, McClelland J, Boysen E, Mountford V, Glennon D, Schmidt U. The FREED project (first episode and rapid early intervention in eating disorders): service model, feasibility and acceptability. Early Interv Psychiatry. 2018;12(2): 250–7. https://doi.org/10.1111/eip.12382.

21. McClelland J, Hodsoll J, Brown A, Lang K, Boysen E, Flynn M, et al. A pilot evaluation of a novel first episode and rapid early intervention service for eating disorders (FREED). Eur Eat Disord Rev. 2018;26(2):129–40. https://doi.org/10.1002/erv.2579.

22. National Institute for Health and Care Excellence (NICE). Eating disorders: recognition and treatment. 2017.

23. Fairburn CG, Beglin SJ. Eating disorder examination questionnaire (6.0). In: Fairburn CG, editor. Cognitive behaviour therapy and eating disorders. New York: Guilford Press; 2008.

24. Mond JM, Myers TC, Crosby RD, Hay PJ, Rodgers B, Morgan JF, et al. Screening for eating disorders in primary care: EDE-Q versus SCOFF. Behav Res Ther. 2008;46(5):612–22. https://doi.org/10.1016/j.brat.2008.02.003.

25. Lovibond PF, Lovibond SH. The structure of negative emotional states: comparison of the depression anxiety stress scales (DASS) with the beck depression and anxiety inventories. Behav Res Ther. 1995;33(3):335–43. https://doi.org/10.1016/0005-7967(94)00075-U.

26. Bohn K, Fairburn CG. The clinical impairment questionnaire (CIA 3.0). In: Fairburn CG, editor. Cognitive behvioural therapy and eating disorders. New York: Guilford Press; 2008.

27. Cole JD, Kazarian SS. The level of expressed emotion scale: a new measure of expressed emotion. J Clin Psychol. 1988;44(3):392–7. https://doi.org/10.1002/1097-4679(198805)44:3<392::AID-JCLP2270440313>3.0.CO;2-3.

28. Van de Schoot R. Latent growth mixture models to estimate PTSD trajectories. Eur J Psychotraumatol. 2015;6(1):27503. https://doi.org/10.3402/ejpt.v6.27503.

29. Clark SL, Muthén B. Relating latent class analysis results to variables not included in the analysis; 2009.

30. Herle M, Micali N, Abdulkadir M, Loos R, Bryant-Waugh R, Hübel C, et al. Identifying typical trajectories in longitudinal data: modelling strategies and interpretations. Eur J Epidemiol. 2020;35(3):205–22. https://doi.org/10.1007/s10654-020-00615-6.

31. Jennings KM, Gregas M, Wolfe B. Trajectories of change in body weight during inpatient treatment for anorexia nervosa. J Am Psychiatr Nurses Assoc. 2018;24(4):306–13. https://doi.org/10.1177/1078390317726142.

32. Attia E, Kaplan AS, Walsh BT, Gershkovich M, Yilmaz Z, Musante D, et al. Olanzapine versus placebo for out-patients with anorexia nervosa. Psychol Med. 2011;41(10):2177–82. https://doi.org/10.1017/S0033291711000390.

33. Tchanturia K, Giombini L, Leppanen J, Kinnaird E. Evidence for cognitive remediation therapy in young people with anorexia nervosa: systematic review and meta-analysis of the literature. Eur Eat Disord Rev. 2017;25(4): 227–36. https://doi.org/10.1002/erv.2522.

34. Dalton B, Bartholdy S, McClelland J, Kekic M, Rennalls SJ, Werthmann J, et al. Randomised controlled feasibility trial of real versus sham repetitive transcranial magnetic stimulation treatment in adults with severe and enduring anorexia nervosa: the TIARA study. BMJ Open. 2018;8(7):e021531. https://doi.org/10.1136/bmjopen-2018-021531.

35. Park J, Yu H-T. Recommendations on the sample sizes for multilevel latent class models. Educ Psychol Meas. 2018;78(5):737–61. https://doi.org/10.1177/0013164417719111.

12

A Pilot Study Exploring the Effect of Repetitive Transcranial Magnetic Stimulation (rTMS) Treatment on Cerebral Blood Flow and its Relation to Clinical Outcomes in Severe Enduring Anorexia Nervosa

Bethan Dalton[1]*[iD], Erica Maloney[2], Samantha J. Rennalls[2], Savani Bartholdy[1], Maria Kekic[1], Jessica McClelland[1], Iain C. Campbell[1], Ulrike Schmidt[1,3] and Owen G. O'Daly[2]

Abstract

Background: Repetitive transcranial magnetic stimulation (rTMS) is a novel treatment option for people with severe enduring anorexia nervosa (SE-AN), but associated neurobiological changes are poorly understood. This study investigated the effect of rTMS treatment on regional cerebral blood flow (CBF) and whether any observed changes in CBF are associated with changes in clinical outcomes in people with SE-AN.

Methods: As part of a randomised sham-controlled feasibility trial of 20 sessions of high-frequency rTMS to the left dorsolateral prefrontal cortex, 26 of 34 trial participants completed arterial spin labelling (ASL) functional magnetic resonance imaging (fMRI) to quantify regional and global resting state CBF before (pre-randomisation baseline) and after real or sham treatment (1-month post-randomisation). A group of healthy females ($n = 30$) were recruited for baseline comparison. Clinical outcomes, including BMI, and depression and anxiety symptoms, were assessed at baseline, 1-, 4-, and 18-months post-randomisation.

Results: No group differences in regional CBF were identified between the SE-AN and healthy comparison participants. A significant treatment-by-time interaction in a medial temporal lobe cluster with the maximal peak in the right amygdala was identified, reflecting a greater reduction in amygdala CBF following real rTMS compared to sham. Participants with the greatest rTMS-related reduction in amygdala CBF (i.e., between baseline and 1-month post-randomisation) showed the greatest sustained weight gain at 18-months post-randomisation. Higher baseline CBF in the insula predicted greater weight gain between baseline and 1-month post-randomisation and between baseline and 4-months post-randomisation.

* Correspondence: bethan.dalton@kcl.ac.uk
[1]Section of Eating Disorders, Department of Psychological Medicine, Institute of Psychiatry, Psychology & Neuroscience, King's College London, London, UK
Full list of author information is available at the end of the article

Conclusions: This exploratory pilot study identified rTMS treatment related changes in CBF in adults with SE-AN and these were associated with changes in weight. Our preliminary findings also suggest that CBF (as measured by ASL fMRI) may be a marker of rTMS treatment response in this patient group. Future rTMS studies in AN should employ longitudinal neuroimaging to further explore the neurobiological changes related to rTMS treatment.

Plain English summary

Repetitive transcranial magnetic stimulation (rTMS) is a novel treatment option for people with severe enduring anorexia nervosa (SE-AN). However, little is known about the neurobiological effects of this treatment. This study explored the effect of rTMS treatment on regional cerebral blood flow (CBF) and whether any observed changes in CBF are associated with changes in clinical outcomes in people with SE-AN. Participants completed arterial spin labelling (ASL) functional magnetic resonance imaging (fMRI) before and after receiving 20 sessions (over 4 weeks) of real or sham rTMS. We found a greater reduction in amygdala CBF following real rTMS compared to sham rTMS. Participants with the greatest rTMS-related reduction in amygdala CBF showed the greatest sustained weight gain at an 18-month follow-up. Higher baseline CBF in the insula predicted greater weight gain during treatment and at a 4-month follow-up. This suggests that CBF (as measured by ASL fMRI) may be a marker of rTMS treatment response in this patient group. Future rTMS studies in AN should use longitudinal neuroimaging to further explore the neurobiological changes related to rTMS treatment.

Keywords: Anorexia nervosa, Cerebral blood flow, Arterial spin labelling, Functional magnetic resonance imaging, Repetitive transcranial magnetic stimulation, Eating disorders

Introduction

Anorexia nervosa (AN) is a disabling and deadly disorder associated with physical and psychological morbidity and impaired quality of life [1]. Psychological therapy is often the treatment of choice for adults with AN; however, with these best available treatments, recovery rates are 13–50% at 1–2 years follow-up [2]. Approximately 20–30% of AN patients develop a chronic form of the disorder [3, 4], termed severe enduring AN (SE-AN, [5]), and after 3–5 years of illness, outcomes become significantly poorer [1, 6]. Thus, treatment innovations are needed. Research into the neural underpinnings of AN have provided a rationale for the investigation of targeted brain-directed interventions [7, 8]. Repetitive transcranial magnetic stimulation (rTMS) has shown potential as a treatment for SE-AN (e.g., [9, 10]). rTMS is a non-invasive form of brain stimulation that can promote (using high-frequency) or inhibit (using low-frequency) cortical activity in a target brain area and produces effects that exceed the duration of the initial stimulation period [11]. As rTMS appears to increase neuroplasticity [12], it is thought to be of value in chronic illnesses, such as SE-AN, which are likely to be associated with changes in neurocircuitry. However, despite the initial promise of this brain-directed intervention in this patient group, neurobiological changes associated with rTMS, and their relationship to clinical outcomes, have only been explored in a few studies of people with eating disorders (EDs) [13, 14]. Such studies will be important for developing an understanding of the

mechanisms and predictors of response underlying rTMS treatment in this patient group.

We recently completed a randomised controlled feasibility trial of 20 sessions of real versus sham high-frequency (10 Hz) rTMS to the left dorsolateral prefrontal cortex (DLPFC) in 34 women with SE-AN (the TIARA trial, [15]). Outcomes provided preliminary evidence for the therapeutic potential of rTMS in SE-AN [16, 17]. Specifically, real rTMS, relative to sham treatment, showed moderate to large effects on anxiety and mood outcomes between baseline (pre-randomisation) and 4-months post-randomisation. The positive effects on mood were maintained at an open 18-month post-randomisation follow-up. These persistent improvements in affective symptoms replicated the findings from a small case series that explored rTMS treatment in SE-AN [18]. In the TIARA trial, there also appeared to be an rTMS effect on body mass index (BMI) change between baseline and 18-months post-randomisation, with greater weight gain in those originally allocated to the real, compared to sham, rTMS group. While neurobiological changes associated with rTMS have yet to be explored in SE-AN, they have been investigated in two small studies of people with EDs characterised by binge-eating and purging. In these, rTMS was associated with reductions in haemoglobin concentrations (assessed using near-infrared spectroscopy) in the rTMS-target brain area [14] and changes in functional connectivity [13]. The latter study also explored predictors of rTMS response and found that participants who responded to rTMS, compared to non-responders, showed baseline hypoconnectivity from the DMPFC to other cortical and subcortical regions, including those involved in emotion generation and regulation (e.g., insula) and significantly greater rTMS-related increases in frontostriatal and fronto-insular connectivity [13]. This highlights the potential of neuroimaging as a tool to optimise rTMS treatment.

Cerebral blood flow (CBF), an indirect marker of neuronal activity, has been explored as a neural correlate of the effects of rTMS in neuroimaging studies in healthy individuals (e.g., [19, 20]) and people with depression (e.g., [21]). This research has reported that CBF is altered during and following rTMS treatment. High-frequency rTMS to the left DLPFC has been associated with increased CBF in this region (e.g., [21–24]), and rTMS targeted at frontal regions has also been reported to lead to more widespread changes in CBF. For example, increases in CBF following rTMS targeted at the prefrontal cortex have been observed in the hippocampus, left amygdala, and bilateral insula [20, 24]. However, the direction of these more distal effects of DLPFC-targeted rTMS on CBF varies, possibly owing to differences in sample characteristics and data pre-processing. Preliminary research has also shown that CBF is associated with rTMS treatment efficacy, though findings are mixed (e.g., [25–27]). For example, baseline CBF in the insular cortex has been negatively [25] and positively [26] correlated with early response to rTMS treatment in patients with depression. Taken together, CBF may be a valuable neural correlate and marker of rTMS treatment effects.

Imaging studies have shown that CBF is altered in people currently unwell with AN (compared to healthy individuals) in posterior cingulate gyrus and temporal areas [28, 29]. However, some studies have identified increases (e.g., [29]) and others identified reductions (e.g., [30]) in CBF in these areas, compared to healthy individuals. Preliminary research also suggests that CBF changes in response to weight gain and recovery in AN [28], e.g., following weight gain, CBF has been reported to increase in the right DLPFC, posterior and anterior cingulate cortex and the parietal lobe, and to decrease in the right amygdala [31–33]. Given these findings in people with AN, along with the reported effects of rTMS on CBF, an exploration of the effect of rTMS on CBF in people with SE-AN and whether this is associated with clinical outcomes is warranted.

The DLPFC plays a key role in self-regulatory control mechanisms and has been implicated in AN, which has been described as a disorder of excessive self-control [34]. The DLPFC has been associated with cognitive control processes in AN, including inhibitory control, food choice, emotion regulation, reward processing, among other processes [7, 35, 36]. The DLPFC is heavily interconnected with limbic regions, including the amygdala and insula, and dysregulation in this fronto-limbic circuit (including the anterior cingulate cortex) has been associated with behavioural and emotional regulation and responses in AN [37]. Taken together, rTMS targeting the left DLPFC may therefore alter the top-down control of the DLPFC to fronto-limbic regions associated with maladaptive emotion regulation strategies (e.g., dietary restraint), and subsequently improve ED and affective symptoms.

In our TIARA trial, before and after completion of 4 weeks of rTMS treatment, we performed at rest arterial spin labelling (ASL) functional magnetic resonance imaging (fMRI), a non-invasive method that provides a quantitative measure of CBF. This pilot analysis aimed to investigate (a) the effect of rTMS treatment on regional CBF at post-treatment (1-month post-randomisation); (b) whether any rTMS-related changes in CBF were associated with change in clinical outcomes at post-treatment (1-month post-randomisation) and follow-up (4- and 18-months post-randomisation); and (c) whether baseline CBF could predict clinical outcomes in the shorter- and longer-term. A secondary aim was to investigate group differences in CBF between SE-AN and healthy comparison participants. Analyses were performed from an exploratory whole brain perspective and also focussed on four regions of interest (bilateral DLPFC, amygdalae, anterior cingulate cortices, insular cortices).

Methods

This study used data collected as part of a double-blind, parallel group, two-arm, sham-controlled randomised feasibility trial (Trial Registration: ISRCTN14329415, registered 23rd July 2015, https://www.isrctn.com/ISRCTN14329415). Methodological details have been described in Bartholdy, McClelland et al. [15] and clinical outcomes reported in Dalton, Bartholdy, McClelland, et al. [16] and Dalton et al. [17]. Ethical approval was obtained from London - City Road & Hampstead Research Ethics Committee (Ref: 15/LO/0196).

Participants

Thirty-four female adults with a current Diagnostic and Statistical Manual of Mental Disorders (DSM)-5 [38] diagnosis of AN and a BMI > 14 kg/m^2 were recruited. Participants had a severe enduring form of AN (defined as illness duration ≥3 years and completion of at least one previous specialist treatment for their ED). Participants were recruited from a specialist Eating Disorder Service in London, through online advertisements (e.g., Beat, the UK national ED charity) and social media, and via participation in previous studies.

Healthy comparison (HC) women (n = 30; ≥18 years), with a BMI in the healthy range (20–25 kg/m^2), were recruited via online and poster advertisements at King's College London (KCL) to provide a comparison group. Exclusion criteria were current/past psychiatric illness or a family history of an ED. HCs completed the baseline assessment only.

Exclusion criteria for all participants included left-handedness, MRI contraindications (e.g., metallic implants), current and/or history of neurological illness, and additionally for SE-AN participants, TMS contraindications (e.g., seizures). Participants completed a telephone screening to confirm their eligibility. This included the TMS Adult Safety Screen for SE-AN participants only; an MRI safety screen questionnaire developed at KCL; the Eating Disorder Diagnostic Scale [39] to assess the presence/absence of ED symptoms in the SE-AN and HC groups, respectively; the researcher version of the Structured Clinical Interview for DSM-IV Axis I Disorders Screening Module [40] to confirm the absence of any psychiatric disorders in the HC participants; and a short inclusion/exclusion screen specific to this study. Written informed consent was obtained from all participants.

Procedure

All participants completed a baseline assessment consisting of weight and height measurements, a questionnaire pack, neuropsychological computer tasks, and a one-hour MRI scan. Following the baseline assessment, SE-AN participants were randomly allocated to receive 20 sessions (every weekday for 4 weeks) of real or sham neuro-navigated rTMS targeting the left DLPFC (Talairach co-ordinates x = − 45, y = 45, z = 30, as used by [41]). The left DLPFC was selected as the target brain area for rTMS in this trial for several reasons: (a) the DLPFC is involved in a number of cognitive processes that have been implicated in AN e.g., emotion regulation, self-control (as described in [7, 42]); (b) high-frequency rTMS to the left DLPFC has shown efficacy and acceptability in the treatment of related psychiatric disorders, including depression [43]; and (c) for practical accessibility reasons. rTMS was administered by trained researchers using the Magstim Rapid device (Magstim®, Whitland, Wales, UK) and Magstim d70-mm-air-cooled real/sham figure-of-eight coil. Participants received 20 min of high-frequency (10 Hz) rTMS consisting of 20 five-second trains with 55-s intervals at 110% of participants' resting motor threshold. Participants allocated to the sham group received rTMS at the same parameters using a sham coil. These stimulation parameters were selected based on protocols used in other ED related rTMS research by our group [44, 45] and were in

accordance with safety and application guidelines for rTMS [11].

SE-AN participants repeated the baseline assessment within 1 week of completing rTMS treatment (post-treatment; 1-month post-randomisation) and at a short-term follow-up (4-months post-randomisation; without the neuroimaging component) prior to unblinding. After this, sham treatment completers were given the opportunity to receive real rTMS treatment (identical protocol and rTMS parameters to those used in the main trial) if they remained eligible. Participant flow through the trial is shown in the Supporting Information (S1: Figure 1). At an open follow-up (18-months post-randomisation), SE-AN participants completed a short questionnaire pack and reported their current BMI.

Clinical outcome measures

BMI and depression and anxiety were selected as clinical outcome measures of interest in the present analyses due to the observed rTMS treatment effects on these variables in the trial. In relation to BMI, we reported a medium between-group effect size for BMI change from baseline to 18-months post-randomisation, favouring those originally allocated to real rTMS over sham, and also a greater rate of weight recovery (BMI ≥18.5 kg/m^2) in the real compared to original sham rTMS group [46]. In relation to depression and anxiety, we reported moderate to large effect sizes for changes in these outcomes from baseline to 4-months post-randomisation and it was concluded that general psychopathology should serve as a primary outcome for future rTMS trials in AN [16]. We also identified somewhat higher depression scores in the trial, compared with other treatment trials in AN [47, 48]. More broadly, both depression and anxiety are highly comorbid with AN [49] and comorbid depression has been associated with poor quality of life in SE-AN [50].

BMI was calculated as weight (in kilograms) divided by height (in metres) squared. Depression and anxiety were measured using the relevant subscales of the Depression, Anxiety and Stress Scales – Version 21 (DASS-21 [51]). The DASS-21 is widely used and has been reported to have acceptable to excellent internal consistency and concurrent and divergent validity in clinical and non-clinical samples [52]. Data on other clinical outcomes are presented elsewhere [16, 17].

Arterial spin labelling functional magnetic resonance imaging

Scanning procedures were carried out at the Centre for Neuroimaging Sciences, Institute of Psychiatry, Psychology & Neuroscience, KCL, using a General Electric MR750 3.0 T scanner.

Pseudo-continuous arterial spin labelling (pCASL) was used to non-invasively obtain a quantitative measure of CBF. Blood water protons are magnetically labelled as the blood flows through the carotid artery to the brain. This is achieved by applying a long radio-frequency pulse to invert the magnetization of the arterial blood water which acts as a diffusible tracer or contrast agent [53–55]. Two whole volume images are acquired: one with and one without the labelled arterial blood. The pairwise subtraction of these images indicate the volume of blood perfused into the cerebral tissue during the time between labelling and image acquisition.

CBF at rest was measured in each participant using pseudo continuous flow-driven adiabatic inversion scheme [56]. Fifty-six slices were acquired with a thickness of 3 mm and a slice gap of 3 mm using the following parameters: 240 mm FoV, 512×8 acquisition matrix, TR/TE of 5135 ms/11.088 ms and flip angle of 111O. The inversion time (TI) between the pulse labelling and the beginning of the readout was 2025 ms for all subjects. CBF maps were calculated in real time on the MRI scanner. A proton density scan was acquired employing the same parameters and was used as a reference image when calibrating the CBF map [57]. A structural T1-weighted (MP-RAGE) scan was performed and used as a co-registration of each individual's imaging data into a common space for processing and analysis, using the following sequence parameters: FoV 270 mm; flip angle $11°$; matrix size 256×256; 196 slices with a slice thickness and slice gap of 1.2 mm; TR = 7.312; TE = 3.016; voxel size $1.1 \times 1.1 \times 1.2$. The MP-RAGE scan was also used in the localisation of the left DLPFC for rTMS treatment.

Image processing and analysis

CBF was processed and analysed voxel-by-voxel using Statistical Parametric Mapping software version 12 (SPM12, Wellcome Trust Centre for Neuroimaging, London, UK) running under Matlab 8.2.0 (MathWorks Inc., Natick, MA, USA). Structural images were manually reoriented so that the image origin was set at the anterior commissure (AC), providing better normalisation to the MNI (Montreal Neurological Institute) space and controlling for unintentional subject movement. Structural scans of all participants were segmented into grey matter (GM), white matter (WM) and cerebrospinal fluid (CSF) probability maps. Based on GM segmentations, a population-based template was created using Diffeomorphic Anatomical Registration using Exponentiated Lie Algebra (DARTEL) to improve registration of structural images. Participants with AN have been found to have reduced brain size and structural brain changes when compared with age-matched healthy controls [58–60] and based on this, it was decided a study-specific

template would be created. DARTEL allows for enhanced accuracy of inter-subject alignment by modelling the shape of each brain using three parameters for each voxel [61].

Rigid-body parameters to align the CBF images to the MP-RAGE image were calculated via co-registration of the proton density image, which is in perfect register with the CBF map, to the structural T1-weighted image. Parameters were then applied to the CBF maps to bring them into register with the MP-RAGE image. Following this, the flow fields created by the DARTEL template were applied to the CBF maps and from there, the images were normalized to MNI (standard) space. The CBF scans were then smoothed using an 8 mm full width at half maximum (FWHM) Gaussian Kernel.

To determine if any regional difference (between groups) or changes (over time) in CBF simply reflect changes in underlying tissue volume, a voxel-based morphometry analysis was carried out. The data were pre-processed in accordance with the published methodology [62]. In brief, T1-weighted structural images underwent unified segmentation, and the resultant GM and WM segmentations were up-sampled (to 1.5 mm × 1.5 mm × 1.5 mm) and used to generate the study-specific DARTEL template mentioned earlier. The tissue segmentations were normalized to standard space via the intermediate template and again smoothed by an 8 mm FWHM smoothing kernel. Total intracranial volume (TIV) was calculated using an in-house script.

Exploratory whole-brain analyses

For GM, WM and CBF data, whole brain analyses were implemented in SPM. To test for baseline group-differences in GM, WM and CBF between the HC and SE-AN group, independent sample t-tests were used. To test for rTMS-related effects in the SE-AN group, a flexible-factorial ANOVA was implemented. This permits modelling with appropriate control for between-subjects' variance when testing for a treatment-by-time interaction. Finally, to determine whether baseline CBF might be a predictive marker of subsequent rTMS treatment response, we conducted regression analyses to explore the relationship between baseline CBF and the change (either from pre-treatment baseline to 1-month post-randomisation or from pre-treatment baseline to 4-months post-randomisation) in those participants who received real rTMS. These regression analyses focussed on three parameters: BMI, and anxiety and depression (as measured by the DASS-21). Given evidence of further weight gain at the 18-month post-randomisation follow-up [17], we also tested whether baseline and treatment-related change in regional CBF predicted sustained change in these variables.

For the independent samples t-test, age and BMI were included as covariates of no interest. For the AN-specific ANCOVA and regression analyses, AN type (AN-restricting [AN-R] / AN-binge-eating/purging [AN-BP]) and the number of hospitalisations (as a proxy measure for disease severity/chronicity) were included as nuisance covariates. For all VBM analyses, the TIV was included as an additional covariate of no interest, whereas for the CBF analysis, the global GM CBF was calculated (using SPM global calculation) and included as a nuisance covariate using the ANCOVA option under global normalization.

For all exploratory whole-brain analysis, results were considered significant if they survived whole-brain familywise error correction on the basis of cluster extent with a critical corrected alpha of 0.05 (i.e., pFWE < 0.05).

Regions of interest (ROI) definition and analysis

Regions of interest (ROI) analysis was conducted for the primary contrast of interest. All ROIs were defined using the WFUPickAtlas toolbox (SCR_007378; RRID: nif-0000-00358) [63] available in SPM. Selection of ROIs was based on *a priori* assumptions and literature detailing the involvement of these structures in prominent behaviours and characteristics associated with AN [7, 36]. All structures were defined using the Automated Anatomical Labelling (AAL) library [64]. The resultant bilateral masks for the amygdalae, anterior cingulate cortices, and insular cortices were combined with bilateral DLPFC ROIs based on the site of rTMS delivery. Specifically, a 15 mm sphere was centred extra-cerebrally on the Talairach coordinate targeted during rTMS ([x = − 45 y = 45 z = 30]) and its mirror contralaterally. The intersection between these spheres and the GM mask (thresholded at 20% probability of mask) served as the DLPFC mask. The final combined mask (see Fig. 1) was used to spatially constrain familywise error correction for hypothesis-led analyses (i.e., small volume correction) with significance defined as a corrected p-value of pFWE< 0.05 on the basis of response amplitude.

Results

Cross-sectional comparison of baseline cerebral blood flow

At baseline, MRI data were available for 30 HC and 26 SE-AN participants (see Table 1 for demographics). Data from eight SE-AN participants were excluded due to incomplete scans and datasets. Specifically, $n = 3$ SE-AN participants only completed the scanning procedure required for neuronavigation in the rTMS treatment for safety reasons, $n = 1$ did not complete the ASL scan due to technical issues, and the remaining $n = 4$ were excluded due to data quality issues.

Hypothesis-led ROI analysis

The hypothesis-led analysis of baseline data found no differences in regional CBF between the HC participants and those with SE-AN (all familywise error corrected p-values (pFWE > 0.409).

Exploratory whole-brain analysis

We found no evidence for significant regional differences in baseline CBF between HC participants and those with SE-AN.

Confirmatory structural analyses

Neither hypothesis-led nor exploratory voxel-brain analyses revealed any regional difference between the HC and SE-AN groups either in GM (all p-values > 0.52) or WM (all p-values > 0.396). However, using the mask of the bilateral amygdala only, we found evidence of less WM volume in a region of the right amygdala in the SE-AN group compared to the HC group (pFWE$_{SVC}$ = 0.044, Z = 3.55, [32–4 -28]; see Supporting Information S2: Table 1 for effect sizes).

Effect of rTMS on cerebral blood flow and the association with clinical outcomes

Twenty-four SE-AN participants ($n = 14$ real rTMS, $n = 10$ sham rTMS) had complete MRI scans and datasets at both baseline and post-treatment (1-month post-randomisation). Table 2 shows the baseline

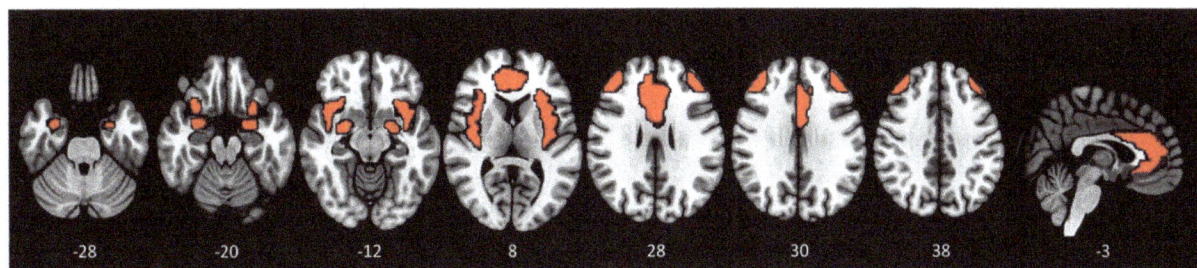

Fig. 1 Brain mask used for all hypothesis-led analyses, including all voxels for the amygdala, insula and anterior cingulate cortices bilaterally and the rTMS-targeted region of the DLPFC and its contralateral mirror

Table 1 Baseline demographics and clinical characteristics for the healthy comparison and severe enduring anorexia nervosa participants

	HC ($n = 30$)	SE-AN ($n = 26$)
Age [years] (mean ± SD)	25.57 ± 4.02	27.62 ± 9.11
Illness duration [years] (mean ± SD)		13.02 ± 9.81
AN-R/AN-BP [n]		16 / 10
EDE-Q Global (mean ± SD)	0.42 ± 0.43	4.17 ± 1.13
BMI [kg/m^2] (mean ± SD)	21.87 ± 1.55	16.06 ± 1.40
DASS-21 Depression (mean ± SD)	1.93 ± 3.70	26.85 ± 10.08
DASS-21 Anxiety (mean ± SD)	1.53 ± 1.87	15.69 ± 10.24

Abbreviations: *HC* healthy comparison, *SE-AN* severe enduring anorexia nervosa, *SD* standard deviation, *AN-R* anorexia nervosa restricting type, *AN-BP* anorexia nervosa binge-eating/purging type, *EDE-Q* Eating Disorder Examination Questionnaire, *BMI* body mass index, *DASS-21* Depression, Anxiety and Stress Scale –Version 21

demographics and clinical characteristics for these SE-AN participants by rTMS treatment arm. Of those who received real rTMS, all ($n = 14$) also had clinical data available at 4-months post-randomisation and $n = 11$ (except for BMI where $n = 10$) at 18-months post-randomisation for the exploratory analyses on the association between CBF and clinical outcomes.

For effect sizes and post-hoc power analyses for the following significant results, see the Supporting Information S2: Table 1.

rTMS effects on regional cerebral blood flow

Hypothesis-led ROI analysis Testing for changes in regional CBF from baseline to the post-treatment scan (i.e., 1 month later) revealed a significant treatment-by-time interaction in a medial temporal lobe cluster with the maximal peak in the right amygdala (pFWE$_{SVC}$ =

Table 2 Baseline demographics and clinical characteristics for severe enduring anorexia nervosa participants included in the present analyses, presented for each treatment group (real and sham) separately

	Real rTMS ($n = 14$)	Sham rTMS ($n = 10$)
Age [years] (mean ± SD)	28.79 ± 10.17	26.20 ± 8.19
Illness duration [years] (mean ± SD)	13.96 ± 11.58	11.70 ± 7.72
AN-R/AN-BP [n]	8 / 6	6 / 4
EDE-Q Global (mean ± SD)	3.95 ± 1.38	4.38 ± 0.76
BMI [kg/m^2] (mean ± SD)	15.93 ± 1.67	16.47 ± 0.73
DASS-21 Depression (mean ± SD)	26.43 ± 10.14	26.40 ± 11.23
DASS-21 Anxiety (mean ± SD)	14.86 ± 8.80	16.40 ± 13.16

Abbreviations: *rTMS* repetitive transcranial magnetic stimulation, *SD* standard deviation, *AN-R* anorexia nervosa restricting type, *AN-BP* anorexia nervosa binge-eating/purging type, *EDE-Q* Eating Disorder Examination Questionnaire, *BMI* body mass index, *DASS-21* Depression, Anxiety and Stress Scale –Version 21

0.014, Z-score = 4.26, peak at [33 –3 -26]). This reflected a significantly greater reduction in amygdala CBF following real rTMS compared to sham (see Fig. 2). The same analysis also revealed an interaction in the anterior cingulate cortex, which did not survive familywise error correction (pFWE$_{SVC}$ = 0.074, Z = 3.78, [– 9 32 20]).

Exploratory whole-brain analysis No regional treatment-by-time interactions were observed in CBF. All whole-brain CBF analyses were constrained by a GM mask, generated by thresholding SPMs GM tissue probability map to include only voxels with at least a 20% probability of being classified as GM.

Confirmatory structural analyses We found no evidence for treatment-by-time interaction in GM (pFWE$_{SVC}$ > 0.762) or WM (pFWE$_{SVC}$ > 0.322; pFWE$_{SVC}$ = 0.158 using amygdala mask only) that survived familywise error correction.

Association between rTMS-related changes in cerebral blood flow and change in clinical outcomes

Hypothesis-led ROI analysis We first explored the relationship between changes in CBF (baseline to post-treatment scan at 1-month post-randomisation) and change in our three clinical outcomes of interest (BMI, anxiety and depression) both from baseline to 1-month post-randomisation and from baseline to the 4-month post-randomisation follow-up. No significant associations using a bilateral mask in three of our ROIs (anterior cingulate cortex, amygdala and insula) (all pFWE$_{SVC}$ > 0.31) were identified. However, when using a bilateral amygdala mask only, a regional change in left amygdala CBF was weakly associated with the change in anxiety over the treatment window (baseline to 1-month post-randomisation) (pFWE$_{SVC}$ = 0.051, Z = 3, [– 21 –9 -10]).

Based on findings from the 18-month post-randomisation follow-up [17], we explored whether rTMS-related change in CBF (post-treatment [1-month post-randomisation] minus baseline) predicted change in BMI, anxiety and depression over this longer time-period in a subset ($n = 11$, except for BMI where $n = 10$) of participants who received real rTMS and responded to this follow-up. The change in BMI between baseline and 18-months post-randomisation was significantly negatively correlated with rTMS-related change in amygdala regional CBF (pFWE$_{SVC}$ = 0.033, Z = 4.56, [28–9 -12]; see Fig. 3) i.e., those with the greatest rTMS-related reduction in amygdala regional CBF showed the greatest sustained weight gain measured at 18-months post-randomisation. However, the association between BMI change and change in regional CBF in the insular

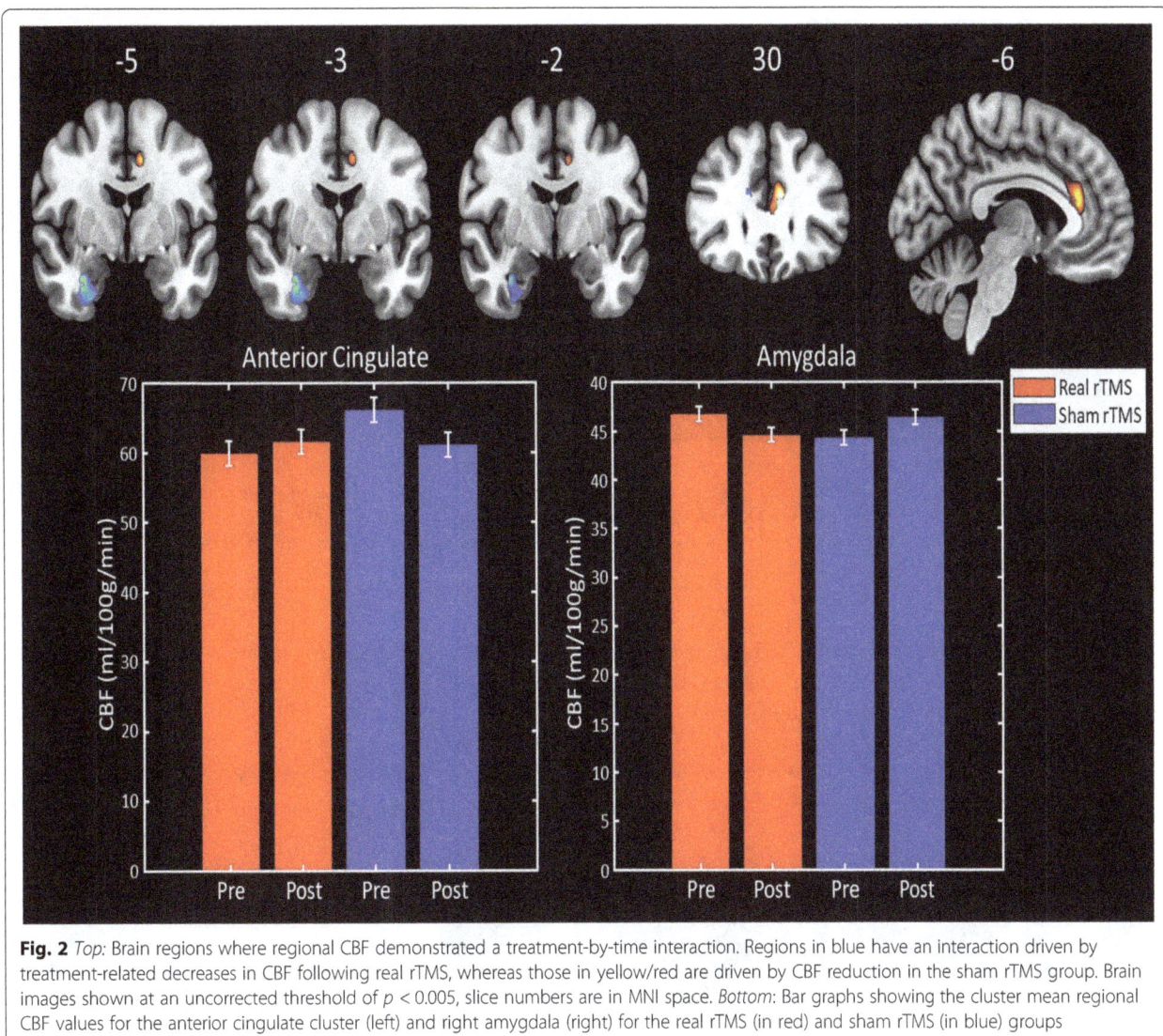

Fig. 2 *Top:* Brain regions where regional CBF demonstrated a treatment-by-time interaction. Regions in blue have an interaction driven by treatment-related decreases in CBF following real rTMS, whereas those in yellow/red are driven by CBF reduction in the sham rTMS group. Brain images shown at an uncorrected threshold of *p* < 0.005, slice numbers are in MNI space. *Bottom:* Bar graphs showing the cluster mean regional CBF values for the anterior cingulate cluster (left) and right amygdala (right) for the real rTMS (in red) and sham rTMS (in blue) groups

cortex did not survive FWE correction (pFWE$_{SVC}$ = 0.096, Z = 4.07, [− 36−16 -3]). To confirm the regional specificity, we tested each region separately using separate bilateral ROIs for the amygdala (pFWE$_{SVC}$ = 0.003) and the insular cortex (pFWE$_{SVC}$ = 0.048). Changes in CBF were not associated with changes in either anxiety or depression.

Association between baseline CBF and short- and longer-term clinical outcomes

Hypothesis-led ROI analysis Regression analyses demonstrated that baseline CBF in the insula positively predicted the change in BMI seen over the one-month treatment period (i.e., 1-month post-randomisation minus baseline; pFWE$_{SVC}$ = 0.019, z = 4.51, [40 10 6]; see Fig. 4A) and also the difference from baseline to the 4-month post-randomisation follow-up (i.e., follow-up minus baseline; pFWE$_{SVC}$ = 0.025, Z = 4.43, [39 9 8]).

With respect to anxiety, the change from baseline to 1-month post-randomisation was positively correlated with the baseline CBF in the left (pFWE$_{SVC}$ = 0.008, Z = 4.79, [− 20−8 -12]; see Fig. 4B), but not the right (pFWE$_{SVC}$ < 0.323, Z = 3.49, [20−2 -14]), amygdalae, unless a bilateral amygdala mask was used (pFWE$_{SVC}$ = 0.034). However, baseline CBF in the left amygdala was no longer significantly associated with anxiety when the change from baseline to the 4-month post-randomisation assessment was examined (pFWE$_{SVC}$ = 0.811; pFWE$_{SVC}$ = 0.149 using bilateral amygdala mask only). No results were significant for depression (all p-values> 0.51).

We also explored whether baseline CBF predicted change in BMI, anxiety and depression from baseline to 18-months post-randomisation (n = 11, except for BMI

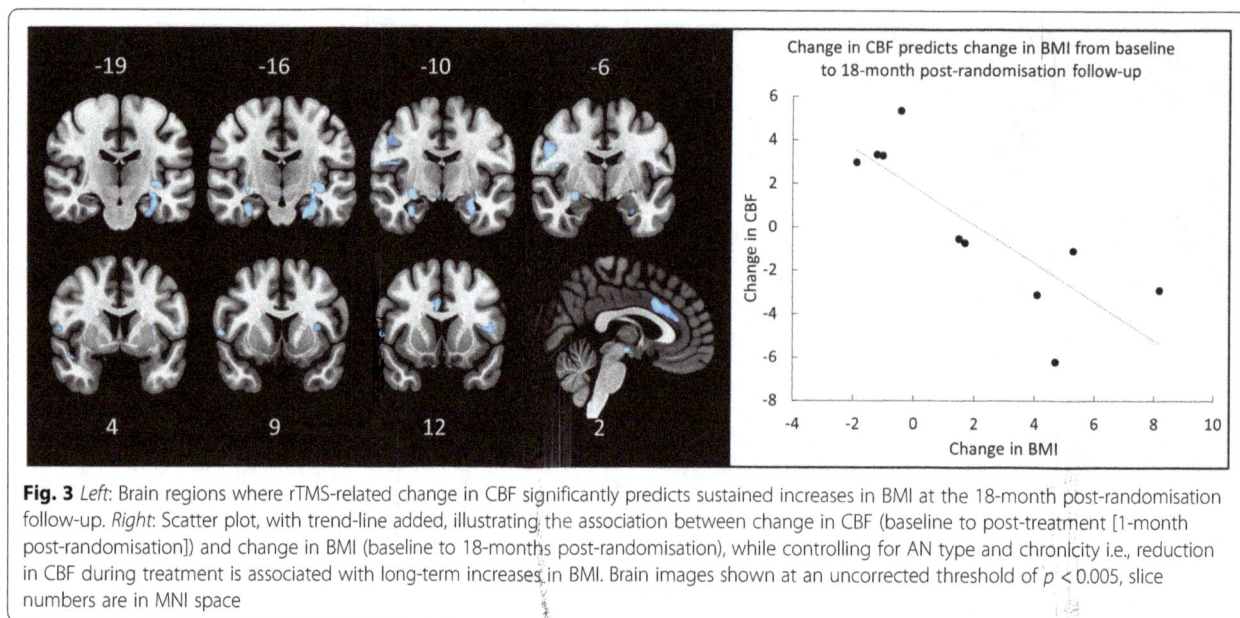

Fig. 3 *Left*: Brain regions where rTMS-related change in CBF significantly predicts sustained increases in BMI at the 18-month post-randomisation follow-up. *Right*: Scatter plot, with trend-line added, illustrating the association between change in CBF (baseline to post-treatment [1-month post-randomisation]) and change in BMI (baseline to 18-months post-randomisation), while controlling for AN type and chronicity i.e., reduction in CBF during treatment is associated with long-term increases in BMI. Brain images shown at an uncorrected threshold of $p < 0.005$, slice numbers are in MNI space

where $n = 10$). We found no significant relationship between baseline CBF and changes in the outcomes of interest at 18-month post-randomisation (all pFWE > 0.637).

Exploratory whole-brain analysis We found no additional associations between baseline CBF and change in

any of the three measures of interest in those that received real rTMS.

Discussion

In this exploratory study, we examined changes in CBF, quantified using pseudo-continuous ASL fMRI,

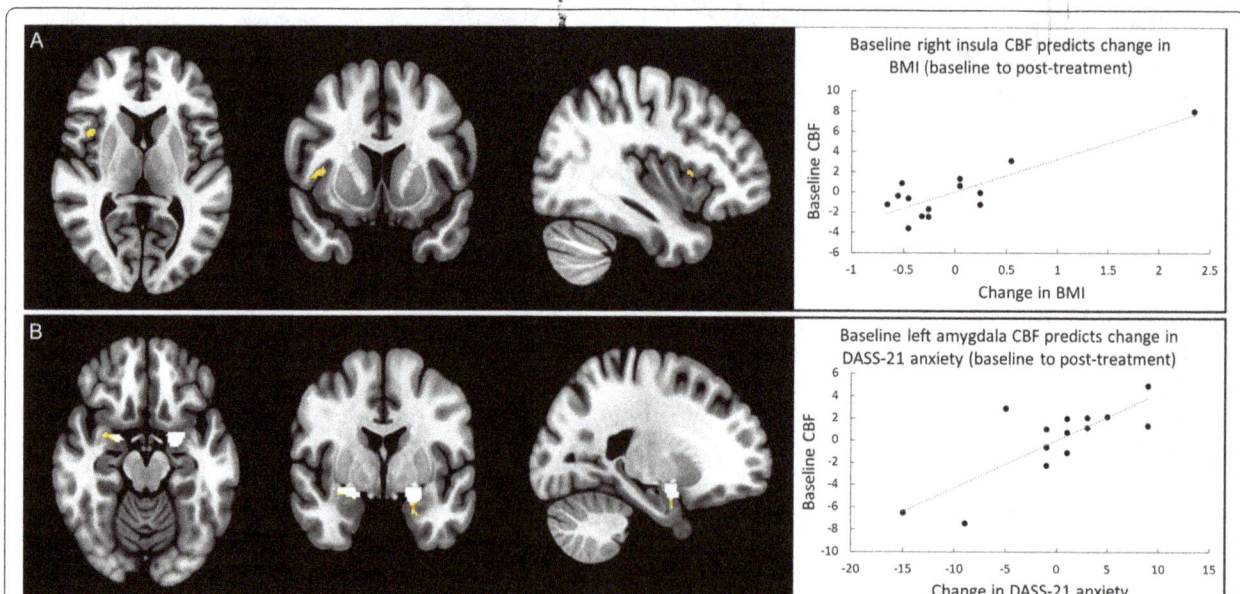

Fig. 4 A *Left*: Brain regions where baseline CBF significantly predicts change in BMI between baseline and post-treatment (1-month post-randomisation). *Right*: Scatter plot, with trend-line added, illustrating the association between baseline CBF and change in BMI, while controlling for AN type and chronicity i.e., lower baseline right insula CBF is associated with increases in BMI. **B** *Left*: Brain regions where baseline CBF significantly predicts change in DASS-21 anxiety between baseline and post-treatment (1-month post-randomisation). *Right*: Scatter plot, with trend-line added, illustrating the association between baseline CBF and change in anxiety, while controlling for AN type and chronicity i.e., lower baseline left amygdala CBF is associated with a reduction in anxiety. Brain images shown at an uncorrected threshold of $p < 0.005$, slice numbers are in MNI space

following high-frequency rTMS to the left DLPFC in people with SE-AN. We also considered how any CBF changes were associated with changes in clinical outcomes and explored whether baseline CBF may be a potential marker of rTMS treatment response. As part of this, we investigated differences in CBF between SE-AN and HC participants, identifying no group differences. This is consistent with findings from two studies that quantified CBF using positron emission topography (PET) [65, 66].

Unlike previous rTMS studies, we found no evidence of increased CBF at the stimulation site following rTMS treatment [21–24]. In studies of CBF in depression [67], the DLPFC has been implicated in rumination, as opposed to a distracted condition, and such resting ruminative activity may explain the evidence for TMS-related modulation of "resting" CBF in that region. For the SE-AN group in our study, in the absence of symptom-provoking stimuli, the DLPFC may not be recruited in a sufficiently sustained manner to change the mean CBF over the scan window (ASL produces an image of average CBF over approximately five-minutes). We did, however, find that amygdala CBF significantly reduced following real rTMS, compared to sham treatment. Although the SE-AN group had less WM in a similar region of the right amygdala, compared to HC participants at baseline, we found no evidence for significant treatment-related structural changes and no association between illness duration and the observed amygdala effects (see Supporting Information S3 and S3: Figure 2). Reasons for reduced perfusion in the right amygdala following real rTMS are unclear, particularly as high-frequency (i.e., excitatory) rTMS was applied to the left DLPFC. Although we did not identify any rTMS related changes in CBF in the DLPFC, this is a densely connected neural hub and so, stimulation to this area could cause widespread changes across brain networks. Indeed, it has been proposed that the DLPFC has indirect projections to the amygdala (e.g., [68, 69]) and rTMS studies targeting the DLPFC in the treatment of depression have reported distal effects on CBF in the amygdala [70]. However, the lateralisation, contralateral effects, and direction (i.e., reduction) of our findings is somewhat contradictory to previous findings in a small study of people with depression i.e., high-frequency left DLPFC rTMS was associated with increased left amygdala CBF [24]. In our study, rTMS to the DLPFC may be altering the efficiency of, or enhancing the "normal" regulation of the DLPFC on tonic amygdala activity, but the lateralisation was unexpected. In addition, no treatment-related changes in left amygdala CBF were observed, even at a liberal uncorrected threshold. Direct electrical stimulation of the right amygdala has been reported to elicit exclusively negative emotions, whereas left amygdala stimulation elicits both positive and negative emotional experiences [71]. Moreover, in healthy controls, harm avoidance traits have been more significantly associated with the strength of right amygdala resting-state connectivity with left hemispheric structures (including the left superior frontal gyrus [BA9] and basal ganglia) than was the left amygdala's connectivity with those regions [72]. It may be that rTMS applied to the DLFPC in a clinical population characterised by high levels of avoidant behaviour, might modulate the resting activity of the contralateral amygdala.

Changes in amygdala CBF were not associated with changes in anxiety or depression. This is surprising given the central role of the amygdala in emotional processing and regulation. While the observed amygdala CBF changes were not associated with any shorter-term clinical changes, participants with the greatest rTMS-related reduction in amygdala regional CBF (i.e., between baseline and 1-month post-randomisation) showed the greatest sustained weight gain at 18-months post-randomisation. Research suggests hyper-activation of the amygdala is associated with fearful emotional processing of body images [73] and importantly, when at rest, elevated amygdala activity is associated with mental health disorders characterised by chronic anxiety (e.g., AN, generalised anxiety disorder, obsessive compulsive disorder). Therefore, it could be considered that a reduction in amygdala activity may be associated with an increased ability to tolerate uncomfortable physical and emotional sensations related to the body, which may in turn influence weight gain.

The above proposal is in accord with our data exploring whether baseline CBF could be used as a predictor of rTMS treatment response. Identifying such predictors may help to optimise treatment and identify appropriate patients for future studies [74]. We found that lower baseline CBF in the right amygdala was associated with a greater reduction in anxiety from baseline to 1-month post-randomisation, but this relationship did not persist. In contrast, higher baseline CBF in the insula predicted greater weight gain between baseline and 1-month post-randomisation and between baseline and 4-months post-randomisation. The insula has an essential role in monitoring body state, interoceptive awareness, and regulation of appetite and eating, and has been implicated in AN [75]. Furthermore, insula hyperactivity has been implicated in anxiety, and it has been proposed that self-starvation and the associated weight loss/low body weight may serve to regulate aversive emotions, such as anxiety, in AN (e.g., [76]), e.g., perhaps by blunting anxiogenic interoceptive and somatic signals processed in the insula. As early weight gain may predict longer-term treatment outcome in AN [77], it is possible that those with relatively preserved insula function are most likely to benefit from even a temporary TMS-induced blunting of the affective reactivity to interoceptive and emotional signals elicited by food perception or consumption. Alternatively, insula-mediated processes may directly underpin weight-gain following rTMS, but this seems less likely. Given the potential value of developing markers of treatment responses that could be assessed prior to investing in such a demanding rTMS treatment programmes, these preliminary findings warrant further investigation to establish the specificity of the association and clarify the underpinning mechanisms.

Strengths and limitations

Our study is the first to explore rTMS effects on CBF in people with SE-AN, as part of a double-blind randomised controlled feasibility trial. ASL is a quantitative neuroimaging method with excellent/good test-retest reliability [78, 79]. In our analyses, we controlled for AN type and ED chronicity. However, a significant number of patients had to be discounted from the analyses due to incomplete datasets, rendering a relatively small patient group overall and particularly for the sham rTMS group and also for analyses on the predictors of long-term rTMS response using data from the 18-month post-randomisation follow-up. In addition, our sample only consisted of female participants but was heterogeneous across several other demographic and clinical parameters. As participants were community dwelling, we were unable to implement several factors that may be relevant for the reliability and clinical usefulness of our results e.g., standardised pre-scan meal, limit pre-scan exercise [80].

Conclusions

In this exploratory study, we identified rTMS treatment related changes in amygdala CBF in adults with SE-AN. Participants receiving real rTMS showed greater reductions in amygdala CBF and this was associated with long-term weight gain. It may be that rTMS applied to the left DLFPC modulates the resting activity of the contralateral amygdala in a clinical population characterised by high levels of avoidant behaviour. Higher baseline CBF in the insula was also associated with greater weight gain between baseline and short-term follow-up and possible explanations are discussed above. Future rTMS investigations in AN should employ longitudinal neuroimaging to confirm and extend our findings.

Abbreviations

AC: Anterior commissure; AN: Anorexia nervosa; AN-BP: Anorexia nervosa binge-eating/purging type; AN-R: Anorexia nervosa restricting type; ASL: Arterial spin labelling; BMI: Body mass index; BN: Bulimia nervosa; CBF: Cerebral blood flow; CSF: Cerebrospinal fluid; DASS-21: Depression Anxiety and Stress Scales – Version 21; DLPFC: Dorsolateral prefrontal cortex; DMPFC: Dorsomedial prefrontal cortex; DSM: Diagnostic and Statistical Manual of Mental Disorders; ED: Eating disorder; EDE-Q: Eating Disorder Examination Questionnaire; fMRI: Functional magnetic resonance imaging; GM: Grey matter; HC: Healthy comparison; KCL: King's College London; pCASL: Pseudo-continuous arterial spin labelling; PET: Positron emission topography; ROI: Region of interest; rTMS: Repetitive transcranial magnetic stimulation; SE-AN: Severe enduring anorexia nervosa; TI: Inversion time; TIV: Total intracranial volume; WM: White matter

Acknowledgements

We would like to thank the individuals who participated in this study for their time and commitment and our patient and public involvement advisors for their valuable feedback. The authors also wish to thank the National Institute for Health Research (NIHR) Biomedical Research Centre (BRC) at the Maudsley and the Wellcome Trust for their continued support of neuroimaging research at our institution.

Authors' contributions

US and OGO conceived the study. Data collection was performed by BD, SJR, SB, MK and JM. OGO analysed and interpreted the data. BD drafted and prepared the manuscript. EM and OGO assisted with drafting the manuscript. All authors critically reviewed and approved the final manuscript.

Funding

This paper presents independent research funded by the National Institute of Health Research (NIHR) under its Research for Patient Benefit (RfPB) Programme (Grant Reference Number PB-PG-1013-32049). This work was also supported by Infrastructure Support for Pilot studies from the NIHR Biomedical Research Centre at South London and Maudsley (SLaM) NHS Foundation Trust and King's College London (KCL). This study was also supported by the United Kingdom Clinical Research Collaboration-registered King's Clinical Trials Unit at King's Health Partners, which is part-funded by the NIHR BRC for Mental Health at SLaM NHS Foundation Trust and KCL and the NIHR Evaluation, Trials and Studies Coordinating Centre.
OGO receives salary support from an NIHR Infrastructure grant for the Wellcome Trust/King's College London Clinical Research Facility. Ulrike Schmidt is supported by an NIHR Senior Investigator Award. Ulrike Schmidt and Iain C. Campbell receive salary support from the NIHR Mental Health BRC at SLaM NHS Foundation Trust and King's College London. Savani Bartholdy and Samantha J. Rennalls were supported by studentships awarded by the NIHR Mental Health BRC at SLaM. Maria Kekic was supported by an Institute of Psychiatry, Psychology and Neuroscience/Medical Research Council Excellence Studentship.
The views expressed are those of the authors and not necessarily those of the NHS, the NIHR or the Department of Health.

Competing interests

The authors declare that they have no competing interests.

Author details

[1]Section of Eating Disorders, Department of Psychological Medicine, Institute of Psychiatry, Psychology & Neuroscience, King's College London, London, UK. [2]Department of Neuroimaging, Institute of Psychiatry, Psychology & Neuroscience, King's College London, London, UK. [3]South London and Maudsley NHS Foundation Trust, Maudsley Hospital, London, UK.

References

1. Treasure J, Duarte TA, Schmidt U. Eating disorders. Lancet. 2020;395(10227): 899–911. https://doi.org/10.1016/S0140-6736(20)30059-3.

2. Brockmeyer T, Friederich HC, Schmidt U. Advances in the treatment of anorexia nervosa: a review of established and emerging interventions. Psychol Med. 2018;48(8):1228–56. https://doi.org/10.1017/s0033291717002604.

3. Dobrescu SR, Dinkler L, Gillberg C, Råstam M, Gillberg C, Wentz E. Anorexia nervosa: 30-year outcome. Br J Psychiatry. 2020;216(2):97–104. https://doi.org/10.1192/bjp.2019.113.

4. Eddy KT, Tabri N, Thomas JJ, Murray HB, Keshaviah A, Hastings E, et al. Recovery from anorexia nervosa and bulimia nervosa at 22-year follow-up. J Clin Psychiatry. 2017;78(02):184–9. https://doi.org/10.4088/JCP.15m10393.

5. Hay PJ, Touyz S, Sud R. Treatment for severe and enduring anorexia nervosa: a review. Aust N Z J Psychiatry. 2012;46(12):1136–44. https://doi.org/10.1177/0004867412450469.

6. Ambwani S, Cardi V, Albano G, Cao L, Crosby RD, Macdonald P, et al. A multicenter audit of outpatient care for adult anorexia nervosa: symptom trajectory, service use, and evidence in support of "early stage" versus "severe and enduring" classification. Int J Eat Disord. 2020;53(8):1337–48. https://doi.org/10.1002/eat.23246.

7. Dunlop KA, Woodside B, Downar J. Targeting neural endophenotypes of eating disorders with non-invasive brain stimulation. Front Neurosci. 2016; 10:30. https://doi.org/10.3389/fnins.2016.00030.

8. Schmidt U, Campbell IC. Treatment of eating disorders can not remain "brainless": the case for brain-directed treatments. Eur Eat Disord Rev. 2013; 21(6):425–7. https://doi.org/10.1002/erv.2257.

9. Dalton B, Bartholdy S, Campbell IC, Schmidt U. Neurostimulation in clinical and sub-clinical eating disorders: a systematic update of the literature. Curr Neuropharmacol. 2018;16(8):1174–92. https://doi.org/10.2174/1570159X16666180108111532.

10. Duriez P, Bou Khalil R, Chamoun Y, Maatoug R, Strumila R, Seneque M, et al. Brain stimulation in eating disorders: state of the art and future perspectives. J Clin Med. 2020;9(8):2358. https://doi.org/10.3390/jcm9082358.

11. Rossi S, Hallett M, Rossini PM, Pascual-Leone A. Safety, ethical considerations, and application guidelines for the use of transcranial magnetic stimulation in clinical practice and research. Clin Neurophysiol. 2009;120(12):2008–39. https://doi.org/10.1016/j.clinph.2009.08.016.

12. Cirillo G, Di Pino G, Capone F, Ranieri F, Florio L, Todisco V, et al. Neurobiological after-effects of non-invasive brain stimulation. Brain Stimul. 2017;10(1):1–18. https://doi.org/10.1016/j.brs.2016.11.009.

13. Dunlop KA, Woodside B, Lam E, Olmsted M, Colton P, Giacobbe P, et al. Increases in frontostriatal connectivity are associated with response to dorsomedial repetitive transcranial magnetic stimulation in refractory binge/ purge behaviors. Neuroimage: Clin. 2015;8:611–8. https://doi.org/10.1016/j.nicl.2015.06.008.

14. Sutoh C, Koga Y, Kimura H, Kanahara N, Numata N, Hirano Y, et al. Repetitive transcranial magnetic stimulation changes cerebral oxygenation on the left dorsolateral prefrontal cortex in bulimia nervosa: a near-infrared spectroscopy pilot ztudy: neural mechanism of rTMS on food craving in bulimia nervosa. Eur Eat Disord Rev. 2016;24(1):83–8. https://doi.org/10.1002/erv.2413.

15. Bartholdy S, McClelland J, Kekic M, O'Daly OG, Campbell IC, Werthmann J, et al. Clinical outcomes and neural correlates of 20 sessions of repetitive transcranial magnetic stimulation in severe and enduring anorexia nervosa (the TIARA study): study protocol for a randomised controlled feasibility trial. Trials. 2015;16(1):548. https://doi.org/10.1186/s13063-015-1069-3.

16. Dalton B, Bartholdy S, McClelland J, Kekic M, Rennalls SJ, Werthmann J, et al. Randomised controlled feasibility trial of real versus sham repetitive transcranial magnetic stimulation treatment in adults with severe and enduring anorexia nervosa: the TIARA study. BMJ Open. 2018;8(7):e021531. https://doi.org/10.1136/bmjopen-2018-021531.

17. Dalton B, Lewis YD, Bartholdy S, Kekic M, McClelland J, Campbell IC, et al. Repetitive transcranial magnetic stimulation (rTMS) treatment in severe, enduring anorexia nervosa: an open longer-term follow-up. Eur Eat Disord Rev. 2020;28(6):773–81. https://doi.org/10.1002/erv.2766.

18. McClelland J, Kekic M, Campbell IC, Schmidt U. Repetitive Transcranial magnetic stimulation (rTMS) treatment in enduring anorexia nervosa: a case series. Eur Eat Disord Rev. 2016;24(2):157–63. https://doi.org/10.1002/erv.2414.

19. Park E, Kang MJ, Lee A, Chang WH, Shin Y-I, Kim Y-H. Real-time measurement of cerebral blood flow during and after repetitive transcranial magnetic stimulation: a near-infrared spectroscopy study. Neurosci Lett. 2017;653:78–83. https://doi.org/10.1016/j.neulet.2017.05.039.

20. Shang Y-Q, Xie J, Peng W, Zhang J, Chang D, Wang Z. Network-wise cerebral blood flow redistribution after 20 Hz rTMS on left dorso-lateral prefrontal cortex. Eur J Radiol. 2018;101:144–8. https://doi.org/10.1016/j.ejrad.2018.02.018.

21. Kito S, Fujita K, Koga Y. Changes in regional cerebral blood flow after repetitive Transcranial magnetic stimulation of the left dorsolateral prefrontal cortex in treatment-resistant depression. J Neuropsychiatry Clin Neurosci. 2008;20(1):74–80. https://doi.org/10.1176/jnp.2008.20.1.74.

22. Catafau AM, Perez V, Gironell A, Martin JC, Kulisevsky J, Estorch M, et al. SPECT mapping of cerebral activity changes induced by repetitive transcranial magnetic stimulation in depressed patients. A pilot study. Psychiatry Res Neuroimaging. 2001;106(3):151–60. https://doi.org/10.1016/S0925-4927(01)00079-8.

23. Knoch D, Treyer V, Regard M, Müri RM, Buck A, Weber B. Lateralized and frequency-dependent effects of prefrontal rTMS on regional cerebral blood flow. Neuroimage. 2006;31(2):641–8. https://doi.org/10.1016/j.neuroimage.2005.12.025.

24. Speer AM, Kimbrell TA, Wassermann EM, D. Repella J, Willis MW, Herscovitch P, et al. Opposite effects of high and low frequency rTMS on regional brain activity in depressed patients. Biol Psychiatry. 2000;48(12):1133–41. https://doi.org/10.1016/S0006-3223(00)01065-9.

25. Iwabuchi SJ, Auer DP, Lankappa ST, Palaniyappan L. Baseline effective connectivity predicts response to repetitive transcranial magnetic stimulation in patients with treatment-resistant depression. Eur Neuropsychopharmacol. 2019;29(5):681–90. https://doi.org/10.1016/j.euroneuro.2019.02.012.

26. Mottaghy FM, Keller CE, Gangitano M, Ly J, Thall M, Parker JA, et al. Correlation of cerebral blood flow and treatment effects of repetitive transcranial magnetic stimulation in depressed patients. Psychiatry Res Neuroimaging. 2002;115(1-2):1–14. https://doi.org/10.1016/S0925-4927(02)00032-X.

27. Shinba T, Kariya N, Matsuda S, Matsuda H, Obara Y. Increase of frontal cerebral blood volume during transcranial magnetic stimulation in depression is related to treatment effectiveness: a pilot study with near-infrared spectroscopy. Psychiatry Clin Neurosci. 2018;72(8):602–10. https://doi.org/10.1111/pcn.12680.

28. Gianni AD, De Donatis D, Valente S, De Ronchi D, Atti AR. Eating disorders: do PET and SPECT have a role? A systematic review of the literature. Psychiatry Res: Neuroimaging. 2020;300:111065. https://doi.org/10.1016/j.pscychresns.2020.111065.

29. Sheng M, Lu H, Liu P, Thomas BP, McAdams CJ. Cerebral perfusion differences in women currently with and recovered from anorexia nervosa. Psychiatry Res. 2015;232(2):175–83. https://doi.org/10.1016/j.pscychresns.2015.02.008.

30. Yonezawa H, Otagaki Y, Miyake Y, Okamoto Y, Yamawaki S. No differences are seen in the regional cerebral blood flow in the restricting type of anorexia nervosa compared with the binge eating/purging type. Psychiatry Clin Neurosci. 2008;62(1):26–33. https://doi.org/10.1111/j.1440-1819.2007.01769.x.

31. Kojima S, Nagai N, Nakabeppu Y, Muranaga T, Deguchi D, Nakajo M, et al. Comparison of regional cerebral blood flow in patients with anorexia nervosa before and after weight gain. Psychiatry Res Neuroimaging. 2005; 140(3):251–8. https://doi.org/10.1016/j.pscychresns.2005.08.002.

32. Komatsu H, Nagamitsu S, Ozono S, Yamashita Y, Ishibashi M, Matsuishi T. Regional cerebral blood flow changes in early-onset anorexia nervosa before and after weight gain. Brain and Development. 2010;32(8):625–30. https://doi.org/10.1016/j.braindev.2009.09.022.

33. Matsumoto R, Kitabayashi Y, Narumoto J, Wada Y, Okamoto A, Ushijima Y, et al. Regional cerebral blood flow changes associated with interoceptive awareness in the recovery process of anorexia nervosa. Prog Neuro-Psychopharmacol Biol Psychiatry. 2006;30(7):1265–70. https://doi.org/10.1016/j.pnpbp.2006.03.042.

34. Fairburn CG, Shafran R, Cooper Z. A cognitive behavioural theory of anorexia nervosa. Behav Res Ther. 1999;37(1):1–13. https://doi.org/10.1016/S0005-7967(98)00102-8.

35. Val-Laillet D, Aarts E, Weber B, Ferrari M, Quaresima V, Stoeckel LE, et al. Neuroimaging and neuromodulation approaches to study eating behavior and prevent and treat eating disorders and obesity. Neuroimage Clin. 2015; 8:1–31. https://doi.org/10.1016/j.nicl.2015.03.016.

36. Simon JJ, Stopyra MA, Friederich H-C. Neural processing of disorder-related stimuli in patients with anorexia nervosa: a narrative review of brain imaging studies. J Clin Med. 2019;8(7):1047. https://doi.org/10.3390/jcm8071047.

37. Kaye W. Neurobiology of anorexia and bulimia nervosa. Physiol Behav. 2008; 94(1):121–35. https://doi.org/10.1016/j.physbeh.2007.11.037.

38. American Psychiatric Association. Diagnostic and statistical manual of mental disorders. 5th ed. Arlington: American Psychiatric Publishing; 2013.

39. Stice E, Telch CF, Rizvi SL. Development and validation of the eating disorder diagnostic scale: a brief self-report measure of anorexia, bulimia, and binge-eating disorder. Psychol Assess. 2000;12(2):123–31. https://doi.org/10.1037/1040-3590.12.2.123.

40. First MB, Spitzer RL, Gibbon M, Williams JB. Structured clinical interview for DSM-IV-TR Axis I disorders, Research Version, Non-Patient Edition: SCID-I/NP. New York State: Psychiatric Institute; 2002.

41. Fitzgerald PB, Hoy K, McQueen S, Maller JJ, Herring S, Segrave R, et al. A randomized trial of rTMS targeted with MRI based neuro-navigation in treatment-resistant depression. Neuropsychopharmacology. 2009;34(5): 1255–62. https://doi.org/10.1038/npp.2008.233.

42. McClelland J, Kekic M, Bozhilova N, Nestler S, Dew T, Van den Eynde F, et al. A randomised controlled trial of neuronavigated repetitive transcranial magnetic stimulation (rTMS) in anorexia nervosa. PLoS One. 2016;11(3): e0148606. https://doi.org/10.1371/journal.pone.0148606.

43. Mutz J, Edgcumbe DR, Brunoni AR, Fu CHY. Efficacy and acceptability of non-invasive brain stimulation for the treatment of adult unipolar and bipolar depression: a systematic review and meta-analysis of randomised sham-controlled trials. Neurosci Biobehav Rev. 2018;92:291–303. https://doi.org/10.1016/j.neubiorev.2018.05.015.

44. Uher R, Yoganathan D, Mogg A, Eranti SV, Treasure J, Campbell IC, et al. Effect of left prefrontal repetitive transcranial magnetic stimulation on food craving. Biol Psychiatry. 2005;58(10):840–2. https://doi.org/10.1016/j.biopsych.2005.05.043.

45. McClelland J, Bozhilova N, Nestler S, Campbell IC, Jacob S, Johnson-Sabine E, et al. Improvements in symptoms following neuronavigated repetitive transcranial magnetic stimulation (rTMS) in severe and enduring anorexia nervosa: findings from two case studies. Eur Eat Disord Rev. 2013;21(6):500–6. https://doi.org/10.1002/erv.2266.

46. Dalton B, Lewis YD, Bartholdy S, Kekic M, McClelland J, Campbell IC, et al. Repetitive transcranial magnetic stimulation treatment in severe, enduring anorexia nervosa: an open longer-term follow-up. Eur Eat Disord Rev. 2020; 28(6):773–81. https://doi.org/10.1002/erv.2766.

47. Byrne S, Wade T, Hay P, Touyz S, Fairburn CG, Treasure J, et al. A randomised controlled trial of three psychological treatments for anorexia nervosa. Psychol Med. 2017;47(16):2823–33. https://doi.org/10.1017/S0033291717001349.

48. Schmidt U, Magill N, Renwick B, Keyes A, Kenyon M, Dejong H, et al. The Maudsley outpatient study of treatments for anorexia nervosa and related conditions (MOSAIC): comparison of the Maudsley model of anorexia nervosa treatment for adults (MANTRA) with specialist supportive clinical management (SSCM) in outpatients with broadly defined anorexia nervosa: a randomized controlled trial. J Consult Clin Psychol. 2015;83(4):796–807. https://doi.org/10.1037/ccp0000019.

49. Ulfvebrand S, Birgegård A, Norring C, Högdahl L, von Hausswolff-Juhlin Y. Psychiatric comorbidity in women and men with eating disorders results from a large clinical database. Psychiatry Res. 2015;230(2):294–9. https://doi.org/10.1016/j.psychres.2015.09.008.

50. Arkell J, Robinson P. A pilot case series using qualitative and quantitative methods: biological, psychological and social outcome in severe and enduring eating disorder (anorexia nervosa). Int J Eat Disord. 2008;41(7): 650–6. https://doi.org/10.1002/eat.20546.

51. Lovibond SH, Lovibond PF. Manual for the depression anxiety stress scales. Sydney: Psychology Foundation of Australia; 1995.

52. Antony MM, Bieling PJ, Cox BJ, Enns MW, Swinson RP. Psychometric properties of the 42-item and 21-item versions of the depression anxiety stress scales in clinical groups and a community sample. Psychol Assess. 1998;10(2):176–81. https://doi.org/10.1037/1040-3590.10.2.176.

53. Mato Abad V, García-Polo P, O'Daly O, Hernández-Tamames JA, Zelaya F. ASAP (automatic software for ASL processing): a toolbox for processing arterial spin labeling images. Magn Reson Imaging. 2016;34(3):334–44. https://doi.org/10.1016/j.mri.2015.11.002.

54. Nezamzadeh M, Matson GB, Young K, Weiner MW, Schuff N. Improved pseudo-continuous arterial spin labeling for mapping brain perfusion. J Magn Reson Imaging. 2010;31(6):1419–27. https://doi.org/10.1002/jmri.22199.

55. Petcharunpaisan S. Arterial spin labeling in neuroimaging. World J Radiol. 2010;2(10):384–98. https://doi.org/10.4329/wjr.v2.i10.384.

56. Dai W, Garcia D, de Bazelaire C, Alsop DC. Continuous flow-driven inversion for arterial spin labeling using pulsed radio frequency and gradient fields: pulsed continuous arterial spin labeling. Magn Reson Med. 2008;60(6):1488–97. https://doi.org/10.1002/mrm.21790.

57. Dai W, Robson PM, Shankaranarayanan A, Alsop DC. Sensitivity calibration with a uniform magnetization image to improve arterial spin labeling perfusion quantification: perfusion quantification with a uniform magnetization image. Magn Reson Med. 2011;66(6):1590–600. https://doi.org/10.1002/mrm.22954.

58. Katzman DK, Lambe EK, Mikulis DJ, Ridgley JN, Goldbloom DS, Zipursky RB. Cerebral gray matter and white matter volume deficits in adolescent girls with anorexia nervosa. J Pediatr. 1996;129(6):794–803. https://doi.org/10.1016/S0022-3476(96)70021-5.

59. Kohn MR, Ashtari M, Golden NH, Schebendach J, Patel M, Jacobson MS, et al. Structural brain changes and malnutrition in anorexia nervosa. Ann N Y Acad Sci. 1997;817(1 Adolescent Nu):398–9. https://doi.org/10.1111/j.1749-6632.1997.tb48238.x.

60. Titova OE, Hjorth OC, Schiöth HB, Brooks SJ. Anorexia nervosa is linked to reduced brain structure in reward and somatosensory regions: a meta-analysis of VBM studies. BMC Psychiatry. 2013;13(1):110. https://doi.org/10.1186/1471-244X-13-110.

61. Zhang W, Song L, Yin X, Zhang J, Liu C, Wang J, et al. Grey matter abnormalities in untreated hyperthyroidism: a voxel-based morphometry study using the DARTEL approach. Eur J Radiol. 2014;83(1):e43–8. https://doi.org/10.1016/j.ejrad.2013.09.019.

62. Ashburner J. VBM Tutorial 2010. https://www.fil.ion.ucl.ac.uk/~john/misc/VBMclass10.pdf.

63. Maldjian JA, Laurienti PJ, Kraft RA, Burdette JH. An automated method for neuroanatomic and cytoarchitectonic atlas-based interrogation of fMRI data sets. NeuroImage. 2003;19(3):1233–9. https://doi.org/10.1016/S1053-8119(03)00169-1.

64. Tzourio-Mazoyer N, Landeau B, Papathanassiou D, Crivello F, Etard O, Delcroix N, et al. Automated anatomical labeling of activations in SPM using a macroscopic anatomical Parcellation of the MNI MRI single-subject brain. NeuroImage. 2002;15(1):273–89. https://doi.org/10.1006/nimg.2001.0978.

65. Bailer UF, Frank GK, Henry SE, Price JC, Meltzer CC, Mathis CA, et al. Exaggerated 5-HT1A but Normal 5-HT2A receptor activity in individuals ill with anorexia nervosa. Biol Psychiatry. 2007;61(9):1090–9. https://doi.org/10.1016/j.biopsych.2006.07.018.

66. Frank GKW, Bailer UF, Meltzer CC, Price JC, Mathis CA, Wagner A, et al. Regional cerebral blood flow after recovery from anorexia or bulimia nervosa. Int J Eat Disord. 2007;40(6):488–92. https://doi.org/10.1002/eat.20395.

67. Cooney RE, Joormann J, Eugène F, Dennis EL, Gotlib IH. Neural correlates of rumination in depression. Cogn Affect Behav Neurosci. 2010;10(4):470–8. https://doi.org/10.3758/CABN.10.4.470.

68. Ghashghaei HT, Barbas H. Pathways for emotion: interactions of prefrontal and anterior temporal pathways in the amygdala of the rhesus monkey. Neurosci. 2002;115(4):1261–79. https://doi.org/10.1016/s0306-4522(02)00446-3.

69. Siegle GJ, Thompson W, Carter CS, Steinhauer SR, Thase ME. Increased amygdala and decreased dorsolateral prefrontal BOLD responses in unipolar depression: related and independent features. Biol Psychiatry. 2007;61(2): 198–209. https://doi.org/10.1016/j.biopsych.2006.05.048.

70. Philip NS, Barredo J, Aiken E, Carpenter LL. Neuroimaging mechanisms of therapeutic Transcranial magnetic stimulation for major depressive disorder. Biolg Psychiatry: Cogn Neurosci Neuroimaging. 2018;3(3):211–22. https://doi.org/10.1016/j.bpsc.2017.10.007.

71. Lanteaume L, Khalfa S, Régis J, Marquis P, Chauvel P, Bartolomei F. Emotion induction after direct intracerebral stimulations of human amygdala. Cereb Cortex. 2007;17(6):1307–13. https://doi.org/10.1093/cercor/bhl041

72. Baeken C, Marinazzo D, Van Schuerbeek P, Wu G-R, De Mey J, Luypaert R, et al. Left and right amygdala - mediofrontal cortical functional connectivity is differentially modulated by harm avoidance. PLoS One. 2014;9(4):e95740. https://doi.org/10.1371/journal.pone.0095740.

73. Gaudio S, Quattrocchi CC. Neural basis of a multidimensional model of body image distortion in anorexia nervosa. Neurosci Biobehav Rev. 2012; 36(8):1839–47. https://doi.org/10.1016/j.neubiorev.2012.05.003.

74. Walton E, Turner JA, Ehrlich S. Neuroimaging as a potential biomarker to optimize psychiatric research and treatment. Int Rev Psychiatry. 2013;25(5): 619–31. https://doi.org/10.3109/09540261.2013.816659.

75. Nunn K, Frampton I, Gordon I, Lask B. The fault is not in her parents but in her insula—a neurobiological hypothesis of anorexia nervosa. Eur Eat Disord Rev. 2008;16(5):355–60. https://doi.org/10.1002/erv.890.

76. Brockmeyer T, Holtforth MG, Bents H, Kämmerer A, Herzog W, Friederich H-C. Starvation and emotion regulation in anorexia nervosa. Compr Psychiatry. 2012;53(5):496–501. https://doi.org/10.1016/j.comppsych.2011.09.003.

77. Nazar BP, Gregor LK, Albano G, Marchica A, Coco GL, Cardi V, et al. Early response to treatment in eating disorders: a systematic review and a diagnostic test accuracy meta-analysis: early response to eating disorder treatment. Eur Eat Disord Rev. 2017;25(2):67–79. https://doi.org/10.1002/erv.2495.

78. Jiang L, Kim M, Chodkowski B, Donahue MJ, Pekar JJ, Van Zijl PCM, et al. Reliability and reproducibility of perfusion MRI in cognitively normal subjects. Magn Reson Imaging. 2010;28(9):1283–9. https://doi.org/10.1016/j.mri.2010.05.002.

79. Wu B, Lou X, Wu X, Ma L. Intra- and interscanner reliability and reproducibility of 3D whole-brain pseudo-continuous arterial spin-labeling MR perfusion at 3T. J Magn Reson Imaging. 2014;39(2):402–9. https://doi.org/10.1002/jmri.24175.

80. Frank GKW, Favaro A, Marsh R, Ehrlich S, Lawson EA. Toward valid and reliable brain imaging results in eating disorders. Int J Eat Disord. 2018;51(3): 250–61. https://doi.org/10.1002/eat.22829.

"I'm still here, But no One Hears You": A Qualitative Study of Young Women's Experiences of Persistent Distress Post Family-based Treatment for Adolescent Anorexia Nervosa

Janet Conti[1]* , Caroline Joyce[2], Simone Natoli[2], Kelsey Skeoch[2] and Phillipa Hay[3]

Abstract

Background: Family-based treatment (FBT) is the current treatment of choice for adolescent AN based on positive outcomes that include weight restoration in around two-thirds of adolescents. Nevertheless around a quarter drop-out from treatment, particularly in the earlier phases, and a notable proportion of treated adolescents are reported to experience ongoing psychological distress during and post-treatment. This study explores the under-researched experiences of these adolescents.

Method: Fourteen participants from Australia, New Zealand and the United Kingdom were interviewed about their experiences of FBT. An inductive thematic analysis of interview transcript data generated key themes related to their experiences, identity negotiations and the discursive materials these used to construct these.

Results: The participants identified working as a family unit as key to their recovery, highlighting the importance of family therapy interventions for adolescent AN. However, they perceived an almost exclusive focus on weight restoration in the first phase of FBT was associated with experiences that included a relative neglect of their psychological distress and a loss of voice. Key within these experiences were processes whereby the adolescent engaged in identity negotiation and (re)claiming of their voice and implicit in their family standing with them in the treatment was that their life was worth saving. What was noted as most helpful was when therapists advocated and took into consideration their unique needs and preferences and tailored treatment interventions to these.

Conclusions: There is a need to develop and research treatments that address, from the outset of treatment, the adolescents' psychological distress (including as experienced in the context of their weight restoration). This should be with priority accorded to the adolescent's voice and identity negotiations, as they and their families take steps to address the physical crisis of AN and in doing so, support more holistic and durable recovery.

Keywords: Adolescent anorexia nervosa, Maudsley family therapy, Family-based treatment, Experience, Identity, Qualitative

*Correspondence: j.conti@westernsydney.edu.au
[1] School of Psychology and Translational Research Institute, Western Sydney University, Locked Bag 1797, Penrith 2751, Australia
Full list of author information is available at the end of the article

Plain English summary

Family-Based Treatment (FBT) is a well-established, intensive approach to the treatment of adolescent anorexia nervosa (AN). The first phase of treatment focuses on eating and weight restoration, where parents are given responsibility for the adolescent's home-based refeeding. This is followed by handing over of this responsibility to the adolescent with the final-phase a focusing on adolescent-specific psychological issues. While the majority of adolescents gain weight with this treatment, a substantive proportion experience ongoing psychological distress and around a quarter of families drop out in the first phase. Little is known about these adolescents' experiences.

In this project, we interviewed 14 individuals who, with their family, had either dropped out of FBT and/or experienced ongoing psychological distress post-treatment. The participants noted that their parents' stance in supporting them was life-saving and contributed to a sense that their life was worth saving. However, they also noted a relative absence of focus on their psychological distress, particularly in the early stages of treatment. Most helpful for participants was when therapists took into consideration and tailored treatments to them. Future treatments need to consider ways to support an adolescent's psychological distress more comprehensively, prioritise their voice and support them in finding an identity outside of the AN identity.

Background

Anorexia Nervosa (AN) is characterised by significantly low weight and an obsessional fear of gaining weight [1], frequent onset in the adolescent years [2] and mortality of 6–15%, with half of all deaths resulting from suicide [3–6]. A complexity for the treatment of AN is the egosyntonicity of the AN symptoms, many of which are valued by the experiencing person that contribute to a reluctance to engage in treatment [7]. For those who do engage in treatment, drop-out rates are high, including 23–73% in outpatient settings [8].

Family Based treatment (FBT) [9] has been reported to have positive treatment outcomes, particularly on eating disorder (ED) symptomatology, including in those adolescents assessed with higher ED symptomatology [10]. FBT has been proposed as the first line, 'gold-standard' evidence-based treatment for adolescent AN [11]. Through a number of randomized controlled trials (RCTs), FBT has been found to be associated with earlier weight restoration and reduced ED symptomatology and lower hospitalizations (and hence treatment cost), compared with adolescent focused individual therapy [12] and family therapy that addressed systemic concerns rather than eating related behaviours [13]. Further RCTs have found parent focused treatment (PFT) to be more efficacious than standard FBT; PFT being where treatment consists of the FBT therapist meeting with the parents separately to the adolescent who meets with a specialist nurse [14]. There is also evidence to indicate that when parental expressed emotion is higher, PFT results in higher rates of remission in the adolescent [15]. Early weight gain, a specific focus of FBT, has also been found to predict improved outcomes for the adolescent, particularly when there is a corresponding early focus on addressing negative emotion, parental criticism and the therapeutic alliance early in FBT and PFT treatments [16]. Furthermore,

therapeutic alliance, as measured by an independent researcher-rater using the Working Alliance Inventory Observer Version (WAI-o) [17], has been found to be 'achievable' [18, 19] and 'generally strong' [20] in FBT. However, this measure of therapeutic alliance in these studies did not find a significant relationship and treatment outcome of remission of AN symptoms [18].

FBT is a three phase manualized treatment that begins with a focus on supporting parents to take responsibility for their child's eating and weight restoration, progressing to phase 2 where this responsibility is re-allocated to the adolescent once they have increased their food intake and sustained reliable weight gain. The final phase commences when the adolescent maintains at least 95% of their ideal body weight, and is focused on re-establishing autonomy and developing a healthy identity [21, 22]; psychological processes and relational problems are not specifically addressed until this final phase of treatment [23, 24]. These phases of treatment are estimated to be delivered over 12 months over 20 sessions. Recent evidence in clinical settings has demonstrated that for those who do not meet remission by session 20, that further FBT sessions resulted in lower number of days in hospital and improved rates of remission compared to those who sought out alternative treatments to FBT [25].

A Cochrane review of 25 published and unpublished randomised controlled trials that compared family therapy interventions, including FBT, with other AN treatments [26] has found some evidence of a small effect size of FBT related to weight gain post-treatment, however, little evidence of differences between outcomes for groups across all comparisons of treatments, including in ED symptomatology (weight, ED psychopathology), drop out, relapse or family functioning measures at post-intervention or at follow-up. This review concluded that there currently exists insufficient evidence that family therapy interventions were superior to educational interventions and other types of psychological interventions for adolescent anorexia nervosa at long term follow up. There was also insufficient evidence of (1) outcomes outside symptom remission with only two trials of 21 reporting outcomes based on a return to normal functioning; and (2) whether one type of family therapy was more effective than others. Furthermore, the lack of detailed information about individuals and their families who drop out of adolescent AN treatments may have contributed to "the effect of artificially inflating the effectiveness of the interventions reviewed" [26].

Overall, results from RCTs show that FBT works well for less than half of the adolescents and their families who engage in this treatment [27]. Outside of this group for whom this intervention works well: (1) up to 27 percent of families drop out from FBT [28]; (2) 40% of adolescents continue with ongoing psychological distress despite weight restoration [29]; and (3) comorbid symptomology has a negative impact on treatment outcomes and increases rates of attrition [30–32]. In response to these findings, and given some promising findings for enhanced cognitive behavior therapy (CBT-E) adapted for adolescent AN [33, 34], CBT-E has recently been compared with FBT in a non-randomised effectiveness trial [35]. Findings indicated that greater early weight gain in FBT that by 6 to 12 months was indistinguishable between the two groups. Both treatments resulted in similar weight gains in general measures of psychopathology and clinical impairment; keeping in mind that the group who elected CBT-E were older and more unwell. Those who fared less well with these treatments reported a history of abuse and, specifically in the lower weight cohort, reported higher internalization, a presence of comorbid psychopathology, and prior mental health treatment.

A meta-synthesis of qualitative research into the experiences of family therapy for AN [36] has found three of 15 papers analysed adolescent and family experiences of FBT with one consisting of data generated from open-ended survey questions [37]. Two of these studies [37, 38] found that the most helpful aspect of FBT was parental support and understanding and the third study [39] found that the authoritative stance of therapists having an oversight of their eating behavior to be helpful. Less helpful was the neglect of issues other than AN [37, 39] and the adolescents' unmet preferences for individual therapy [37]. There is increasing evidence to support the need for ED treatment interventions to focus on more rapid relief of the psychological dimensions of AN [40]. Furthermore, research into treatment experiences of those with a lived AN experience has identified a need for treatments to more directly address questions of identity,

including the rebuilding a sense of identity outside of the ED identity [41, 42].

Overall there have been few studies that have focused on the experiences and identity struggles of those whose families either drop out of FBT and/or adolescents who continue with substantive psychological distress post-treatment [29]. This study sought to address this gap and give voice to those who experience persistent distress post FBT.

The current study

The current study utilised a qualitative framework to give voice to the person with a lived adolescent AN experience with a focus on participant:

1) Experiences of Family-Based Treatment for adolescent AN in those who were interested in participating in research to improve the intervention; and
2) Identity negotiations in the context of this treatment intervention.

The aim of this study is to explore how these participant experiences and identity negotiations might inform future augmentations and transformative treatments for adolescent AN.

Methods
Design

This study was an inductive thematic analysis [43] with the understanding of themes as constructed within an interpersonal context. Analysis of data that comprised the themes/subthemes focused on some of the ways participants negotiated their identities through the discursive materials or language forms available to them at the time, the semantic and latent meanings they ascribed to the experiences of FBT and some of the dilemmas they faced [44] in the context of their recollection of experiences of FBT for adolescent AN. This study was also part of a larger study that explored the experiences and perspectives of parents who had experienced FBT [45] and clinicians who reported being trained and having practiced as FBT practitioners [46].

Participants

A purposive sampling technique was utilised to invite participants to talk about their experiences of FBT and generate a context through which they could voice aspects of the treatment that was both helpful and their ideas of ways the intervention could be improved. These participants responded to advertisements via Australian clinicians; and after indicating their interest on completion of an eating disorders (ED) treatment experiences survey advertised through Facebook (see "Appendix A" for the wording of the research advertisement).

Fourteen participants aged 14–27 years ($M = 18.58$, $SD = 3.20$), who reported being diagnosed with AN and treated with FBT for adolescent AN on average 4 years earlier (range 1–14 years) were interviewed (in person or online/telephone). See Table 1 for further demographics and FBT treatment details. Half of the participants reported weight restoration post-treatment (with one later relapsing); all the participants reporting ongoing ED symptoms and psychological distress post-FBT. Eleven participants reported additional treatments for co-morbid psychological problems prior to or post FBT with three of these participants reporting psychological counselling whilst also engaging in FBT (see Table 2 for details).

Procedure and materials

This study was approved by the Western Sydney University Human Research Ethics Committee (approval number: H11303).

Semi-structured interviews were carried out by two researchers (JC, SC) (see "Appendix B" for interview format) that were audio recorded, transcribed verbatim and de-identified with participants' chosen pseudonyms. Transcripts were then given to participants to member check for accuracy and the removal of further identifying information for confidentiality.

Analysis

The analysis was data-driven and inductive with all themes generated from the dataset [43]. Throughout the analytic process, themes were constructed through the explicit language used by participants, and an analysis of implicit meanings in their narratives, as language in this instance is assumed to construct a version of the participants' experiences and meaning-making processes [47]. Three authors (KS, SN, JC) familiarised themselves with the data by reading and re-reading transcripts, coding meaningful units of raw data into draft themes and subthemes. Two authors (CJ, JC) also coded raw data into 'nodes' using QSR NVivo-12 qualitative data analysis software, examined the nodes for similarities and differences and grouped data related to the research question into categories. These categories of data were then collated and contrasted with the earlier drafted themes/sub-themes before being analysed for any further relationships and grouped together to generate overarching themes and a thematic map that addressed the research questions through in-depth analysis of exemplar data within each theme/sub-theme (JC, CJ, PH). Analysis by the researchers (see "Appendix C" for researcher

Table 1 Demographic and treatment details

Participant Pseudonym	Family structure	Age at interview	Age at diagnosis	FBT age	FBT mths	Individual therapy + FBT	Phase completed	Weight restored after treatment
Abbey	Parents + 3C	27	13	13	12	Yes psychiatrist & psychologist	3	Yes
Amy	Parents + 4C	18	16	16	24	Psychologist-depression/anxiety	3	No (recent AN hospitalization)
Beth	Parents + 2C	16	14	14	7–8	No	1 (D/C)	No
Charlotte	Parents + 3C	19	16	16/17	12	Psychiatrist	2 (D/C)	No
Harley	Parents + 3C	17	14	14	6	No	2 (D/C)	Yes (temporary) then lapsed
Hayley	Parents + 2C	14	10	11	24	CBT (at end FBT)	2 then lapsed (D/C)	No
Jessica	Parents separated + 3C	16	14	14	12	No	1 (D/C)	Yes
Kate	Parents separated + 3 C	18	17	17/18	3–4	No	1 (D/C)	No
Kaylee	Parents + C	20	16	16	6	No	1 (D/C)	Yes
Lydia	Parents + 3C	19	14/15	15	12	No	1 (D/C)	No
Maisy	Parents + 2C	19	14	14	24	CBT, mindfulness, Psychiatrist	3	Yes
Nora	Parents + 2C	21	14/15	15		No	1 (D/C)	No
Phoenix	Parents + 2C	18	15/16	15/16	7	No	3	Yes
Rachel	Parents + 2C	20	17	17	6–8	No	1 (D/C)	Yes

C children, D/C discontinued, ED eating disorder

Table 2 Additional treatments for Eating Disorder (ED) and other psychological problems

Participant Pseudonyms	Other eating disorder treatments	Eating disorder behaviours	Treatment for other problems
Abbey	Psychological therapy (including during FBT) Inpatient (P), BN day program	Restriction, over-exercise	Group Dialectical Behaviour Therapy
Amy	3 inpatient admissions (P), about to recommence hospital treatment, individual therapy(including during FBT)	Restriction, overexercise, Purging and binge eating	Psychiatrists/psychologists/school counsellor (P) for Depression, anxiety (included anti-depressants)
Beth	Nil	Restriction, over-exercise	Nil
Charlotte	Inpatient, psychiatrist	Restriction, purging	Nil
Harley	Inpatient then FBT (P), outpatient, multi-family therapy (P)	Restriction, overexercise, Purging	Psychiatrist/psychologist (C): Self-harm, Conversion Disorder, depression with psychosis: medication including SSRI's, Seroquel (+ "atypical antipsychotics")
Hayley	Psychologist (Narrative Therapy) (C) Inpatient admission (P)	Restriction, overexercise	Psychologist (C): Anxiety
Jessica	Inpatient then FBT (P)	Restriction, over-exercise,	Saw Psychologist as a child (unsure why)
Kate	Psychologist (Narrative Therapy), dietitian, psychiatrist (C)	Restriction, overexercise	Psychologist and Psychiatrist (C): Anxiety; Family counselling before ED (P)
Kaylee	Inpatient then FBT (P) then inpatient	Restriction, over-exercise, Prior AN: purging, binge eating	Parent reported diagnosis ASD ("Asperger's"), depression
Lydia	Inpatient then FBT (P) then inpatient (total 8 admissions), ED day program (C)	Restriction, over-exercise,	Nil
Maisy	Psychological therapy (including during FBT) + ED support group	Purging-reported once	Psychiatrist OCD—current treatment lithium, recently ceased escitalopram
Nora	Psychologist and psychiatrist (C) Inpatient admissions (P)	Restriction, overexercise, Purging	Psychologist and psychiatrists for depression, OCD (C)
Phoenix	Psychologists (P&C), paediatrician, dietitian, school counsellor	Restriction, overexercise Purging, binging	Depression, OCD
Rachel	Outpatient Psychologist and Dietitian, Group Therapy	Restriction	Counsellor for OCD (age 10 years), current anti-depressants

C current, *P* past, *OCD* obsessive compulsive disorder

positioning statements) traced some of the discursive materials these participants used to piece together key experiences and dilemmas associated with components of FBT and including patterns of identity negotiation [44, 48, 49].

The draft analysis was given to participants to member check for the purposes of validity (see "Appendix D" for member feedback provided by 4 participants) and to align analysis with participant feedback.

Results

Analysis traced these participants' experiences of key dimensions of the FBT intervention and ways they engaged in identity negotiations within these treatment contexts, including the reclaiming of identity and voice in matters related to their treatment (see thematic map, Fig. 1).

Theme 1: Therapeutic focus

Participants recounted being both supported and distressed by the focus of Phase 1 of treatment on eating and weight restoration and handing control of these over to

their parents. Of the 4 participants who reported completing the three phases of FBT, 3 concurrently had treatment with an individual therapist (Abbey, Amy & Maisy) and one participant retrospectively described being "taught" strategies by psychologists and dietitians during treatment to assist her with managing distress (Phoenix). Participant narratives highlighted that although FBT was preferred to inpatient treatment for most, when the therapeutic focus was predominantly on AN symptom reduction their emotional distress was obscured and further escalated.

Subtheme 1(a): Focus on the visible

Ten participants' narratives indicated that the early treatment focus of FBT, where their parents took responsibility for their eating, was experienced as a relief, albeit it was also a distressing experience.

EXTRACTS 1

Pheonix: *[...] As much as I hated it, and as much as I just wished for it to be over, it (FBT) did save*

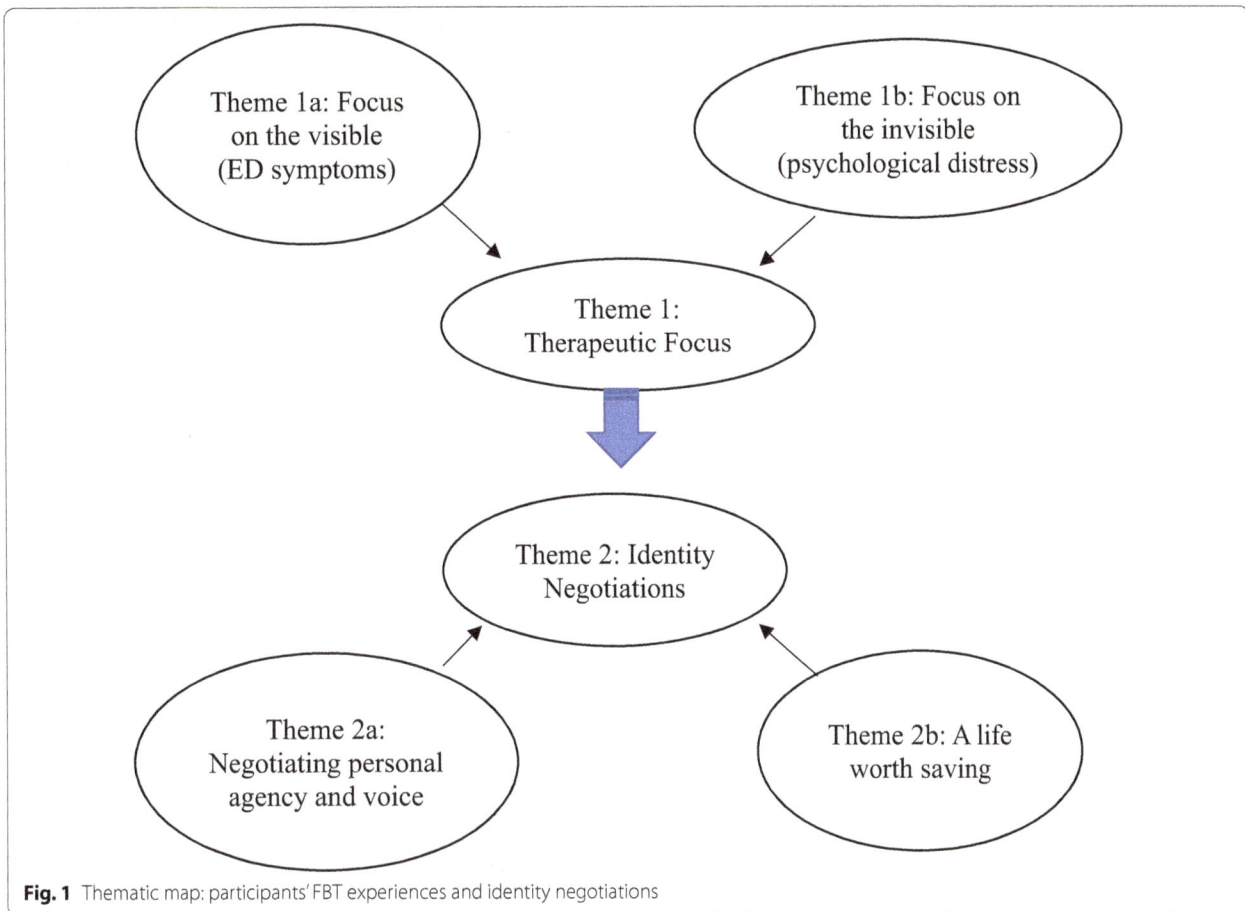

Fig. 1 Thematic map: participants' FBT experiences and identity negotiations

me. *The first few months were extremely distressing [...] Knowing that I had no control whatsoever. [Later in interview] it was sort of down to business, let's do this as quick as possible to get your life back.*

Kate: *It was helpful...that saved my life. 100%. Going to that first appointment, they put me on eating plan. [...] I'm glad that they got someone to be my eyes in that sense because I would not be here today.*

Kaylee: *The whole control aspect, it was, my parents had full control which made me feel real safe.*

Abbey: *[...] cause there was part of me that was, obviously I was fighting it but there was part of me that was like, "Oh thank god" like "I can't get away with it. I just have to like sit and eat this"*

The allocation of responsibility for their eating to their parents was experienced as life-saving for these participants. The marking out of a boundary by which they were no longer responsible for their eating

cultivated for some, a sense of relief and safety (e.g. Kaylee) and the possibility of getting "your life back" from AN, despite also being "extremely distressing" (Phoenix). Furthermore, the sense that others could "be my eyes" (Kate) indicated that these participants valued not only the support but also the alternative perspectives of others in assisting them to take steps to diminish the influence of AN on their lives. This included parents being supported by treatment teams to engage in nutritional nourishment despite a divided sense of self ("part of me ... fighting it"; Abbey). Identified as helpful was when their parents were experienced as a steady support, informed yet understanding, cultivating safety whilst taking control over their eating that contributed to a containment of their distress in the context of the challenging time of nutritional restoration.

Alongside FBT being a life-saving treatment that addressed the medical crisis of AN, the participants also recounted parallel experiences of distress during and post FBT irrespective of extent of their eating and weight restoration and all of them acknowledged the significance of support by others for this distress, including family members.

Theme 1(b): Focus on the invisible

Thirteen of the 14 participants argued that there was a lack of treatment focus on their experiences of psychological distress during FBT, including co-morbid psychological problems (see Table 2). The remaining participant (Maisy) reported FBT was experienced as "extremely pivotal to me getting better" and tailored to her preferences where her siblings attended only the first session. Individual therapy in addition to FBT was experienced for her as both an opportunity to "challenge my thoughts", "learn how to self-soothe" through mindfulness techniques and a motivational intervention that worked "to convince me that recovery was a good thing". She also highlighted the significance of seeing an individual therapist in addition to FBT who was "an outside person [...] different from my parents".

For ten of the participants who reported dropping out prematurely from FBT, an absence of focus on addressing emotional distress and interpersonal struggles was cited as a major contributor to this decision. For example;

EXTRACTS 2

Harley: *Because they never really addressed the underlying problems, it was all so much harder than it probably should have been, because I was still battling with the thoughts and battling with the guilt and all that.*

Charlotte: *My mum does have issues with her eating [...] just made me feel like I was doing the wrong thing as a woman and as a female. [...] my sadness and how much I was hurting would also be expressed as anger[...] a lot of the times I would find it so difficult that I would ask to sit outside [of FBT sessions]. [...] They[parents] hated seeing me so sad and I hated seeing them so sad, and it was just very confronting to have to bring that all up in family therapy and then not really take it further [...] Like we opened old wounds and then they never really got closed and healed.*

Beth: *[...] [...] I never really got a chance to properly, like talk out, like my anger, like with people. Like I never got to just express how I was really feeling, which is probably why I was so angry, because it was all, like building up inside, because I never got to express how I was feeling.*

The inadvertent effect of prioritizing of physical safety in phase 1 of FBT meant that these participants' psychological safety was obscured with the implicit meaning

taken from what was "going on inside" (Hayley) did not matter. For Charlotte, the structure of FBT meant the "old wounds" were opened and not healed, including the parallel process of eating difficulties of women in her family being left unaddressed contributing to an identity conflict where she was left questioning herself and to feelings of "sadness". Implicit in these participants' experiences of anger, was their valued stance and desire for openness within their family systems. They recollected their anger being responded to by being positioned as outsiders to their own therapy, losing their voice with systemic family issues left substantively unaddressed.

Within this context, a different sort of safety issue arose with six of the 14 adolescents reporting suicidal ideation during and/or post FBT treatment.

EXTRACTS 3

Kate: *[...] I never got to the point where I could really end my life but there were feelings of just wanted to end it because it's easier than the voices that are in your head (crying, quite upset) and then you go into these sessions and they're supposed to be sessions where you can let yourself speak your mind and you get time with the psychologist and it's almost like, you just need to sit there and be quiet while everyone talks around you. They're talking about you too (emotional).*

Beth: *I think I didn't, like make it clear how, like depressed I was, and like the feelings of, like wanting to just end it all really. And I would never dare to say that in front of my mum, so I never did. And that's, like kind of one of the things I was struggling with and struggled with it for a long time. And I thought I just never spoke up about it.*

Harley   (further   quote   from   member
checking):*[...] Still to this day because of FBT if there's a situation where I feel like there are links or similarities with control related or people talking at or about me like they did in FBT, my suicidal ideations are triggered. The focus on the impact of my family—which was a big aspect of FBT—as a result of the anorexia contributed to feelings of being a burden and secondarily, at times I wanted to kill myself because the FBT highlighted the damage I was doing to everyone around me.*

These participants argued that nutritional and weight restoration alone did not reduce their psychological distress; distress that continued largely unaddressed for them during the FBT intervention. Kate recollected experiences of a loss of voice where she was recruited into need(ing) "to sit there and be quiet"; Beth actively hid her distress, particularly from her mother; and Harley's feedback on the analysis of her transcript (member checking) emphasized the lasting impression of treatment where being talked "at" or "about" continued to trigger "suicidal ideations" with continued identity associations of herself as a "burden" on others. These participants were active in their arguments that AN treatments need a greater focus on enabling the voicing, holding and processing of their and their family members' emotional distress.

Parallel to the adolescent's distress was family distress and conflict that was also experienced in the context of parents taking responsibility for their eating and weight restoration.

EXTRACTS 4

Rachel: *It [meals] just ended up being hard, plates smashed, tables turned, me punching, kicking and screaming, [...] and then at the end of the time and it'd be like four hours later and we'd both be exhausted; no food would've been eaten.*

Kaylee: *[...] I didn't know who to listen to or who to follow (my parents or my urges) and so those were the destructive ways I dealt with them. For my parents, they wouldn't have known why I was acting out either, as I couldn't verbalise what was happening internally. So they responded to my outburst with screaming and anger and physical restraint towards me because I assume in their eyes, I was just being difficult about eating. Their reaction made the stress in my head even worse and made me even more suicidal, but I don't blame them for how they responded.*

Increased conflict in the family was evident in the participant narratives, with examples cited including angry outbursts with four participants disclosing anger that was physically expressed through parental restraint such as being held down or against a wall. Kaylee clarified that she was not blaming her parents for their responses at the time, that included physical restraint, however, she also recounted how these responses contributed to further distress, including suicidal ideation.

On the other hand, some of the participants talked about their experiences of FBT therapists advocating for them and mobilizing their parental support in ameliorating a sense of being "alone" in addressing AN.

EXTRACTS 5

Amy: *[...] in comparison to me going alone to therapy, my parents are actually getting an insight of where I'm at, [...] the therapist, just to bounce off what I've said, from her conclusion, and what she feels is okay and what's not okay, and um just I guess, in my best interests, what I should be doing, for her then to talk to my parents about it. Like that was—that was good.*

Kaylee: *[...] it definitely did teach my family them some things, and it definitely educated them on what would be helpful for me and what wouldn't be helpful. And I think it was nice not to feel alone; it was nice to have my family there. So, it wasn't just, like by myself.*

Charlotte: *[...] it taught them a lot about the tricks and the way that I was managing my eating disorder and keeping up with hiding food and water loading and making sure that I'd gained such and such amount of weight before the next appointment, [...] and how it manifested itself in different ways, and different habits, and so then they were then able to become a lot more on top of it.*

These extracts exemplify key components of the therapeutic alliance that included FBT therapist advocacy, scaffolding insight into themselves and others' understanding of their experiences (Amy) and ameliorating a sense of being alone in treatment through engagement with families in the intervention (Beth), including in standing together against AN (Charlotte).

Theme 2: Identity negotiations

Alongside the participants' treatment experiences were their parallel identity negotiations that were shaped by their experiences of personal agency and voice throughout treatment and their engagement in the FBT practice of externalisation of the illness (theme 2a). Furthermore, the implicit meanings ascribed to their parents' support was that their life was worth living (theme 2b).

Theme 2(a): Negotiating personal agency and voice

All the participants, at some point in their narratives, talked about struggles to negotiate personal agency and voice in their treatment, particularly in the first phase of FBT where their parents were allocated responsibility for their eating restoration.

EXTRACTS 6

Phoenix: *Because at stage one I definitely felt like a*

Kate: *monkey in a cage and I had no control. My
parents were doing everything for me.*

*[...] I felt tiny. I felt like everyone was over-
powering to me and it was, I would just shut
up and shut down. [...] I just didn't feel like a
person. [...] You feel like you're getting treated
like just someone who's sick...it's not the way
you want to be seen.*

These extracts exemplify the identity negotiations of
participants as they ascribed meaning to their parents
being asked to take responsibility for their eating in the
first phase of FBT. Phoenix's use of the metaphor of a
"monkey in a cage" depicted her experiences of a loss of
personal agency, being monitored and unable to escape.
The participants ascribed a number of negative identity
conclusions in the context of their parents taking responsibility for their eating—for example for Kate this reinforced the identity of herself as a "sick" person that did
not fit with who she understood herself to be.

Furthermore, parent's taking responsibility for their
eating had real effects on some of the participant's relationships with their parents that had unintended impacts
on their sense of themselves as a daughter.

EXTRACTS 7

Lydia: *[...] it [treatment] really fractured our relationship [...] at that point, there was such a
high level of conflict all the time, mutual distrust. [...] , I think I lost my sense of that [self as
person and daughter] and it's almost as though
I regressed and I was um, I was acting how I
was being treated.*

Harley (member checking):

*FBT ruined a previously strong relationship
and caused my parents and siblings their own
psychological unease and detriment. This contributed to a loss of myself and my identity
and resulted in further destructive behaviours.*

A loss of voice was recounted by eight participants in
the context of externalisation of the illness where they
too experienced themselves as externalised with the AN.

EXTRACTS 8

Nora: *[...] just the fact that you had an eating disorder meant they were dismissive of any-
thing you say, they believed anything you
say was completely motivated by the eating disorder [...] I was very distressed by
that because I thought I'm still me, I'm still*

*here, I can recognise that I have anxiety and
unhelpful thoughts but I can still communicate as a person. [...] I'm still me.*

Lydia: *I think to a certain degree, the treatment
team had drilled into them [parents] that
um I was not a person, I was an eating
disorder and giving the reins to an eating
disorder.*

Charlotte: *I was just infuriated that, you know, I'm
trying to say something or have a conversation with my mum, and she's referring
to like anorexia and not Charlotte, telling
Charlotte to come back whenever. Um, and
I was like, "No, listen, like listen to me. I'm
trying to tell you something"—that was very
difficult—I've never really used that separation terminology until probably now, [...] my
eating disorder was me, [...] That was my
talent, that was what I was good at, that's
what I excelled in because I'd lost a lot of
my identity, so I felt that that was my identity. So when—when people would refer to
not say that they were talking to Charlotte
I'd be like, "Are you kidding me?" But now I
can see that that's different and I can see the
difference.*

These extracts exemplify the potential effects of the
FBT practice of externalisation of the illness that led
to the person's voice being assumed by others to be the
AN/ED. This misappropriation of the person's sense of
self ("I'm still me"; Nora) to the disorder by others ("I
was an eating disorder"; Lydia) contributed further to
a loss of voice and exacerbation of distress. Charlotte
traced the problem of externalization when built on
the assumption that it is possible to achieve "separation" of the person from the ED when their identity is
invested in the egosyntonic dimensions of the experience ("I felt that was my identity"). These extracts highlight the unintended consequences and struggles when
the practice of externalization of the illness aimed to
completely separate AN from the person and neglected
to take into consideration the identity investments into
the egosyntonicity of AN.

On the other hand, five of the participants found
the process by which their therapists engaged them to
externalize AN/ED to connect with a sense of identity
outside the AN.

EXTRACTS 9

Phoenix: *[...] as I was restoring weight and as I was
getting better and given more privileges and*

so on that I got to really find out who I was. [...] they made us draw a Venn diagram with two circles. And they named one side "Phoenix" and one side anorexia and then throughout treatment they would make me draw where I thought the circles were overlapping and there was definitely a correlation between the distance of those circles and the amount of weight I restored. As I got healthier, the circles grew further apart and anorexia was separated from me

Rachel: *They just called it, "the eating disorder." [...] And they'd be like, "What would your eating disorder say to this? Now sit in this chair and it'd be like, what would you say to this?" [...] that was helpful, but they just didn't do it enough. Like, it was just so much about food but they needed to care about my feelings.*

Kate: *[...] the other good thing about the FBT method was, they did really try and separate the person from the eating disorder. So you weren't ever talking about, like, you could tell when someone was talking through the voice of the eating disorder or talking through their own voice. That's what they tried to really distinguish.*

Abbey: *The anorexia. This is me genuinely saying something to you. Um, and also just for my own identity, um, and seeing the shift and the balance go. Like my identity increase and that decrease um, that was, that was really helpful. But mainly it was expressing my opinion to others that it was most, most helpful.*

Emerging across these participant narratives was their preference for a person-centred approach where the practice of externalization was focused on the person's identity outside of the AN rather than primarily on elimination of the AN. Phoenix recounted a process of "finding out who I was" through the process of being given "privileges" as she gained weight and tracing her shifting relationship with AN as both individual and overlapping entities. Rachel was invited through a chair technique to have a dialogue with AN to enable her to reclaim her voice and preferences from AN; she argued that her preference was to do more of this work that indicated care for her feelings than being centred on eating. Kate outlined how therapy sought to enable her to distinguish between the voice of the ED and her own voice and Abbey talked

about how externalization enabled her to reclaim both her voice and identity outside of the AN identity.

Theme 2(b): Life is worth saving—"No one was ever going to give up on me"

Interwoven in participant narratives was a process of ascribing meaning to their parent's commitment to their recovery.

EXTRACTS 10

Hayley: *I think I don't want to forget um, (pause), ah how much care I have seen shine through people in this, like my parents have been supportive the whole time and shows how great they are.*

Phoenix: *My parents are really good with supporting me. They keep reassuring me that it's okay. Like, if I'm struggling, they'll be really understanding and they won't force me to do anything that I don't want to do. But they will— they will encourage me.*

Kate: *[...] even though I was really angry and did not want to eat anything, mum would still just sit me down and wait*

Jessica: *[...] your parents do try to—they try their best to like understand what you're going through but it's difficult for them to do that.*

Maisy: *[...] how hard it must have been for my parents and how—what a good job they did to persevere and get me to where I am today.*

The participants ascribed a range of meanings to their parents' support during their treatment, including taking responsibility for their eating in the early phases of FBT. Recollections ranged from parental support and reassurance (Phoenix) and parents' capacity to be with them when emotionally distressed (Kate). Reflecting back, Jessica connected with her parents' efforts to "understand" her experience of AN and Maisy with her parents' perseverance to "get me to where I am today". Furthermore, three participants (Kate, Maisy & Abbey) specifically remembered their parents taking up this role in treatment to avoid them requiring inpatient treatment. These participant experiences highlight the importance of parental support in AN treatments.

For participants who discontinued FBT in the earlier phases, parental support was also noted in their parents' active collaboration with them to find alternative AN treatments that met their needs and preferences, including treatments that focused on addressing their psychological distress.

EXTRACTS 11

Lydia: *I had some serious conversations with my parents and I think that I began to sort of get through to them and I think they to some extent also realised that this really wasn't working, and I needed a different sort of treatment, a different sort of support than what I was receiving.*

Nora: *[...] I would say that our relationship [with her mother] now is better than ever and we are able to reflect on the experience and how traumatic it was and how much we both believe the more sick I am is quite harmful to our family and how great it was when we did get individual psychologists.*

Implicit in both these extracts was the significance of these participants being validated in their treatment needs and preferences and specifically for Nora in "how traumatic" AN and its treatment with FBT and hospitalisations were for her and her family. Furthermore, all the participants talked about the significance of their parents standing for them as a person in the face of AN and its treatment.

EXTRACTS 12

Maisy: *[...] my parents [...] were always there telling me that I would get through this and that I was a strong person and—and that no one was ever going to give up on me.*

Kate: *Oh, she's [Mum] just awesome! Like, she is always advocating for my best interest.*

Charlotte: *I don't want to forget that even though, ah, it was very, very traumatising for me, um, that I still have my family and they still stand by me and I stand by them, and even though we went through such a terrible and awful time, um, we still love each other and have each other's backs during the worst and best periods of our lives. That's what I—what I wouldn't want to forget".*

Amy: *Accept the changes that are necessary because ultimately, at the end of the day, people just care about you and they care so much about you that they're going to put you through this. And it's going to be hard, it's going to be really hard, but as soon as you come out the other side and start living your life again and being healthy, the thoughts go away.*

These narratives highlight the significance of the parents standing for these individuals in cultivating a sense

of teamwork (Abbey), care (Amy, Phoenix), and that they were not alone (Beth, Jessica). Implicit in all the adolescent narratives was that their parents' commitment to them and their treatment was hope for their futures and the sense that their lives were worth saving—for example, as depicted by Maisy—"no one was going to give up on me".

Discussion

Family-Based Treatment continues to be the frontline treatment for adolescent AN in Australia, although the evidence for it's effectiveness in addressing both the physical and psychological symptoms of AN is incomplete. This study sought to understand and give voice to the experiences of adolescents who had either dropped out of FBT or continued to be distressed post-treatment to inform future treatment interventions and research. These young women reported that family support in the context of the treatment was instrumental in saving their lives and contributed to the sense that they were not alone and mattered as a person. Nutritional restoration is non-negotiable [50] in the early stages of any AN intervention to prevent potentially adverse medical outcomes [51]; however, this study has highlighted that delaying interventions to address the individuals' psychological distress, including in the early stages of treatment, contributed to a loss of voice and/or an exacerbation of their distress. This is consistent with more recent FBT research that has demonstrated the imperative of early treatment focus on not only adolescent weight gain, but also the therapeutic addressing of difficult emotions, criticism of parents towards their child and the alliance between the adolescent/family and the FBT therapist [16].

The current study found the majority of the participants experienced a loss of voice, particularly in the early stages of FBT. This was evident in contexts where their voice was assumed to be the voice of the illness/AN (by parents and/or therapists) thereby externalizing their identities with the AN [24]. Notable in this process, was a disordering of their identities where they were assumed to be incapable of having a valid voice or perspective on their own lives. Furthermore, the neglect of any substantive focus on their psychological distress in the early stages of treatment set the precedent that their internal struggles were of lesser significance. This lack of focus on their psychological distress was cited as a major reason for treatment drop out. Other responses included anger and disengagement from treatment with the sense of themselves as outsiders to their own treatment. This concern has been echoed by Greg Dring [23]:

[...] if the therapist spends the first sixteen sessions of the work discouraging the discussion of feelings,

relationship issues and developmental difficulties in a personal way, then it may be very difficult to revive such discussion at a later stage when, in any case, the work is about to be concluded (p. 66).

The participants' narratives also exemplified how the early treatment focus of FBT on adolescent nutritional restitution inadvertently risked obscuring not only the young persons' distress but also their family's systemic distress, which had a recursive effect on their emotional distress. The efforts of parents (as supported by therapists) to encourage their child's nutritional restoration therefore, at times, unintentionally may have diverted their focus away from holding their child's less visible, emotional distress. Furthermore, the participants recounted distress and interpersonal strain on their family relationships in the context of parents taking responsibility for their nutritional restoration. It is important to note that some of the parental responses reported by the participants are contraindicated and proscribed in FBT (for example, parental physical restraint). Some of the participants' experiences highlight possible challenges of parents taking responsibility for their adolescent child's eating, including whether the ends of adolescent weight gain justify the therapeutic means by which this may be achieved [24], and the imperative of FBT therapists prioritizing the building of a therapeutic alliance [16]. Important in this alliance is a safe context for adolescents and their families to disclose interpersonal difficulties, and that therapists have skills in addressing family conflict, should this arise. Furthermore, in prioritizing the therapeutic alliance, the implementation of the intervention may align more closely with the adolescents preferences for a greater therapeutic focus on addressing intra and inter-personal distress throughout treatment.

Contrary to expectations, the therapeutic alliance, measured by the researcher-rating of the therapeutic alliance (WAI-o), has not been found to be related to AN symptom remission with FBT in previous research [18, 19]. This is a counterintuitive finding when considered with other areas of psychological research where the therapeutic alliance has been shown to predict psychotherapy outcomes more broadly in children and adolescents [52]. The therapeutic alliance is a complex construct and the WAI-o instrument may have been measuring an aspect of the treatment alliance that is not associated with outcomes for FBT with adolescents experiencing AN. At this stage we do not know. It is an interesting finding that needs further research. However, in keeping with others who have highlighted the importance of listening to a person's preferences out of respect for their 'rights and dignity' and to optimise treatment outcomes [53], this present study indicated that participants valued

a strong therapeutic alliance, albeit this may not translate into outcomes that requires additional research. Therefore, the differences between this and these previous FBT studies may be the methods of assessing and reporting therapeutic alliance and perhaps the construct itself.

Furthermore, the present study findings are consistent with Sibeoni et al. [54] who found that for 15 adolescents who had engaged in both outpatient and inpatient treatment for AN, the therapeutic alliance was facilitated by: the adolescent perception of the treatment team as authentic where they felt heard and understood, themselves and their parents playing an active role in their treatment, time to develop trust with the treatment team with the adolescent-parent relationship as 'the central element of the therapeutic alliance'. These findings are similar to the experiences of the adolescents in this study, including the importance of a safe therapeutic context to voice their experiences and concerns and to address these, including family difficulties and conflict, should these arise.

The findings of this study are also consistent with Medway and Rhodes' [36] meta-synthesis into adolescent experiences of family therapy for AN who concluded that psychological interventions for adolescent AN would benefit from scope for interventions that focus more comprehensively on underlying adolescent and family issues. This may go some way to ameliorate the ongoing psychological distress post treatment reported in the current and prior studies [29] and may also prevent the progression on to severe and enduring AN for some [55].

Aspects of the FBT experience were also cited as important in participant recovery journeys. These included parental understanding of their AN experience and standing for them as a person, being treated outside of an inpatient setting, and clarifying a sense of identity outside of the AN identity or "find(ing) out who I was" (Phoenix). These participant experiences highlight the importance of addressing questions of identity in AN treatments [41, 42] and how externalization as an intervention may, in some contexts, facilitate this process. On the other hand, in contexts where the adolescent themselves was excluded from the process of discernment and naming of the AN, externalisation was experienced as invalidating rather than having the intended effect of empowering the person to reclaim their identity from AN [56].

A number of adolescents in this current study reported comorbid depression, anxiety, and/or OCD and all the participants reported experiencing ongoing psychological difficulties irrespective of weight restoration. This is in contrast to recent research that has shown a significant reduction in co-morbid major depressive disorder, generalized anxiety disorder and panic disorder; proposed in those for whom these conditions are likely to be secondary to malnutrition [57]. Notably, a third of participants retrospectively reported escalating suicide risk during the treatment intervention. This is of concern, given the findings that half of all deaths in AN result from suicide [3, 4]. Consistent with previous research [36] and an Australian Broadcasting Commission medical report in 2017 (https://www.abc.net.au/news/2017-05-04/australian-health-system-failing-patients-with-eating-disorders/8485300), the participants in this study argued for more holistic approaches to AN treatments and that, in their experiences, there was limited scope for FBT to be tailored to their individual needs and preferences, thereby contributing to the decision for some of the participants to cease treatment prematurely and/or continuance of ongoing psychological distress post-treatment.

The importance of addressing an adolescents' psychological distress has been increasingly recognized over the past decade with a number of FBT treatment augmentations being proposed and researched. These have included multi-family therapy [58, 59], parent-to-parent consultations [60], separated-family therapy [61], addition of psychological interventions such as CBT [62] and Dialectical Behavior Therapy (DBT) [63] and therapist guided internet chat rooms [64]. These augmentations have tended to focus on changing the context of treatment, providing additional or novel means of support in addition to treatment as usual, particularly for parents [65], rather than augmentation to the structure and/or transformation of content of the treatment intervention itself. The structural augmentation to separate parent and adolescent sessions, particularly in phase one of FBT, has found similar weight gain outcomes, irrespective of whether the adolescent is involved in the early phases, with increased retention and remission rates for some adolescents [14]. Furthermore, the majority of augmentations involve phase one only and are reflective of the reluctance to change or 'tamper' with the manualized intervention, despite the call for more 'potent augmentations' to improve outcomes [60]. There continues, however, to be a paucity of researched interventions that have scope to transform the landscape of treatment options for anorexia nervosa.

Clinical questions

This research study has explored the treatment preferences of 14 adolescents who either dropped out or continued with psychological distress post FBT and the following questions need to be interpreted in light of this. These participants' experiences prompt consideration of the following questions by clinicians and researchers in relation to future treatment interventions for adolescent AN:

(1) What is going on for the adolescent, including their emotional life [23]?

(2) How might the adolescent's' voice [23] and personal agency be prioritized as they undertake the challenging task of nutritional restoration in the early stages of treatment within a treatment non-negotiable framework [50]?;

(3) What is going on for the family and how might problematic family dynamics, including family conflict, be addressed?

(4) At what point and how do therapists assess whether the allocation of responsibility to the parents is working and when this intervention might be contraindicated for an individual family?;

(5) How might interventions more comprehensively address complex identity negotiations for adolescents and their family members? [45]; and

(6) To what extent might interventions be flexibly tailored to the adolescent and family needs and preferences within a treatment non-negotiable framework [50] that prioritizes and supports the adolescent's physical and psychological safety?

Furthermore, future treatments might consider what is already becoming increasingly recognized, that family treatments for adolescent AN need to consider behavioural, psychological symptomology and family functioning in parallel and to map treatment effectiveness to these outcome measures [26].

Study strengths and limitations

The current study recruited a population of whom the majority had either dropped out and/or continued with ongoing psychological distress post treatment with FBT. Qualitative papers are, by design, in-depth investigations of small samples. However, it is usual to continue to interview or seek data until thematic saturation is reached. As the wording of the advertisement indicated inclusion of those who had discontinued FBT, this may have inadvertently excluded participants who continued to experience psychological distress post FBT suggesting that further research on this group is indicated. With this targeted recruitment of participants there exists a risk of negative bias in participants' recollection of their FBT treatment experiences in the event that participants subsequently engaged in more positively experienced treatments. On the other hand, this study goes some way in mitigating against the risk of positive bias in participant recollection of their treatment experiences that may arise in the context of a positive outcome and recovery. Another strength of the study was two author extraction of data to reduce the risk of bias in interpretation of the transcript data. Furthermore, the scope of this study is in the development of a better understanding of why FBT does work for all and why.

Negative experiences in a treatment intervention are important to understanding, however, empirical study of methods of change are required to suggest modifications to treatment that may lead to improved outcomes. It is not possible to know whether, if these adolescents' treatment preferences had been met at the time of treatment with FBT, treatment outcomes would have been improved. Also unknown were the skills and training of the FBT therapists' who delivered the individual interventions, including their capacity to build a therapeutic alliance and address the adolescent and/or family's distress.

What is known, is that the findings would suggest further research is needed to test, and find ways to test, the clinical questions that have been raised in this paper in regard to improving both treatment engagement and outcomes for adolescent AN. Future research may also seek to conduct similar research to explore the experiences and perspectives from a more diverse group of adolescents with a lived experience of adolescent AN. Further research would benefit from qualitative data triangulation (from multiple sources including adolescent, parent and clinician experiences of FBT) for completeness, convergence and dissonance of the key themes identified in this paper.

Concluding remarks

This current study highlights the complexity that is involved in the treatment of adolescent AN and consideration of systemic family issues, adolescent psychological distress and identity formation in family-based treatments. Many adolescents experience physical and psychological symptom improvement with FBT. Nevertheless, the need for greater focus on addressing psychological distress, in all phases of treatment, was identified by all the adolescents in this study as putative changes that would improve experiences and outcomes in AN treatments. Further research is needed to extend the current findings, including the tailoring of treatment to the adolescent and family needs and preferences [66] and addressing more comprehensively questions of identity, and how they may be applied in the development and evaluation of transformative AN treatment interventions.

Appendix A
Research study advertisement

This study is interested in hearing the voices of those who have experienced Family-based therapy for anorexia nervosa and decided for whatever reason to not continue in this treatment. We are interested in hearing what it was like for you and your family to experience Family-Based

Therapy for anorexia nervosa as we believe that your experiences are important to consider when developing new ways of treating anorexia.

Appendix B
Interview schedule
A selection of questions will be used with each participant and questions will scaffold between.

- Experience (e.g. Can you tell me about ...?)
- Meaning (What does ... mean to you?)
- Identity (e.g. How does ... have you seeing yourself as a person, what does this say to you about what matters to you as a parent/what is important to you/what you value?)
- Positioning on experience/identity conclusion (e.g. is this OK for you or not? Why?)

(A) Interview will be augmented with a timeline for narrative/discourse

1. Can you tell me your story of anorexia?
2. When did anorexia start to have an impact on your life? What was this like for you as a person? And as a child in your family? How did this have you seeing yourself as a person? Was this helpful or not? Why?
3. As you look back on your experiences of anorexia*, which events stand out in your mind?
4. As you look even further back before anorexia*, which events stand out in your mind?
5. Can you tell me a bit about your relationship with anorexia now? How does this affect your life? Relationships? How you see yourself as a person/child?
6. Do you consider your relationship with anorexia* to be problematic for you now? If so, how? If not, why?
7. What does having experienced anorexia mean to you as a person?
8. Has your life changed with your experience of anorexia*? What have you got in touch with yourselves as a person/daughter/son?

(B) Experiences of Family-Based treatment

1. How did you come to be involved in Family-Based treatment (FBT)?
2. Can you tell me about your experiences of FBT?
3. What was most helpful about FBT? Why?
4. What was least helpful about FBT? Why?
5. Did you complete FBT? Why or why not?
6. Did FBT assist you to shift your relationship with anorexia?

7. Overall, what stands out for you if you reflect on what impacts FBT had on you? Was this helpful or not? Why?
8. How has participating in the FBT affected how you see yourself as a person? Is this helpful or not? Why?

Then ask questions from (C) OR (D)
(C) If the adolescent/family completed FBT

1. When did you finish FBT?
2. What has your relationship with anorexia been like since you completed FBT? How has this been for you as a person and as a family since discontinuing FBT?

OR
(D) If the adolescent/family discontinued FBT

1. At what phase of FBT did you discontinue treatment?
2. What has your relationship with anorexia been like since then? How has this been for you as a person and as a family since discontinuing FBT?
3. Can you tell us about the circumstances/your experiences that led you to no longer continue with FBT?
4. Looking back how do you make sense of why you chose not to continue with FBT?
5. Are you settled with the decision or not? Why?
6. Did you have any fears/concerns about what might happen if you were to continue or discontinue with FBT?
7. What were you hoping for as you made the decision to cease FBT?

(E) Questions to all participants regardless of whether completed or discontinued FBT

1. What do you want to not forget about yourself from the FBT?
2. What might be important for another person/family to know as they commence FBT?
3. What advice might you give to a person or family who is about to start FBT?
4. What would you like more of in future treatments for anorexia? What would you like less of in future treatments for anorexia nervosa? What does this say to you about what matters for you/your child/ your family?
5. Do you have hopes for future treatment/therapy in terms of the sort of work you would like to engage in? What does this say to you about what you value as a person?
6. Has our conversation today been helpful or unhelpful or both? Why?

7. What has stood out for you from our conversation today?
8. What might be important for us not to forget as we analyse the data from this interview?

Appendix C
Researcher positioning statements
Janet Conti: I am a Clinical Psychologist, Dietitian and academic in Clinical Psychology. My research and clinical work seeks to prioritise the voice of the experiencing person to inform the development of a greater number of effective treatment inteventions for AN that are tailored to the needs and preferences of the experiencing person and their family. This research is one arm of a larger research project that is aimed to give voice to adolescents, parents and the clinicians who treat them about their experience of FBT as the first line of treatment for adolescent AN in Australia.

Caroline Joyce: I am an academic in medicine with a background in Health Psychology. My research explores the impact of psychosocial factors on people adjusting to illness and chronic diseases. I am particularly interested in how psychological distress impacts treatment adherence and recovery from illness to better understand more effective treatments.

Simone Natoli: I am a Clinical Psychologist currently working in private practice with a number of clients diagnosed with eating disorders. I have an interest in understanding the best treatments available and how to maximise treatment outcomes. Understanding the factors contributing to poor treatment outcomes is an important part of this approach.

Kelsey Skeoch: I am a Clinical Psychologist currently working in a Child and Adolescent Mental Health Service for the National Health Service (NHS) in the United Kingdom. I have a keen interest in the mental health of children and young people, and in particular how the systems in which young people live and access, can both promote and hinder treatmemt outcomes.

Phillipa Hay: I am an academic Psychiatrist with long-standing clincial and research experience in the treatment of people with anorexia nervosa. I am very interested to explore and understand better how to improve treatments, reduce distress during treatment, and in particular to better understand why some people have poor outcomes.

Appendix D
Participant member check feedback (participant pseudonyms)
Lydia: I have read over the paper and am happy with the way my testimony has been used. Thank you for keeping

it authentic. I eagerly await publication of the final paper. I feel it will prove instructive for my parents, going forward.

Harley: Addition to extract 2: "The FBT Program in my opinion has a narrow focus on food and weight restoration, rather than overall psychological wellbeing. For me it was harder than what it should have been because FBT unmasked other psychological issues which the anorexia had been used to deal with. The 'manualised' program approach failed to accommodate individual needs".

Amy: It looks great though, very interesting report.

Charlotte: I am happy with the paper and would be most grateful to receive a copy of the paper if published. Thank you very much for including me in the study.

(Note: Some participants were unable to be contacted).

Abbreviations
AN: Anorexia Nervosa; ED: Eating Disorder; DBT: Dialectical Behavior Therapy; FBT: Family-Based Treatment; OCD: Obessive Compulsive Disorder.

Acknowledgements
The authors would like to acknowledge the collaborative work of the following researchers who contributed to the paper by Conti et al. (2017) that formed a foundation for the analysis of this paper: Dr. Daphne Hewson (formerly Macquarie University), Professor Tanya Meade (Western Sydney University), Dr Jamie Calder (Australian Catholic University), A/Professor Paul Rhodes (Sydney University) Sara Cibralic (SC) (formerly Western Sydney University) and Emma Sheens (formerly University of Sydney).

Authors' information
JC is a Senior Lecturer in Clinical Psychology at Western Sydney University, CJ is a Lecturer in the School of Medicine at Western Sydney University , SN is a Clinical Psychologist working in private practice, KS is a Clinical Psychologist working in the NHS, UK, and PH is a Professor of Medicine at Western Sydney University.

Authors' contributions
Each of the authors have made substantive contributions to this paper. JC conceived this research, interviewed participants, analysed the data, co-wrote and edited the manuscript. CJ analysed the data and contributed to the discussion, SN and KS analysed the data and contributed some of the sections of the paper, PH contributed to all sections of the paper including final editing. All authors read and approved the final manuscript.

Competing interests
The authors declares that they have no competing interests.

Author details
[1] School of Psychology and Translational Research Institute, Western Sydney University, Locked Bag 1797, Penrith 2751, Australia. [2] School of Psychology, Western Sydney University, Penrith, Australia. [3] Chair of Mental Health, School of Medicine, Translational Health Research Institute, Western Sydney University, Penrith, Australia.

References
1. American Psychiatric Association. Diagnostic and statistical manual of mental disorders. 5th ed. Washington: American Psychiatric Association; 2013.
2. Keski-Rahkonen A, Hoek HW, Susser ES, Linna MS, Sihvola E, Raevuori A, et al. Epidemiology and course of anorexia nervosa in the community. Am J Psychiatry. 2007;164(8):1259–65.
3. Arcelus J, Mitchell AJ, Wales J, Nielsen S. Mortality rates in patients with anorexia nervosa and other eating disorders: a meta-analysis of 36 studies. Arch Gen Psychiatry. 2011;6(7):724–31.
4. Crow S, Peterson CB, Swanson S, Raymond N, Specker S, Eckert ED, et al. Increased mortality in bulimia nervosa and other eating disorders. Am J Psychiatry. 2009;166(12):1342–6.
5. Keel PK, Klump K, Miller K, McGue M, Iacono WG. Shared transmission of eating disorders and anxiety disorders. Int J Eat Disord. 2005;38(2):99–105.
6. Steinhausen HC. The outcome of anorexia nervosa in the 20th century. Am J Psychiatry. 2002;159:1284–93.
7. Gregertsen EC, Mandy W, Serpell L. The egosyntonic nature of anorexia: an impediment to recovery in anorexia nervosa treatment. Front Psych. 2017;8:2273.
8. Fassino S, Pierò A, Tomba E, Abbate-Daga G. Factors associated with dropout from treatment for eating disorders: comprehensive literature review. BMC Psychiatry. 2009;9(1–9):67.
9. Lock J, Le Grange D. Treatment manual for anorexia nervosa: a family-based approach. New York: Guilford; 2013.
10. Zeeck A, Herpertz-Dahlmann B, Friederich H, Brockmeyer T, Resmark G, Hagenah U, et al. Psychotherapeutic treatment for Anorexia Nervosa: A systematic review and network meta-analysis. Front Psychiatry. 2018;0:1–14.
11. Murray SB, Thornton C, Wallis A. A thorn in the side of evidence-based treatment for adolescent anorexia nervosa. Aust N Z J Psychiatry. 2012;46(11):1026–8.
12. Lock J, Le Grange D, Agras WS, Moye A, Bryson SW, Jo B. Randomized clinical trial comparing family-based treatment with adolescent-focused individual therapy for adolescents with anorexia nervosa. Arch Gen Psychiatry. 2010;67(10):1025–32.
13. Agras W, Lock J, Brandt H, Bryson S, Dodge E, Halmi K, et al. Comparison of 2 family therapies for adolescent anorexia nervosa: a randomized parallel trial. JAMA Psychiat. 2014;72(11):1279–86.
14. Le Grange D, Hughes EK, Court A, Yeo M, Crosby R, Sawyer SM. Randomized clinical trial of parent-focused treatment and family-based treatment for adolescent anorexia nervosa. J Am Acad Child Adolesc Psychiatry. 2016;55(8):683–92.
15. Allan E, Le Grange D, Sawyer SM, McLean LA, Hughes EK. Parental expressed emotion during two forms of family-based treatment for adolescent anorexia nervosa. Eur Eat Disord Rev. 2017;26(1):46–52.
16. Hughes EK, Sawyer SM, Accurso E, Singh S, Le Grange D. Predictors of early response in conjoint and separated models of family-based treatment for adolescent anorexia nervosa. Eur Eat Disord Rev. 2019;27(3):283–94.
17. Tichenor V, Hill CE. A comparison of six measures of working alliance. Psychotherapy. 1989;26:195–9.
18. Forsberg S, Lo Tempio E, Bryson S, Fitzpatrick KK, Le Grange D, Lock J. Therapeutic alliance in two treatments for adolescent anorexia nervosa. Int J Eat Disord. 2013;46:34–8.
19. Lo Tempio E, Forsberg S, Bryson S, Fitzpatrick KK, Le Grange D, Lock J. Patients' characteristics and the quality of the therapeutic alliance in family-based treatment and individual therapy for adolescents with anorexia nervosa. J Fam Ther. 2013;35:29–52.
20. Pereira T, Lock J, Oggins J. Role of therapeutic alliance in family therapy for adolescent anorexia nervosa. Int J Eat Disord. 2006;39:677–94.
21. Scarborough J. Family-based therapy for pediatric anorexia nervosa: highlighting the implementation challenges. Fam J. 2018;26(1):90–8.
22. Smith A, Cook-Cottone C. A review of family therapy as an effective intervention for anorexia nervosa in adolescents. J Clin Psychol Med Settings. 2011;18(4):323–34.

23. Dring G. Finding a voice: family therapy for young people with anorexia. London: Karnac; 2015.

24. Conti JE, Calder J, Cibralic S, Meade T, Hewson D. "Somebody else's roadmap". Lived experience of Maudsley and Family-Based therapy for anorexia nervosa. Aust N Z J Fam Therapy. 2017;38:405–29.

25. Wallis A, Miskovic-Wheatley J, Madden S, Alford C, Rhodes P, Touyz S. Does continuing family-based treatment for adolescent anorexia nervosa improve outcomes in those not remitted after 20 sessions? Clin Child Psychol Psychiatry. 2018;23(4):592–600.

26. Fisher CA, Skocic S, Rutherford KA, Hetrick SE. Family therapy approaches for anorexia nervosa (Review). Cochrane Datab Syst Rev. 2019(5):Art. No.: CD004780.

27. Dalle Grave R, Eckhardt SG, Calugi S, Le Grange D. A conceptual comparison of family-based treatment and enhanced cognitive behavior therapy in the treatment of adolescents with eating disorders. J Eat Disord. 2019;7(42):1–9.

28. DeJong H, Broadbent H, Schmidt U. A systematic review of dropout from treatment in outpatients with anorexia nervosa. Int J Eat Disord. 2012;45(5):635–47.

29. Lock J, Couturier J, Agras WS. Comparison of long-term outcomes in adolescents with anorexia nervosa treated with family therapy. J Am Acad Child Adolesc Psychiatry. 2006;45(6):666–72.

30. Le Grange D, Lock J, Agras WS, Moye A, Bryson SW, Jo B, et al. Moderators and mediators of remission in family-based treatment and adolescent focused therapy for anorexia nervosa. Behav Res Ther. 2012;50(2):85–92.

31. Lock J, Agras WS, Bryson S, Kraemer HC. A comparison of short-and long-term family therapy for adolescent anorexia nervosa. J Am Acad Child Adolesc Psychiatry. 2005;44(7):632–9.

32. Franko DL, Tabri N, Keshaviah A, Murray HB, Herzog DB, Thomas JJ, et al. Predictors of long-term recovery in anorexia nervosa and bulimia nervosa: data from a 22-year longitudinal study. J Psychiatr Res. 2018;96:183–8.

33. Dalle Grave R, Calugi S, Doll H, Fairburn CG. Enhanced cognitive behaviour therapy for adolescents with anorexia nervosa: an alternative to family therapy? Behav Res Ther. 2013;51(1):R9–12.

34. Dalle Grave R, Sartirana M, Calugi S. Enhanced cognitive behavioral therapy for adolescents with anorexia nervosa: Outcomes and predictors of change in a real-world setting. Int J Eat Disord. 2019;52(9):1042–6.

35. Le Grange D, Eckhardt SG, Dalle Grave R, Crosby RD, Peterson CB, Keery H, et al. Enhanced cognitive-behavior therapy and family-based treatment for adolescents with an eating disorder: a non-randomized effectiveness trial. Psychol Med. 2020:1–11.

36. Medway M, Rhodes P. Young people's expeirence of family thearpy for anorexia nervosa: a qualitative meta-synthesis. Adv Eat Disord Theory Res Pract. 2016;4(2):189–207.

37. Krautter T, Lock J. Is manualized family-based treatment for adolescent anorexia nervosa acceptable to patients? Patient satisfaction at the end of treatment. J Fam Ther. 2004;26(1):66–82.

38. Chen EY, le Grange D, Doyle AC, Zaitsoff S, Doyle P, Roehrig JP, et al. A case series of family-based therapy for weight restoration in young adults with anorexia nervosa. J Contemp Psychother. 2010;40(4):219–24.

39. le Grange D, Gelman T. Patients' perspective of treatment in eating disorders: a preliminary study. S Afr J Psychol. 1998;28(3):182–6.

40. Murray SB, Quintana DS, Loeb K, Griffiths S, Le Grange D. Treatment outcomes for anorexia nervosa: a systematic review and meta-analysis of randomized controlled trials. Psychol Med. 2018;49:535–54.

41. Conti JE, Joyce C, Hay P, Meade T. "Finding my own identity": a qualitative metasynthesis of adult anorexia nervosa treatment experiences. BMC Psychol. 2020;8:110.

42. Espindola CR, Blay SL. Anorexia nervosa treatment from the patient perspective: a metasynthesis of qualitative studies. Ann Clin Psychiatry. 2009;21(1):38–48.

43. Braun V, Clarke V. Using thematic analysis in psychology. Qual Res Psychol. 2006;3(2):77–101.

44. Edley N. Analysing masculinity: interpretative repertoires, ideological dilemmas and subject positions. In: Wetherell M, Taylor S, Yates SJ, editors. Discourse as data: a guide for analysis. London: Sage; 2001. p. 189–224.

45. Wufong E, Rhodes P, Conti JE. "We don't really know what else we can do". When adolescent distress persists after the Maudsley and family-based therapies for anorexia nervosa: parent experiences. J Eat Disord. 2019;7(5):1–18.

46. Aradas J, Sales D, Rhodes P, Conti JE. "As long as they eat?" Therapist experiences, dilemmas and identity negotiations of Maudsley and Family-Based Therapy for Adolescent Anorexia Nervosa. J Eat Disord. 2019;7(26):1–12.

47. Potter J, Wetherell M. Discourse and social psychology: beyond attitudes and behaviour. London: Sage; 1987.

48. Wetherell M. Positioning and interpretative repertoires: conversation analysis and post-structuralism in dialogue. Discourse Soc. 1998;9(3):387–412.

49. Burr V. Social constructionism. New York: Routledge; 2015.

50. Geller J, Srikameswaran S. Treatment non-negotiables: why we need them and how to make them work. Eur Eat Disord Rev. 2006;14:212–7.

51. Tan JOA, Stewart A, Fitzpatrick R, Hope T. Competence to make treatment decisions in anorexia nervosa: thinking and processes and values. Philos Psychiatry Psychol. 2006;13(4):267–82.

52. Karver MC, De Nadai AS, Monahan M, Shirk SR. Meta-analysis of the prospective relation between alliance and outcome in child and adolescent psychotherapy. Psychotherapy. 2018;55(4):341–55.

53. Swift JK, Mullins RH, Penix EA, Roth KL, Trusty WT. The importance of listening to patient preferences when making mental health care decisions. World Psychiatry. 2021;20(3):315–451.

54. Sibeoni J, Verneuil L, Poulmarc'h L, Orri M, Jean E, Podlipski M, et al. Obstacles and facilitators of therapeutic alliance among adolescents with anorexia nervosa, their parents and their psychiatrists: a qualitative study. Clin Child Psychol Psychiatry. 2020;25(1):16–21.

55. Touyz SW, Hay P. Severe and enduring anorexia nervosa (SE-AN): in search of a new paradigm. J Eat Disord. 2015;3(26):1–3.

56. White M. Narrative practice: continuing the conversations. New York: W.W. Norton; 2011.

57. Trainor C, Gorrell S, Hughes EK, Sawyer SM, Burton C, Le Grange D. Family-based treatment for adolescent anorexia nervosa: What happens to rates of comorbid diagnoses? Eur Eat Disord Rev. 2020;28:351–7.

58. Asen E. Multiple family therapy: an overview. J Fam Ther. 2002;24(1):3–16.

59. Dare C, Eisler I. A multi-family group day treatment programme for adolescent eating disorder. Eur Eat Disord Rev. 2000;8(1):856.

60. Rhodes P, Baillee A, Brown J, Madden S. Can parent-to-parent consultation improve the effectiveness of the Maudsley model of family-based treatment for anorexia nervosa? A randomized control trial. J Fam Ther. 2008;30(1):96–108.

61. Eisler I, Simic M, Russell GFM, Dare C. A randomised controlled treatment trial of two forms of family therapy in adolescent anorexia nervosa: a five-year follow-up. J Child Psychol Psychiatry. 2007;48(6):552–60.

62. Hurst K, Read S, Wallis A. Anorexia nervosa in adolescence and Maudsley family-based treatment. J Couns Dev. 2012;90(3):339–45.

63. Johnston JAY, O'Gara JSX, Koman SL, Baker CW, Anderson DA. A pilot study of Maudsley family therapy with group dialectical behavior therapy skills training in an intensive outpatient program for adolescent eating disorders. J Clin Psychol. 2015;71(6):527–43.

64. Binford Hopf RB, Le Grange D, Moessner M, Bauer S. Internet-based chat support groups for parents in family-based treatment for adolescent eating disorders: a pilot study. Eur Eat Disord Rev. 2013;21(3):215–23.

65. Richards I, Subar A, Touyz S, Rhodes P. Augmentative approaches in family-based treatment for adolescents with restrictive eating disorders: a systematic review. Eur Eat Disord Rev. 2018;26:92–111.

66. Norcross JC. Psychotherapy relationships that work: Evidence-based responsiveness. 2nd ed. New York: Oxford University Press; 2011.

14

Challenging Rigidity in Anorexia (Treatment, Training and Supervision): Questioning Manual Adherence in the Face of Complexity

Annaleise Robertson[1]* [ID] and Chris Thornton[2]

Abstract

Background: Anorexia Nervosa is a debilitating illness. While there have been many advancements to treatment protocols and outcomes for people with eating disorders, the field acknowledges there remains considerable room for improvement. This timely Special Edition of the Journal of Eating Disorders has invited those of us in the field to consider a range of topics in aid of this task, including potential modifications and implementation of evidence-based practice, specific and common psychotherapy factors, treatment manuals, adherence and individualising treatment approaches for individuals and families.

Body: In this paper, we briefly outline the key manualised treatments currently available to treat children, adolescents and adults with Anorexia Nervosa, considering the benefits, potential reasons for adaptations and limitations. We then review the current evidence for training strict adherence to treatment manuals which is often a key focus in training and supervision, questioning the association of increased treatment adherence with improved therapeutic outcome. We then summarise some key evidence behind other therapeutic factors which have been demonstrated to affect outcome regardless of which manual is implemented, such as readiness to change and therapeutic alliance.

Conclusion: The paper concludes with implications and considerations for future research, clinical guidelines, training and supervision, highlighting the need to consider the therapeutic relationship and processes alongside manual content to conduct best evidence-informed practice.

Plain English summary

While there have been many advancements to treatment options and recovery rates for people with eating disorders, the field acknowledges there remains a long way to go. The development of treatment manuals for clinicians to use has many benefits, including promoting rigorous research, clear training and clinical guidelines, broader dissemination and accessibility, a common language for professionals, platforms from which to research necessary adaptations, and a set of core treatment principles. While it is often assumed that strict adherence to manuals will lead to the best treatment outcomes, research tells us a different story; that working flexibly and collaboratively with service users in an individually tailored way, focusing on meeting them where they're at, and building trust and understanding between them may actually be the best way to improve treatment experience and outcomes. This paper highlights the need for this way of working to be embraced as a crucial part of evidence-informed practice, with some suggestions for further research, treatment guidelines, training and supervision provided.

*Correspondence: annaleise.robertson@health.nsw.gov.au
The Children's Hospital at Westmead, Sydney, Australia
Full list of author information is available at the end of the article

Keywords: Eating disorders, Anorexia nervosa, Adherence, Manuals, Training, Supervision, Evidence-based practice, Therapeutic alliance

Background

Anorexia Nervosa (AN) is a debilitating illness. While there have been many advancements to treatment protocols and outcomes for people with eating disorders, the field acknowledges there remains considerable room for improvement [1]. Positively, manualised treatments such as Family Based Treatment (FBT) [2, 3] and Enhanced Cognitive Behaviour Therapy (CBT-E) [4, 5] have enabled a wider breadth of outcome research and clinical training to be implemented, and the development of fundamental principles for clinical practice and training standards both nationally [6–8] and worldwide [9, 10]. In this paper, we explore the evidence for training strict adherence to treatment manuals, considering the benefits, potential reasons for adaptations and limitations. We then outline evidence behind other therapeutic factors which have been demonstrated to impact outcome regardless of which manual is implemented, such as readiness to change and therapeutic alliance. We conclude with implications and considerations for current research, clinical guidelines, training and supervision.

Manualised treatments

Key manualised treatments have been developed for the psychological treatment of eating disorders. For children and adolescents, the National Institute for Health and Care Excellence (NICE) guidelines [9] recommend family therapy, of which manualised versions include FBT [3] and Family Therapy for Anorexia Nervosa (FT-AN) [11]. If family therapy is not appropriate, individual options include CBT-E adapted for adolescents [12] or Adolescent-Focused Therapy (AFT) [13].

For adults with AN, the NICE guidelines suggest Cognitive Behaviour Therapy (CBT) [4, 5], Maudsley Anorexia Nervosa Treatment for Adults (MANTRA) [14] or Specialist Supportive Clinical Management (SSCM) [15], all of which have accompanying manuals. While not listed as a first line option, Focal Psychodynamic Therapy [16, 17] is also suggested as an appropriate alternative if the above options are deemed unsuitable or ineffective. There are also other versions of psychotherapy, such as Interpersonal Psychotherapy (IPT), which achieve equivalent outcomes [18]. While there is certainly a sound evidence base from which to continue to research treatment, training and supervision, the quality of this evidence base remains a debated topic [19, 20].

There are clear benefits to the use of treatment manuals within the eating disorders field and within psychology more generally. One key benefit is they promote the ability to engage in more rigorous research, such as randomised controlled trials (RCTs) which, alongside meta-analyses, are considered the highest forms of evidence [21]. Furthermore, manuals provide clear guidelines for training therapists or those inexperienced within the field, and their accessibility enables broader dissemination beyond in-person or on the job training. Similarly to other manuals like the Diagnostic and Statistical Manual of Mental Disorders (DSM) [22], treatment manuals also help professionals to adopt shared language. This is important to aid communication and a consistent approach within and between treatment teams, which is particularly important given the need for multidisciplinary care for those with AN [23].

Adherence and drift in treatment manuals

Therapist adherence is defined as the accuracy with which the specified protocols of a manualised treatment are implemented in the clinical setting [24]. It is argued to be a key component in training and providing evidence-based treatment, and is a large focus in research, training and supervision [25]. However, it is also recognised that therapists commonly deviate substantially from empirically supported protocols in psychotherapy both generally, and within the eating disorders field specifically [26]. Such deviations from the manuals are labelled as non-adherence or therapist drift, which is defined as where therapists either actively decide to ignore or passively avoid key elements of treatment manuals [27–31]. Non-adherence and therapist drift often have negative connotations [28–30]. Non-adherence is cited as a reason for 'failed Family Based Treatment' [29]. An implication of this 'failure' is that non-adherent therapists feel responsible for poor outcome [32] or families feel responsible for being treatment failures [33]. An alternative hypothesis is perhaps that strict application of a treatment manual may lead to treatment failures. Rather than lying with clinicians or families, the problem may lie with how manuals are taught, implemented and supervised.

It has been repeatedly demonstrated that rates of the adoption of evidence-based manuals by clinicians in the eating disorders field are low. For those practitioners that identify as using manuals, adherence to the manual is also low [34–38]. One study of 40 therapists delivering FBT to young people with AN found not one therapist delivered a therapy that was consistently adherent to the FBT manual [34]. Similarly, another study found that around one third of FBT practitioners deviated substantially from manual adherent treatment [39]. Research has shown that CBT for adults with eating disorders is also commonly delivered in ways that deviate substantially from empirically-supported protocols, with fewer than half of self-defined CBT clinicians using core CBT techniques when delivering treatment [27]. These studies do not discuss if non-adherent practitioners have better or worse outcomes than adherent practitioners.

Why do therapists deviate from manuals?

Potential reasons cited for non-adherence and therapist drift include comorbidities in complex cases, when the patient is perceived as treatment resistant, a lack of training and supervision in the protocol, and therapist preference, anxiety, mood or personality [26, 38]. These reasons are often framed as the therapist prioritising their own needs or preferences over those of their patient. However, a difficulty with maintaining strict adherence to manuals is that some research indicates that the inclusion of key aspects of treatment manuals does not necessarily impact outcome, such as including the family meal in session two [40, 41] or siblings attending FBT [42, 43]. One implication of this is that adaption of manuals, rather than strict adherence, need to be considered in our training and supervision of the use of manuals in clinical practice. Research into adaptations of manualised family therapy treatments has demonstrated promising results. For example, Parent-Focused Treatment (PFT) [42], short verses longer form of FBT [44], Multi-family therapy (MFT) [45, 46], Temperament-Based Therapy with Supports (TBT-S) [47], adapted family admissions [48], brief intensive programmes [49] and carer skills training programs [50]. Given full recovery rates at end of FBT (as measured by > 95% BMI and within one standard deviation of average Eating Disorder Examination (EDE) Global scores) are between 22 and 49% [42, 44, 51], with dropout rates of up to 20% [42, 52], the need to continue developing appropriate adaptations to existing manuals is something which the authors of manuals themselves, as well as the field more generally, acknowledge and promote [53, 54].

It is worth noting that most treatment manuals include statements promoting adaptations and acknowledging that this is required to apply the treatment most effectively in an individualised and real-world clinical context. This is important as clinical research needs to have real-world significance in addition to research based significance. While comorbid psychological disorders like anxiety and depression often mean a person may be excluded from a treatment trial, the reality of clinical work is that the majority of patients will present with comorbidities which may, and should, impact treatment

[55–57]. Furthermore, adaptation of treatment manuals is often crucial to respectfully and sensitively embrace different cultural backgrounds of the patient, families, and therapist. More recent research has also identified the need to adapt treatment to better work for various populations, including young people or their families who identify as neurodiverse, such as those diagnosed with Autistic Spectrum Disorder [58], young people engaging in self-harm [59], or those who experience gender diversity or dysphoria [60]. Adaptation is also crucial in working in a trauma informed manner, where issues such as attachment and interpersonal style, self-concept and capacity for mentalisation are important considerations [61].

Interestingly, therapists with greater clinical experience are more likely to deviate from treatment manuals, which may be explained by the finding that some therapists view manuals as too inflexible to apply appropriately to complex cases [62, 63]. This may also be a result of applying evidence-informed practice, which promotes a flexible process of balancing best clinical evidence with therapist experience or clinical opinion and patient values and preferences [64, 65]. Therapists newer to a specific model cite a number of reasons why they are less adherent, including inadequate consideration of comorbid conditions, difficulties engaging parents or members of the multidisciplinary team and insufficient training and supervision [24, 66].

Does adherence lead to better outcomes?

When manual adherence is low, it makes sense that outcomes differ from those found in clinical trials, which inherently require a high degree of manual adherence [28, 67]. A review of the wider psychotherapy literature by those in the eating disorders field allows consideration of whether strict adherence to any treatment manual is of benefit to our patients. In reality, it remains completely unsubstantiated whether or not high levels of adherence are related to therapeutic outcome [68, 69]. A meta-analysis of 36 treatment integrity outcome studies in adults concluded that neither manual adherence nor competence, defined as how well interventions were delivered, displayed an effect on outcome that was significantly different from zero [70]. A review of literature in child and adolescent psychotherapy found a small relationship between adherence and outcome in a meta-analysis of 35 studies [71]. However, the authors note that "the finding of a statistically significant association with outcome is tempered by the fact that the small effect suggests that adherence only accounts for just under one percent of variance in outcomes" (p.426). Importantly, neither therapeutic alliance nor patient readiness for change were considered as potential moderating variables. There is also some data that therapists being flexible in adherence may lead to improved treatment effects, at least within psychodynamic psychotherapy [72, 73].

There is an increasing amount of research on manual adherence relating to treatment efficacy within eating disorders specifically. Loeb et al. [74] found no significant association between adherence and outcome in either CBT or IPT for Bulimia Nervosa (BN). Another study found a complex relationship between adherence and outcome in CBT which changed over time [75]. Initial adherence was high in the behaviourally focused early and middle sessions, with therapists becoming less adherent in later sessions. While higher early adherence was related to less binging behaviour, this correlation decreased over time. There was also a notable correlation between high early adherence and increased drop out [75]. Interestingly, while it is noted that there was significant variation in adherence between the four therapists in the study, it is not reported if the less adherent therapists had poorer outcomes. One limitation of this study is the small sample size, although it does highlight an interesting area for future investigation. There is also a need to research the relationship between adherence and outcome in treatment for AN.

Considering complexity: moderating factors

Perhaps not surprisingly, there appears to be a more complex relationship between adherence and outcome than typically assumed. Potential moderators of the relationship between adherence and outcome may include type of therapy (multisystemic or individual), patient diagnosis, therapist competence, therapeutic alliance and patient readiness to change [76].

Within the general psychotherapy literature, it appears that rigidly implementing a therapy approach is ineffective at best and potentially deleterious to outcomes at worst [77]. This is supported by research which suggests that where therapeutic alliance is poor, strong manual adherence is associated with a poorer outcome [76]. One study found that manual adherence to treat panic disorder was unhelpful when patients had low readiness for change, but was not related to outcome in patients with higher levels of motivation [78]. In evaluating CBT for adults with depression, Snippe et al. [79] found that therapist adherence was not related to positive outcome, particularly when patients were less engaged in treatment. Barber et al. [80] found that therapist adherence when working with people with substance abuse difficulties was less strongly related to outcome when therapeutic alliance was strong. Weck et al. [81] found that in three RCTs for depression, social phobia and hypochondriasis, alliance at session one, but not session two, predicted therapist

adherence in later sessions, but that adherence had no relationship with future alliance. Such studies also demonstrate that therapeutic relationship and adherence are likely interrelated and bidirectional.

The above research highlights the complex interaction between patient readiness to change, manual adherence and outcome. When patients have low readiness to change, strict adherence to an action-based manual is likely to be ineffective [82]. This is especially pertinent to patients with AN, characterised by its ego syntonic nature in which sustained readiness to change is typically low [83]. It follows that an initial focus of treatment may therefore need to be engagement and building therapeutic alliance and increasing a patient's readiness to change, rather than working strictly to a manual [84]. One of the major strengths behind family therapy for eating disorders is that even though young people may not want to engage in treatment, parents are often appropriately concerned and highly motivated. However, this by no means negates the importance of engaging the young person in the process. Strategies to build rapport and engage young people are being developed, such as using psychoeducation on the biological effects of starvation (for example, delayed gastric emptying) [11, 85].

While the relationship between adherence and outcome remains unclear, therapeutic alliance consistently predicts, or is at least correlated with, treatment outcome [86]. Baier et al. [87] reports that there are now over 300 studies of the alliance-outcome relationship, with stronger alliance consistently associated with positive treatment outcome across a range of psychotherapies. It is proposed that alliance is a non-specific mediator of change and is important in all psychotherapies [88], with the impact of the therapist relationship on patient outcome estimated to be between 5 and 8% [89]. Similarly, another study found that 97% of variance between the outcome of individual therapists was due to their ability to form better therapeutic relationships with patients [90]. Of course, it is also likely that alliance and adherence are interrelated and reinforce one another during therapy [89].

Parallel processes are a well-documented phenomenon in which therapists, supervisors, multidisciplinary teams and researchers can unknowingly begin to emulate and repeat the same patterns present for their patients [91, 92]. For an illness such as AN, which is characterised by cognitive and behavioural rigidity, higher threat sensitivity and intolerance of uncertainty, we must be careful as a field that we do not unknowingly fall into the same rigid processes. An example of this may be a specialist treatment team who refuses to provide treatment to a 15 year old patient with AN seeking help without support of their family because they strictly adhere to the idea that family therapy is the only appropriate option, despite the NICE guidelines offering suitable evidence-based alternatives.

Implications for training and supervision

The positive impact of alliance on patient outcome, seemingly over manual adherence, is demonstrated both in the eating disorder and wider psychotherapy literature. Additionally, the importance of readiness to change on the appropriateness of manual adherence is also substantiated. As such, this paper questions the focus on strict manual adherence in training and supervision in the eating disorders field. While there remain numerous benefits to the development and application of treatment manuals as previously mentioned, the field may be better served by shifting the emphasis of training and supervision away from strict adherence to a more flexible, yet empirically consistent approach. Perhaps one can envisage manuals in the eating disorders field as a series of core interventions or tasks that should be included in an eating disorders treatment. Recent practice and training standards [7] have alluded to this way of thinking about treatment. These guidelines highlight that some of the core principles of eating disorder treatment may include developing a therapeutic relationship, assessing motivational status, the use of "evidence-based interventions" which include weighing the patient, a focus on modifying the eating disordered behaviour, developing a clinical case formulation and developing alternative coping strategies, amongst others. These guidelines are clearly based on the existing manuals and evidence base, but perhaps suggest a core principle approach rather than strict manual adherence.

One potential method to move away from a stirictly manualised approach to clinical training and practice has been described through Process Oriented Therapy (POT) [93]. POT proposes that treatment, training and supervision should focus on core clinical processes, including motivational enhancement, behavioural activation, cognitive flexibility and emotional regulation skills, rather than manualised content. In this view, training and supervision should focus on identifying specific patient needs through individual and systemic case formulation, rather than the application of specific manuals. One core process discussed is psychological flexibility, as opposed to rigidity. This seems especially important when working to increase psychological flexibility in people with AN. Further research, clinical work and training is already exploring the importance of promoting flexibility in over-controlled individuals through therapeutic adaptations like Radically Open Dialectical Behaviour Therapy (RO-DBT) [94]. Interestingly, POT also highlights the role of the therapeutic relationship and suggests this may model, instigate and promote the internalisation of an ability to

be within the present moment, accept difficult experiences and engage in valued action [93].

Constantino et al. [76] offer a further suggestion to rethinking our training and supervision process. They describe Context Responsive Psychotherapy Integration (CRPI) as another alternative to strictly adherent manual training. The authors draw on data suggesting that successful management of alliance ruptures predicts treatment outcome [95], and therefore that training and supervision should help a therapist to identify and respond to the dynamic nature of the therapeutic relationship. They suggest that adjusting therapist actions to patients' presenting difficulties, context and non-diagnostic characteristics, including the interpersonal dynamics present during therapy, represents a more skilful and nuanced approach that is well supported within evidence-informed practice. They also suggest replacing long-form trainings on single treatment manuals for specific diagnostic problems with briefer trainings that focus on the main principles underlying the manuals. Training would also dedicate time to teaching the clinicians important contextual markers, such as when to move away from the manual (for example, patient hesitancy to change or need to further develop clinical formulation) and empirically supported interventions appropriate for that circumstance (for example, use motivational enhancement techniques) [84].

Adoption of a more flexible core principle approach to treatment has implications for how adherence is assessed. We are in no way calling for an abandonment of treatment manuals or randomised controlled trials evaluating them. These trials, which need strict adherence to assist replicability, provide important data on which techniques should be included in a core principle approach (for example, weighing the patient). The document produced by Hurst et al. [7] could be modified into a checklist form, so that clinicians can assess their adherence to the core principles in treatment. It may also be important to assess common factors of therapy, such as the therapist's ability to be empathic and to form a therapeutic alliance, as well as specific techniques included in the treatment. Of course, the key assessment is to monitor patient outcome on a regular basis [7]. Assessment of treatment acceptability, in either a strict or flexible form, to both therapist and patient may also be important.

Conclusion

This paper recognises the important advances that treatment manuals have provided our field. Manuals promote rigorous research, provide clear training and clinical guidelines, allow broader dissemination and accessibility, and create a common language and platform from which to research necessary adaptations. Taken together, manuals provide a set of core principles important in the evidence-informed treatment of eating disorders, such as monitoring weight and other markers of health, supporting physical recovery as a means to establish psychological recovery, and utilising a patient's support network. We know that training in the delivery of manualised treatment does make the clinician more adherent to the delivery of that manualised treatment [69]. However, a growing body of literature from both the field of general psychotherapy and within eating disorders specifically indicates that treatment adherence does not consistently predict patient outcomes and may indeed be contraindicated in some cases. We suggest that clinicians be encouraged in their clinical practice, training and supervision to use the treatment manual alongside individual and systemic case formulation, the client's stage of change and the therapeutic relationship, with a focus on resolving therapeutic breaches. In combination, these factors allow a clinician to truly engage in evidence-informed practice. We would recommend future research is undertaken regarding formulation-driven adaptation of manuals, and training and supervision that goes beyond strict adherence to treatment manuals in the field of eating disorders.

Abbreviations
AN: Anorexia Nervosa; FBT: Family-Based Treatment; CBT-E: Enhanced Cognitive Behaviour Therapy; NICE: National Institute for Health and Care Excellence; FT-AN: Family therapy for Anorexia Nervosa; AFT: Adolescent Focused Therapy; CBT: Cognitive Behaviour Therapy; MANTRA: Maudsley Anorexia Nervosa Treatment for Adults; SSCM: Specialist Supportive Clinical Management; FFP: Focal Psychodynamic Psychotherapy; IPT: Interpersonal Psychotherapy; RCT : Randomised Controlled Trial; DSM: Diagnostic and Statistical Manual of Mental Disorders; PFT: Parent-Focused Treatment; MFT: Multi-Family therapy or Multiple Family Therapy; TBT-S: Temperament-Based Therapy with Supports; EDE: Eating Disorder Examination; BN: Bulimia Nervosa; POT: Process Oriented Therapy; ACT: Acceptance and Commitment Therapy; RO-DBT: Radically Open Dialectical Behaviour Therapy; CRPI: Context Responsive Psychotherapy Integration.

Acknowledgements
Not applicable

Authors' contributions
AR and CT co-wrote this article. Both authors read and approved the final manuscript.

Competing interests
The authors declare they have no competing interests.

Author details
[1]The Children's Hospital at Westmead, Sydney, Australia. [2]The Redleaf Practice, Sydney, Australia.

References
1. Treasure J, Duarte TA, Schmidt U. Eating disorders. Lancet. 2020;395:899–911.
2. Lock J, Le Grange D, Agras WS, Dare C. Treatment manual for anorexia Nervosa: a family-based approach. New York, London: Guildford Press; 2000.
3. Lock J, Le Grange D. Treatment manual for anorexia nervosa: a family-based approach. 2nd ed. New York, London: Guilford Press; 2012.
4. Fairburn CG. Cognitive behaviour therapy and eating disorders. New York: Guildford Press; 2008.
5. Waller G, Cordery H, Corstorphine E, Hinrichsen H, Lawson R, Mountford V, Russell K. Cognitive behavioural therapy for eating disorders: a comprehensive treatment guide. Cambridge: Cambridge University Press; 2007.
6. Heruc G, Hurst K, Casey A, et al. ANZAED eating disorder treatment principles and general clinical practice and training standards. J Eat Disord. 2020. https://doi.org/10.1186/s40337-020-00341-0.
7. Hurst K, Heruc G, Thornton C, et al. ANZAED practice and training standards for mental health professionals providing eating disorder treatment. J Eat Disord. 2020. https://doi.org/10.1186/s40337-020-00333-0.
8. Heruc G, Hart S, Stiles G, et al. ANZAED practice and training standards for dietitians providing eating disorder treatment. J Eat Disord. 2020. https://doi.org/10.1186/s40337-020-00334-z.
9. National Institute for Clinical Excellence. Eating disorders: recognition and treatment NG69 2017. Available online: https://www.nice.org.uk/guidance/ng69. Accessed 13 May 2020.
10. Hilbert A, Hoek HW, Schmidt R. Evidence-based clinical guidelines for eating disorders: international comparison. Curr Opin Psychiatry. 2017;30(6):423–37.
11. Eisler I, Simic M, Blessitt E, Dodge L, et al. Maudsley service manual for child and adolescent eating disorders. London: King's College; 2019.
12. Grave RD, Calugi S. Cognitive behaviour therapy for adolescents with eating disorders. New York: Guildford Press; 2020.
13. Lock D. Adolescent-focused therapy for anorexia nervosa: a developmental approach. New York: Guilfod Press; 2020.
14. Schmidt U, Wade T, Treasure J. The Maudsley Model of Anorexia Nervosa Treatment for Adults (MANTRA): development, key features, and preliminary evidence. J Cogn Psychother. 2014. https://doi.org/10.1891/0889-8391.28.1.48.
15. McIntosh VV, Jordan J, Luty SE, Carter FA, McKenzie JM, Bulik CM, Joyce PR. Specialist supportive clinical management for anorexia nervosa. Int J Eat Disord. 2006. https://doi.org/10.1002/eat.20297.
16. Friederich H, Wild B, Zipfel S, Schauenburg H, Herzog W. Anorexia Nervosa: focal psychodynamic psychotherapy. Boston: Hogrefe Publishing; 2019.
17. Zipfel S, Wild B, Gross G, Friederich H, Teufel M, Schellberg D, et al. Focal psychodynamic therapy, cognitive behaviour therapy, and optimised treatment as usual in outpatients with anorexia nervosa (ANTOP study): randomised controlled trial. Lancet. 2014. https://doi.org/10.1016/S0140-6736(13)61746-8.
18. Carter FA, Jordan J, McIntosh VV, Luty SE, McKenzie JM, Frampton CM, Bulik CM, Joyce PR. The long-term efficacy of three psychotherapies for anorexia nervosa: a randomized, controlled trial. Int J Eat Disord. 2011. https://doi.org/10.1002/eat.20879.
19. Murray SB, Quintana DS, Loeb KL, Griffiths S, le Grange D. Treatment outcomes for anorexia nervosa: a systematic review and meta-analysis of randomized controlled trials. Psychol Med. 2019. https://doi.org/10.1017/S0033291718002088.
20. Lock J, Kraemer H, Jo B, Couturier J. When meta-analyses get it wrong: Response to 'treatment outcomes for anorexia nervosa: a systematic

review and meta-analysis of randomized controlled trials.' Psychol Med. 2019. https://doi.org/10.1017/S003329171800329X.

21. Greenhalgh T. How to read a paper: the basics of evidence-based medicine. 4th ed. Chichester: Wiley-Blackwell; 2010.

22. American Psychiatric Association. Diagnostic and statistical manual of mental disorders: DSM-5. Arlington: VA; American Psychiatric Association; 2013.

23. Beumont P, Hay P, Beumont R. Summary Australian and New Zealand clinical practice guideline for the management of Anorexia Nervosa. Australas Psychiatry. 2003. https://doi.org/10.1046/j.1039-8562.2003.00534.x.

24. Waller G. Treatment protocols for eating disorders: clinicians' attitudes, concerns, adherence and difficulties delivering evidence-based psychological interventions. Curr Psychiatry Rep. 2016. https://doi.org/10.1007/s11920-016-0679-0.

25. Cooper Z, Bailey-Straebler S. Disseminating evidence-based psychological treatments for eating disorders. Curr Psychiatry Rep. 2015. https://doi.org/10.1007/s11920-015-0551-7.

26. Waller G, Mountford VA, Tatham M, Turner H, Gabriel C, Webber R. Attitudes towards psychotherapy manuals among clinicians treating eating disorders. Behav Res Ther. 2013. https://doi.org/10.1016/j.brat.2013.10.004.

27. Waller G, Stringer H, Meyer C. What cognitive behavioral techniques do therapists report using when delivering cognitive behavioral therapy for the eating disorders? J Consult Clin Psychol. 2012;80:171–5.

28. Waller G, Turner H. Therapist drift redux: why well-meaning clinicians fail to deliver evidence-based therapy, and how to get back on track. Behav Res Ther. 2016. https://doi.org/10.1016/j.brat.2015.12.005.

29. Lavender KR. Rebooting "failed" family-based treatment. Front Psych. 2020. https://doi.org/10.3389/fpsyt.2020.00068.

30. Mulkens S, de Vos C, de Graaff A, Waller G. To deliver or not to deliver cognitive behavioral therapy for eating disorders: Replication and extension of our understanding of why therapists fail to do what they should do. Behav Res Ther. 2018. https://doi.org/10.1016/j.brat.2018.05.004.

31. Waller G. Evidence-based treatment and therapist drift. Behav Res Ther. 2009. https://doi.org/10.1016/j.brat.2008.10.018.

32. Aradas J, Sales D, Rhodes P, Conti J. "As long as they eat"? Therapist experiences, dilemmas and identity negotiations of Maudlsey and family-based therapy for anorexia nervosa. J Eat Disord. 2019. https://doi.org/10.1186/s40337-019-0255-1.

33. Wufong E, Rhodes P, Conti J. "We don't really know what else we can do": parent experiences when adolescent distress persists after the Maudsley and family-based therapies for anorexia nervosa. J Eat Disord. 2019. https://doi.org/10.1186/s40337-019-0235-5.

34. Couturier J, Kimber M, Jack S, Niccols A, Van Blyderveen S, McVey G. Understanding the uptake of family-based treatment for adolescents with anorexia nervosa: therapist perspectives. Int J Eat Disord. 2013;46:177–88.

35. Tobin DL, Banker JD, Weisberg L, Bowers W. I know what you did last summer (and it was not CBT): a factor analytic model of international psychotherapeutic practice in the eating disorders. Int J Eat Disord. 2007. https://doi.org/10.1002/eat.20426.

36. Wallace LM, von Ranson KM. Perceptions and use of empirically-supported psychotherapies among eating disorder professionals. Behav Res Ther. 2012;50:215–22.

37. Wallace LM, von Ranson KM. Treatment manuals: Use in the treatment of bulimia nervosa. Behav Res Ther. 2011. https://doi.org/10.1016/j.brat.2011.09.002.

38. Simmons AM, Milnes SM, Anderson DA. Factors influencing the utilization of empirically supported treatments for eating disorders. Eat Disord. 2008;16:342–54.

39. Kosmerly S, Waller G, Lafrance RA. Clinician adherence to guidelines in the delivery of family-based therapy for eating disorders. Int J Eat Disord. 2015. https://doi.org/10.1002/eat.22276.

40. Herscovici CR, Kovalskys I, Orellana L. An exploratory evaluation of the family meal intervention for adolescent Anorexia Nervosa. Fam Process. 2017. https://doi.org/10.1111/famp.12199.

41. Agras WS, Lock J, Brandt H, Bryson SW, Dodge E, Halmi KA, Jo B, Johnson C, Kaye W, Wilfley D, Woodside B. Comparison of 2 family therapies for adolescent anorexia nervosa: a randomized parallel trial. JAMA Psychiat. 2014. https://doi.org/10.1001/jamapsychiatry.2014.1025.

42. le Grange D, Hughes EK, Court A, Yeo M, Crosby RD, Sawyer SM. Randomized clinical trial of parent-focused treatment and family-based treatment for adolescent anorexia nervosa. J Am Acad Child Adolesc Psychiatry. 2016;55(8):683–92.

43. Ellison R, Rhodes P, Madden S, Miskovic J, Wallis A, Baillie A, Kohn M, Touyz S. Do the components of manualized family-based treatment for anorexia nervosa predict weight gain? Int J Eat Disord. 2012. https://doi.org/10.1002/eat.22000.

44. Lock J, Agras WS, Bryson S, Kraemer HC. A comparison of short- and long-term family therapy for adolescent anorexia nervosa. J Am Acad Child Adolesc Psychiatry. 2005. https://doi.org/10.1097/01.chi.0000161647.82775.0a.

45. Eisler I. The empirical and theoretical base of family therapy and multiple family day therapy for adolescent anorexia nervosa. J Fam Ther. 2005;27(2):104–31.

46. Eisler I, Simic M, Hodsoll J, Asen E, Berelowitz M, Connan F, Ellis G, Hugo P, Schmidt U, Treasure J, Yi I, Landau SA. Pragmatic randomised multi-centre trial of multifamily and single family therapy for adolescent anorexia nervosa. BMC Psychiatry. 2016. https://doi.org/10.1186/s12888-016-1129-6.

47. Kaye W, Wierenga C, Knatz S, Liang J, Boutelle K, Hill L, Eisler I. Temperament-based treatment for anorexia Nervosa. Eur Eat Disord Rev. 2014. https://doi.org/10.1002/erv.2330.

48. Wallis A, Alford C, Hanson A, Titterton J, Madden S, Kohn M. Innovations in Maudsley family-based treatment for anorexia nervosa at the Children's Hospital at Westmead: a family admission programme. J Fam Ther. 2013;35(S1):68–81.

49. Knatz S, Murray SB, Matheson B, Boutelle KN, Rockwell R, Eisler I, Kaye WH. A brief, intensive application of multi-family-based treatment for eating disorders. Eat Disord. 2015;23(4):315–24.

50. Hodsoll J, Rhind C, Micali N, et al. A Pilot, Multicentre pragmatic randomised trial to explore the impact of carer skills training on carer and patient behaviours: testing the cognitive interpersonal model in adolescent anorexia nervosa. Eur Eat Disord Rev. 2017;25:551–61.

51. Madden S, Miskovic-Wheatley J, Wallis A, Kohn M, Lock J, Le Grange D, Jo B, Clarke S, Rhodes P, Hay P, Touyz S. A randomized controlled trial of inpatient treatment for anorexia nervosa in medically unstable adolescents. Psychol Med. 2015. https://doi.org/10.1017/S0033291714001573.

52. Dejong H, Broadbent H, Schmidt U. A systematic review of dropout from treatment in outpatients with anorexia nervosa. Int J eat Disord. 2012;45:635–47.

53. Lock J, Le Grange D, Agras WS, Moye A, Bryson SW, Jo B. Randomized clinical trial comparing family-based treatment with adolescent-focused individual therapy for adolescents with anorexia nervosa. Arch Gen Psychiatry. 2010;67:1025–32.

54. Lock J, Le Grange D. Family-based treatment: Where are we and where should we be going to improve recovery in child and adolescent eating disorders. Int. J Eating Disord. 2018; https://doi.org/10.1002/eat.22980.

55. Rienecke RD. Family-based treatment of eating disorders in adolescents: current insights. Adolesc Health Med Ther. 2017;8:69–79.

56. Strober M, Johnson C. The need for complex ideas in Anorexia Nervosa: why biology, environment, and psyche all matter, why therapists make mistakes, and why clinical benchmarks are needed for managing weight correction. Int J Eat Disorders. 2012;45:155–78.

57. Hughes EK, Goldschmidt AB, Labuschagne Z, Loeb KL, Sawyer SM, le Grange D. Eating disorders with and without comorbid depression and anxiety: similarities and differences in a clinical sample of children and adolescents. Eur Eat Disord Rev. 2013;21(5):386–94.

58. Kinnaird E, Norton C, Stewart C, Tchanturia K. Same behaviours, different reasons: what do patients with co-occurring anorexia and autism want from treatment? Int Rev Psychiatry. 2019. https://doi.org/10.1080/09540261.2018.1531831.

59. Reilly EE, Orloff NC, Luo T, Berner LA, Brown TA, Claudat K, Kaye WH, Anderson LK. Dialectical behavioral therapy for the treatment of adolescent eating disorders: a review of existing work and proposed future directions. Eat Disord. 2020. https://doi.org/10.1080/10640266.2020.1743098.

60. Diemer EW, Hughto JMW, Gordon AR, Guss C, Austin SB, Reisner SL. Beyond the binary: differences in eating disorder prevalence by gender identity in a transgender sample. Transgender Health. 2018. https://doi.org/10.1089/trgh.2017.0043.

61. Tasca GA. Attachment and eating disorders: a research update. Curr Opin Psychol. 2019. https://doi.org/10.1016/j.copsyc.2018.03.003.

62. Haas HL, Clopton JR. Comparing clinical and research treatments for eating disorders. Int J Eat Disord. 2003;33:412–20.

63. Mountford V, Tatham M, Turner H, Waller G. Complexity in eating disorders: a case for simple or complex formulation and treatment? Cognit Behav Ther. 2017. https://doi.org/10.1017/S1754470X17000162.

64. Sackett DL, Rosenberg WMC, Muir Gray JA, Haynes RB, Richardson W. Evidence based medicine: what it is and what it isn't. BMJ. 1996. https://doi.org/10.1136/bmj.312.7023.71.

65. Nevo I, Slonim-Nevo V. The myth of evidence-based practice: towards evidence-informed practice. Br J Soc Work. 2011. https://doi.org/10.1093/bjsw/bcq149.

66. Couturier J, Kimber M, Jack S, Niccols A, Van Blyderveen S, McVey G. Using a knowledge transfer framework to identify factors facilitating implementation of family-based treatment. Int J Eat Disord. 2014;47(4):410–7.

67. Bearman SK, Schneiderman RL, Zoloth E. Building an evidence base for effective supervision practices: an analogue experiment of supervision to increase EBT fidelity. Adm Policy Ment Health. 2017. https://doi.org/10.1007/s10488-016-0723-8.

68. Perepletchikova F, Kazdin AE. Treatment integrity and therapeutic change: Issues and research recommendations. Clin Psychol Sci Pract. 2005. https://doi.org/10.1093/clipsy.bpi045.

69. Miller SJ, Binder JL. The effects of manual-based training on treatment fidelity and outcome: a review of the literature on adult individual psychotherapy. Psychother Theory Res Pract Train. 2002; https://doi.org/10.1037/0033-3204.39.2.184

70. Webb CA, Derubeis RJ, Barber JP. Therapist adherence/competence and treatment outcome: a meta-analytic review. J Consult Clin Psychol. 2010. https://doi.org/10.1037/a0018912.

71. Collyer H, Eisler I, Woolgar M. Systematic literature review and meta-analysis of the relationship between adherence, competence and outcome in psychotherapy for children and adolescents. Eur Child Adolesc Psychiatry. 2020. https://doi.org/10.1007/s00787-018-1265-2.

72. Katz M, Hilsenroth MJ, Gold JR, Moore M, Pitman SR, Levy SR, Owen J. Adherence, flexibility, and outcome in psychodynamic treatment of depression. J Couns Psychol. 2019. https://doi.org/10.1037/cou0000299.

73. Owen J, Hilsenroth MJ. Treatment adherence: the importance of therapist flexibility in relation to therapy outcomes. J Couns Psychol. 2014. https://doi.org/10.1037/a0035753.

74. Loeb KL, Wilson GT, Labouvie E, Pratt EM, Hayaki J, Walsh BT, Agras WS, Fairburn CG. Therapeutic alliance and treatment adherence in two interventions for bulimia nervosa: a study of process and outcome. J Consult Clin Psychol. 2005. https://doi.org/10.1037/0022-006X.73.6.1097.

75. Folke S, Daniel SIF, Gondan M, Lunn S, Tækker L, Poulsen S. Therapist adherence is associated with outcome in cognitive-behavioral therapy for bulimia nervosa. Psychotherapy (Chic). 2017. https://doi.org/10.1037/pst0000107.

76. Constantino MJ, Coyne AE, Muir HJ. Evidence-based therapist responsivity to disruptive clinical process. Cognit Behav Pract. 2020. https://doi.org/10.1016/j.cbpra.2020.01.003.

77. Castonguay LG. Psychotherapy, psychopathology, research and practice: pathways of connections and integration. Psychother Res. 2011. https://doi.org/10.1080/10503307.2011.563250.

78. Huppert J, Barlow D, Gorman J, Shear K, Woods S. The interaction of motivation and therapist adherence predicts outcome in cognitive behavioral therapy for panic disorder: preliminary findings. Cognit Behav Pract. 2006. https://doi.org/10.1016/j.cbpra.2005.10.001.

79. Snippe E, Schroevers MJ, Tovote KA, Sanderman R, Emmelkamp PMG, Fleer J. Explaining variability in therapist adherence and patient depressive symptom improvement: the role of therapist interpersonal skills and patient engagement. Clin Psychol Psychother. 2019. https://doi.org/10.1002/cpp.2332.

80. Barber J, Gallop R, Crits-Christoph P, Frank A, Thase M, Weiss R, Gibbons M. The role of therapist adherence, therapist competence, and alliance in predicting outcome of individual drug counseling: Results from the National Institute Drug Abuse Collaborative Cocaine Treatment Study. Psychother Res. 2006. https://doi.org/10.1080/10503300500288951.

81. Weck F, Grikscheit F, Jakob M, Höfling V, Stangier U. Treatment failure in cognitive-behavioural therapy: therapeutic alliance as a precondition for an adherent and competent implementation of techniques. Br J Clin Psychol. 2015. https://doi.org/10.1111/bjc.12063.

82. Vitousek K, Watson S, Wilson GT. Enhancing motivation for change in treatment-resistant eating disorders. Clin Psychol Rev. 1998;18:391–420.

83. Bewell CV, Carter JC. Readiness to change mediates the impact of eating disorder symptomatology on treatment outcome in anorexia nervosa. Int J Eat Disord. 2008. https://doi.org/10.1002/eat.20513.

84. Macdonald P, Hibbs R, Corfield F, Treasure J. The use of motivational interviewing in eating disorders: a systematic review. Psychiatry Res. 2012. https://doi.org/10.1016/j.psychres.2012.05.013.

85. Jewell T, Blessitt E, Stewart CS, Simic M, Eisler I. Family therapy for child and adolescent eating disorders: a critical review. Fam Process. 2016;55(3):577–94.

86. Horvath AO, Del Re AC, Flückiger C, Symonds D. Alliance in individual psychotherapy. Psychotherapy. 2011. https://doi.org/10.1037/a0022186.

87. Baier AL, Kline AC, Feeny NC. Therapeutic alliance as a mediator of change: a systematic review and evaluation of research. Clin Psychol Rev. 2020. https://doi.org/10.1016/j.cpr.2020.101921.

88. Bertolino B, Bargmann S, Miller SD. Manual 1: what works in therapy: a primer. Chicago, IL: ICCE Press; 2012.

89. Baldwin SA, Wampold BE, Imel ZE. Untangling the alliance-outcome correlation: exploring the relative importance of therapist and patient variability in the alliance. J Consult Clin Psychol. 2007. https://doi.org/10.1037/0022-006X.75.6.842.

90. Lange AM, van der Rijken RE, Delsing MJ, Busschbach JJ, van Horn JE, Scholte RH. Alliance and adherence in a systemic therapy. Child Adolesc Ment Health. 2017. https://doi.org/10.1111/camh.12172.

91. Mothersole G. Parallel process. Clin Superv. 1999;18(2):107–21. https://doi.org/10.1300/J001v18n02_08.

92. Hamburg P, Herzog D. Supervising the therapy of patients with eating disorders. Am J Psychother. 1990;44(3):369–80.

93. Hayes SC, Hofmann SG, Ciarrochi J. A process-based approach to psychological diagnosis and treatment: the conceptual and treatment utility of an extended evolutionary model. Clin Psychol Rev. 2020. https://doi.org/10.1016/j.cpr.2020.101908.

94. Lynch TR, Hempel RJ, Dunkley C. Radically open-dialectical behavior therapy for disorders of over-control: signaling matters. Am J Psychother. 2015;69(2):141–62.

95. Eubanks CF, Sergi J, Samstag LW, Muran JC. Commentary: Rupture repair as a transtheoretical corrective experience. J Clin Psychol. 2021. https://doi.org/10.1002/jclp.23117.

15

Cost-effectiveness of Specialist Eating Disorders Services for Children and Adolescents with Anorexia Nervosa: a National Surveillance Study

Sarah Byford[1]* [iD], Hristina Petkova[1], Barbara Barrett[1], Tamsin Ford[2], Dasha Nicholls[3], Mima Simic[4], Simon Gowers[5], Geraldine Macdonald[6], Ruth Stuart[1], Nuala Livingstone[7], Grace Kelly[8], Jonathan Kelly[9], Kandarp Joshi[10], Helen Smith[11] and Ivan Eisler[12]

Abstract

Background: Evidence suggests specialist eating disorders services for children and adolescents with anorexia nervosa have the potential to improve outcomes and reduce costs through reduced hospital admissions. This study aimed to evaluate the cost-effectiveness of assessment and diagnosis in community-based specialist child and adolescent mental health services (CAMHS) compared to generic CAMHS for children and adolescents with anorexia nervosa.

Method: Observational, surveillance study of children and adolescents aged 8 to 17, in contact with community-based CAMHS in the UK or Republic of Ireland for a first episode of anorexia nervosa. Data were reported by clinicians at baseline, 6 and 12-months follow-up. Outcomes included the Children's Global Assessment Scale (CGAS) and percentage of median expected body mass for age and sex (%mBMI). Service use data included paediatric and psychiatric inpatient admissions, outpatient and day-patient attendances. A joint distribution of incremental mean costs and effects for each group was generated using bootstrapping to explore the probability that each service is the optimal choice, subject to a range of values a decision-maker might be willing to pay for outcome improvements. Uncertainty was explored using cost-effectiveness acceptability curves.

Results: Two hundred ninety-eight children and adolescents met inclusion criteria. At 12-month follow-up, there were no significant differences in total costs or outcomes between specialist eating disorders services and generic CAMHS. However, adjustment for pre-specified baseline covariates resulted in observed differences favouring specialist services, due to significantly poorer clinical status of the specialist group at baseline. Cost-effectiveness analysis using CGAS suggests that the probability of assessment in a specialist service being cost-effective compared to generic CAMHS ranges from 90 to 50%, dependent on willingness to pay for improvements in outcome.

* Correspondence: s.byford@kcl.ac.uk
[1]Institute of Psychiatry, Psychology & Neuroscience at King's College London, PO24 David Goldberg Centre, De Crespigny Park, London SE5 8AF, UK
Full list of author information is available at the end of the article

Conclusions: Assessment in a specialist eating disorders service for children and adolescents with anorexia nervosa may have a higher probability of being cost-effective than assessment in generic CAMHS.

Plain English summary

Specialist eating disorders services may improve outcomes and reduce hospitalisations for children and adolescents with anorexia nervosa. Reductions in hospitalisation could save money for the NHS and are better for young people because hospitalisation disrupts their home life, social life and education. This study evaluated outcomes and costs of specialist eating disorders services compared to general child and adolescent mental health services (CAMHS) for children and adolescents with anorexia nervosa.

Children and adolescents were identified by contacting child and adolescent psychiatrists in the UK and Ireland and asking them to report any new cases of anorexia nervosa. These psychiatrists identified 298 young people aged 8 to 17 with an anorexia nervosa diagnosis for the first time. The psychiatrists provided information on the health services these young people used and how they were doing when they were first diagnosed and 6 months and 1 year later.

Children and adolescents in specialist services were more severely ill than those in CAMHS when they were first diagnosed. Despite this, care for the young people in specialist services cost about the same as for those diagnosed in CAMHS, and their outcomes after 1 year were similar. This work showed that specialist services may be better value for money than CAMHS.

Keywords: Anorexia nervosa, Cost-effectiveness analysis, Specialist eating disorders services, Child and adolescent mental health services

Background

Anorexia nervosa is an eating disorder associated with severe physical and psychological impairments and a significant cost burden [1–4]. Due to the life-threatening nature of the disorder, a substantial proportion of children and adolescents are admitted to hospital with evidence to suggest that the number of admissions is rising [5, 6]. Admissions are disruptive to family, school and social life, costly to health services and relapse rates following inpatient treatment are high [7, 8]. In the United Kingdom (UK) and Republic of Ireland, children and adolescents with anorexia nervosa are commonly assessed and diagnosed by generic child and adolescent mental health services (CAMHS) or specialist community-based eating disorders services. Few studies have compared the relative benefits of these different models of care but the available evidence suggests specialist outpatient treatment may be more effective than generic CAMHS [9, 10]. Economic evidence also supports the case for specialist services, suggesting that specialist outpatient treatment is cost-effective compared to both inpatient treatment and generic outpatient treatment [11]. However, available data are over 10 years old and service configurations may now be very different. No other economic evaluations of specialist eating disorders services for children and adolescents were identified. A recent systematic review found only nine economic evaluations of treatment interventions for all eating disorders in all ages [12], including the study referred to above [11]. Of

the remainder, seven were carried out in adults or populations 16 years of age and over and age was unclear in one study. If the findings from the earlier study [11] can be shown to be generalisable, investing in specialist eating disorders services could have significant implications for the National Health Service (NHS), with the potential to improve health outcomes and the quality of life of young people and their families, and reduce costs through reduced admissions.

Methods

Aim

The Cost-effectiveness of models of care for young people with Eating Disorders (CostED) study aimed to evaluate the cost-effectiveness of assessment and diagnosis in community-based specialist CAMHS (e.g. specialist eating disorders services) and generic CAMHS for child and adolescent anorexia nervosa. The work presented here is a condensed version of one element of the CostED study, the full details of which are published elsewhere [13].

Design

An observational, surveillance study was undertaken using the Child and Adolescent Psychiatry Surveillance System (CAPSS), a system designed to identify cases of rare childhood mental health conditions through monthly reporting by hospital, community and university-based child and adolescent psychiatrists in the

UK and Republic of Ireland [14]. The CostED study involved monthly reporting of new cases of anorexia nervosa for a period of 8 months from 1st February to 30th September 2015.

Setting
Community-based secondary or tertiary child and adolescent mental health services in the UK and Republic of Ireland.

Procedures
All CAPSS clinicians were sent a study-specific protocol card and reporting instructions for new cases of anorexia nervosa and asked to check boxes to confirm any new cases of anorexia nervosa seen in the preceding month, or to check a "nil return" box if appropriate. The protocol card detailed the case notification definition for DSM5 anorexia nervosa [15] (see Appendix) which aimed to guide clinicians in their decision of whether to report a positive case. A tear-off slip was provided to enable psychiatrists to keep a record of the patients they reported. Positive returns were allocated a unique CAPSS ID number by the CAPSS administrator and notified to the CostED trial manager, who contacted the reporting clinician directly to request completion of a baseline questionnaire.

Participants
Cases were eligible for inclusion if the young person: (1) was aged 8 to 17 years; (2) had no previous episode of anorexia nervosa that had come to the attention of services; (3) received a clinical assessment in the reporting service during the study surveillance period; (4) had not been referred from another secondary health service, to ensure assessment and diagnosis had not happened prior to the surveillance period; (5) were notified by a community-based service; and (6) had the following clinical symptoms reported: "Restriction of energy intake relative to requirements" and "Persistent behaviour that interferes with weight gain, despite low weight". These two symptoms were used to provide an initial assessment of case eligibility and were subsequently checked using a tighter DSM5 analytic definition (see Appendix). Only one case meeting the broad criteria failed to meet the tighter criteria, thus confirming the validity of the broad criteria applied. Cases were excluded if the data were insufficient to assess eligibility.

Data
Data were collected at baseline using questionnaires sent to clinicians notifying a positive case of anorexia nervosa and, if the case was found to be eligible for inclusion, follow-up questionnaires were sent 6 and 12-months after the date the case was assessed and diagnosed, as reported by clinicians in the baseline questionnaires. Clinicians completed all questionnaires from clinical records.

In line with CAPSS procedures and ethics requirements, baseline questionnaires contained a limited set of patient identifiers to describe the sample and identify duplicate notifications. Patient identifiers included NHS or Community Health Index number (unique patient identifiers used in the included regions), hospital number, first half of postcode or town of residence for Republic of Ireland, gender, date of birth and ethnicity (White, Mixed, Asian, Black, Chinese, Other or Unknown). In Northern Ireland, identifiers were further limited to age in years and months (instead of date of birth) and hospital identifier (instead of hospital number), to further reduce the risk of patient identification given the small geographic area. In keeping with the requirements of the Northern Ireland Privacy Advisory Committee, all patient identifiable data from Northern Ireland were retained by the local research team, deduplicated, anonymised and subsequently sent for analysis to the central research team in King's College London.

The management of duplicates was dependent on the outcome for the original notification for which a duplicate had been identified. Four scenarios were considered, and each was assessed in different ways, as follows:

- Duplicates of notifications where the first notification met the study inclusion criteria, were excluded and the original notification retained.
- Duplicates of notifications where the first notification had been excluded due to age (too young) or clinical ineligibility, were assessed as a new case to determine if the case now met eligibility criteria.
- Duplicates of notifications where the first notification had been excluded due to a previous episode of anorexia nervosa, an assessment and diagnosis date prior to the study recruitment period, or referral from another secondary care service were excluded.
- Duplicates of notifications where the first notification contained insufficient information to judge eligibility for inclusion (for example, missing date of birth), were checked to see if the second notification contained the information missing from the first and, if available, the first notification was reassessed for eligibility and the duplicate excluded.

Baseline questionnaires covered characteristics of the notifying service (to enable classification of services as specialist or generic), clinical characteristics of the notified case and outcome measures (to assess eligibility and provide baseline assessments of outcome), and referral pathway information (to ensure assessment and diagnosis had not happened prior to the surveillance period and to determine whether the case had been referred to another service). Follow-up questionnaires included characteristics of the service, clinical characteristics of the notified case, outcome measures, and use of health services.

Incomplete or unreturned questionnaires were pursued via email, post and telephone. Cases where any symptoms required for case definition remained absent despite chasing, were assessed for eligibility by a consultant child and adolescent psychiatrist (MS). Those determined by MS to have too much data missing to assess, were excluded.

Clinical characteristics and outcome measures

Clinical characteristics included weight and height and a range of symptoms to support diagnosis (see Appendix). Weight and height were used to calculate percentage of median expected body mass index (BMI) for age and sex (%mBMI) [16, 17]. In addition, clinicians were asked to report scores for two generic outcome measures: the Children's Global Assessment Scale (CGAS) [18] and the Health of the Nation Outcome Score for Children and Adolescents (HoNOSCA) [19]. The CGAS is completed by clinicians and used to rate emotional and behavioural functioning of young people in the family, school, and social context. Clinicians score the young person on a scale from 1 to 100 using a classification which includes ten categories ranging from 'Extremely impaired' (score 1–10) to 'Doing very well' (score 91–100) [18]. All CostED questionnaires contained a copy of the CGAS classification system, describing each of the ten categories, to support scoring by clinicians. The HoNOSCA is a routine outcome measurement tool rating 13 clinical features on a 5-point severity scale. It assesses behaviours, impairments, symptoms, and social functioning of young people with mental health problems, producing a total score on a scale from 0 to 52, where a higher score indicates a poorer outcome.

Although there is a preference for generic measures of health-related quality of life capable of generating quality adjusted life years (QALYs) in economic evaluations – since this allows for comparison across populations and disorders when making resource allocation decisions – no such measure is routinely collected by NHS clinical services. Given the reliance on data from clinical records, it was therefore not possible to undertake a cost-utility analysis, which uses QALYs as the measure of effect, as is preferred, for example, by the National Institute for Health and Care Excellence which produces clinical guidelines in England [20].

Service use and costs

Since data were collected from clinical records, the perspective of the economic evaluation was limited to health services for which data were likely to be available to clinicians. This included: hospital inpatient admissions (including paediatric, general child/adolescent or adult psychiatry, child/adolescent or adult eating disorders unit, or other), out-patient attendances (including paediatrics, specialist eating disorders service, and other psychiatric service) and day-patient attendances (including paediatrics, specialist eating disorders service, and other psychiatric service). Adult services were included because some adolescents may have transferred to adult services by follow-up.

All costs, in pounds sterling, were for the 2015/16 financial year, in line with the data collection period. Discounting was not necessary as follow-up was not longer than 12-months. Costs for NHS hospital admissions and outpatient and day-patient contacts, including CAMHS contacts, were taken from NHS reference costs [21]. Independent sector costs were provided by a range of independent sector organisations and NHS Trusts via personal communications. Unit costs are summarised in Table 1.

Classification of services

Specialist eating disorders services are not clearly defined, with definitions changing over time [22, 23]. In order to classify services as specialist or generic, an online Delphi survey was undertaken to obtain consensus on the key features of a specialist child and adolescent eating disorders service from a range of stakeholders, including service users and their families, child and adolescent psychiatrists, paediatricians, other eating disorders professionals and service commissioners [13]. Further information regarding the characteristics included in the Delphi survey can be found in the published report [13]. Characteristics meeting pre-defined consensus thresholds to be considered important for the classification of services as specialist eating disorders services included: offering specialist outpatient treatment for eating disorders, providing multi-disciplinary specialist outpatient clinics dedicated to eating disorders and holding weekly multi-disciplinary meetings dedicated to eating disorders. All cases notified by a service meeting all three criteria were classified as specialist; all other services were classified as generic CAMHS.

Data analysis

Analyses compared participants assessed in specialist eating disorders services with those assessed in generic CAMHS. All analyses were adjusted for pre-specified baseline covariates including CGAS, %mBMI, age, sex and region (England, Wales, Scotland, Northern Ireland,

Table 1 Unit costs for health services used

Service	Unit cost	Source
NHS inpatient cost per night		
Eating disorders unit – child/adolescent	510.14	NHS Reference Costs[a]
Eating disorders unit – adult	455.02	NHS Reference Costs[a]
General psychiatry – child/adolescent	633.07	NHS Reference Costs[a]
General psychiatry – adult	197.29	NHS Reference Costs[a]
Paediatric if stay = 1 night	426.99	NHS Reference Costs[a]
Paediatric if stay> 1 night	592.27	NHS Reference Costs[a]
Other NHS	389.10	NHS Reference Costs[a]
Independent sector inpatient cost per night		
Eating disorders unit – child/adolescent	695.00	Personal communication
General psychiatry – child/adolescent	668.00	Personal communication
Outpatient cost per contact		
Eating disorders service	262.12	NHS Reference Costs[a]
Other psychiatry	298.57	NHS Reference Costs[a]
Paediatric	194.36	NHS Reference Costs[a]
Day-patient cost per contact		
Eating disorders service	274.21	NHS Reference Costs[a]
Other psychiatry	326.16	NHS Reference Costs[a]
Paediatric	446.60	NHS Reference Costs[a]

[a]Department of Health. NHS reference costs. 2015

Republic of Ireland). Outcomes and total costs per participant were compared using standard parametric t-tests [24], with the robustness of this approach for costs confirmed using bootstrapping (5000 iterations) [25]. Analyses used complete case data with the impact of missing cost and outcome data over the follow-up period tested in sensitivity analyses using multiple imputations [26]. Alternative approaches to the handling of observational data were considered, such as matching and stratification [27], but small sample sizes, compounded by missing data at baseline and follow-up, and imbalance in the size of the two groups (specialist versus generic) precluded these, and more sophisticated, approaches.

The pre-specified primary measure of effectiveness, as outlined in the original protocol, was the HoNOSCA. The %mBMI was specified as a secondary cost-effectiveness analysis because, although more narrowly focused, data on weight and height were expected to be available for a greater proportion of the sample. From the baseline questionnaires, however, the level of missing HoNOSCA data was substantial (79% missing at baseline) and the protocol was amended replacing the HoNOSCA with the CGAS, for which a greater proportion of data were available (8% missing at baseline).

Cost-effectiveness was explored in a decision-making context, focusing on the probability of one service type being cost-effective compared to the other, given the data available, rather than a focus on statistical significance. This is the recommended approach for economic evaluation in the UK [28]. Cost-effectiveness was assessed using incremental cost-effectiveness ratios (difference in mean cost between two interventions divided by the difference in mean effect) and taking the recommended net benefit approach [29]. Incremental cost-effectiveness ratios were calculated for scenarios where one intervention demonstrates higher costs and better outcomes (it is unnecessary to calculate these ratios where one group shows both lower costs and better outcomes as it 'dominates' the other group). A joint distribution of incremental mean costs and effects for each group was generated using bootstrapping [25] to explore the probability that each service is the optimal choice, subject to a range of values a decision-maker might be willing to pay for outcome improvements (£0 to £30,000). Cost-effectiveness acceptability curves were generated by plotting these probabilities for a range of possible values of the ceiling ratio [30, 31]. These curves are the recommended approach to dealing with uncertainty around the cost and effect estimates and the maximum cost-effectiveness ratio that decision-maker would consider acceptable [28, 31].

Results
Sample
Over the eight-month surveillance period, 6401 case notification cards were sent to clinicians and 3211 were returned (50.16%). Of these, 997 positive cases of anorexia nervosa were reported and 2214 were nil returns. Of the 997 positive returns, 48 (5%) were excluded due to reporting errors or clincans stating that they did not wish to take part in the study (due to lack of time, retirement etc.). Baseline questionnaires were sent to clinicians who reported the remaining 949 positive returns, and 597 (63%) were returned. Of these, 299 (49%) were ineligible (due to age, previous episode of anorexia nervosa, date of assessment outside the surveillance period, referral from another secondary care service, current inpatient, duplicate notification or insufficient information to assess diagnosis). Thus 298 cases were included in the study, 192 (64%) assessed in a specialist eating disorders service and 106 (36%) assessed in generic CAMHS. Clinicians completed and returned follow-up questionnaires for 220 cases at 6-months (74%), 147 specialist (77%) and 73 generic (69%), and 187 cases at 12-months (63%), 137 specialist (71%) and 50 generic (47%). Included cases were referred from a total of 79 services, 50 of which were generic CAMHS (63%) and 29 were specialist eating disorders services (37%).

Demographic and baseline characteristics are reported in Table 2. Mean age (approx. 15 years), proportion female (92%) and ethnicity (92–94% Any White background) were similar between the two groups and in line with evidence of the demographic at risk for anorexia

Table 2 Baseline characteristics of specialist versus generic cases

	Specialist		Generic	
	N	Mean (SD) or %	N	Mean (SD) or %
Age	192	15.09 (1.60)	106	14.84 (1.66)
Sex				
Female	176	91.67%	97	91.51%
Male	16	8.33%	9	8.49%
Ethnicity				
Any White	174	91.58%	95	94.06%
Other	16	8.42%	6	5.94%
Clinical status				
%mBMI	191	82.70 (11.11)	105	83.60 (9.90)
CGAS	174	43.22 (14.40)	99	47.86 (13.29)
HoNOSCA	45	21.04 (8.43)	16	14.88 (5.77)

NB: Not all percentages add up to 100% due to rounding

nervosa [32]. Baseline clinical variables suggest the sample were significantly impaired. Mean %mBMI was approximately 83%, falling within the range expected for a diagnosis of anorexia nervosa (< 85%). Mean CGAS score was approximately 44, falling within the 'obvious problems' range [18], and mean total HoNOSCA score was approximately 19, indicative of a severity similar to that at inpatient admission [9, 33]. Comparing the two groups, %mBMI was similar in the two groups (82.7% versus 83.6%) but differences were evident for CGAS (mean 43 specialist versus 48 generic) and HoNOSCA (mean 21 specialist versus 15 generic).

Service use
Mean use of inpatient, outpatient and day-patient services over the 12-month follow-up is reported in Table 3. Mean number of inpatient admissions and inpatient nights per participant were similar in the two groups, although participants assessed in specialist services spent longer, on average, in eating disorders facilities (20 versus 13 nights) and less time on general psychiatry wards (7 versus 13 nights). The pattern for outpatient attendances was similar, with participants assessed in specialist services having more contacts in eating disorders facilities (27 versus 15 attendances) but fewer general psychiatry contacts (3 versus 12 attendances) and a similar number of contacts in total (30 versus 27 attendances). Day-patient services were accessed by 11% of the specialist group but only 4% of the generic group, with average number of attendances also being higher for the specialist group (5 versus 1 attendance). Most of these contacts were in eating disorders services.

Cost
Cost results are reported in Table 4. Although there were only small observed differences in total costs, adjustment for pre-specified baseline variables made a substantial difference due to baseline differences, particularly in the CGAS. Adjusted analyses suggested large differences in favour of specialist services (costs lower on average), although these differences were not significant. Imputation of missing data made little difference to the results, with costs remaining lower in the specialist group in adjusted analyses.

Outcomes
Outcome results are reported in Table 5. At baseline, %mBMI was not statistically different between the two groups. However, both CGAS and HoNOSCA scores were significantly worse in the specialist group. At the 6-month follow-up, in adjusted analyses, %mBMI was significantly higher in the specialist than the generic group. Although %mBMI remained higher for the specialist group at 12-months, the difference

Table 3 Service use between baseline and 12-month follow-up

Service	Specialist (n = 137)		Generic (n = 50)	
	Mean (SD)	% using	Mean (SD)	% using
Inpatient admissions	0.54 (1.06)	28.47%	0.60 (1.20)	30.00%
Inpatient nights	31.75 (80.03)	28.47%	30.78 (68.65)	30.00%
Paediatric – NHS	2.18 (9.28)	15.33%	4.72 (12.96)	20.00%
Eating disorders – NHS	5.56 (37.72)	2.92%	0.28 (1.98)	2.00%
Eating disorders – Independent	14.28 (57.93)	8.76%	12.84 (49.89)	8.00%
Psychiatry – NHS	5.38 (24.47)	6.57%	11.58 (39.42)	12.00%
Psychiatry – Independent	1.39 (12.43)	2.19%	1.36 (9.62)	2.00%
Other – NHS	0.53 (6.15)	1.46%	0.00 (0.00)	0.00%
Outpatient attendances	29.98 (17.70)	98.54%	27.14 (32.62)	96.00%
Paediatric	0.07 (0.34)	5.11%	0.98 (2.46)	28.00%
Eating disorders	27.11 (18.11)	92.70%	14.58 (32.07)	56.00%
Psychiatry	2.80 (8.94)	17.52%	11.58 (13.55)	68.00%
Day patient attendances	4.61 (16.60)	10.95%	0.86 (5.66)	4.00%
Paediatric	0.00 (0.00)	0.00%	0.06 (0.42)	2.00%
Eating disorders	4.25 (16.13)	10.22%	0.80 (5.66)	2.00%
Psychiatry	0.37 (4.27)	0.73%	0.00 (0.00)	0.00%

was no longer significant. No significant differences were identified for CGAS or HoNOSCA at either follow-up. Imputation of missing data made little difference, with imputed results being similar to complete case results.

Cost-effectiveness

Using the CGAS (primary measure of effect) at 12-months (primary endpoint), adjusted total costs per participant were lower and adjusted CGAS scores slightly lower (poorer outcomes) in the specialist than the

Table 4 Total cost per participant between baseline and 12-month follow-up

Service	Specialist Mean £ (SD)	Generic Mean £ (SD)	Unadjusted[a] Mean difference (95% CI)	p-value	Adjusted[ab] Mean difference (95% CI)	p-value
Baseline to 6 months	n = 147	n = 73				
Inpatient	11105 (28877)	11179 (29050)				
Outpatient	4764 (2866)	4310 (3975)				
Day-patient	947 (3468)	299 (1708)				
Total	16817 (28469)	15789 (28184)	1028 (– 6979 to 9036)	0.801	– 3586 (–11999 to 4827)	0.402
Six to 12 months	n = 137	n = 50				
Inpatient	8153 (24763)	8224 (20894)				
Outpatient	3103 (3058)	3279 (5775)				
Day-patient	306 (1703)	44 (310)				
Total	11562 (24905)	11547 (22133)	14 (– 7875 to 7903)	0.997	– 2785 (– 11241 to 5670)	0.516
Baseline to 12 months	n = 137	n = 50				
Inpatient	19462 (49946)	19755 (44677)				
Outpatient	7955 (4722)	7470 (8499)				
Day-patient	1284 (4608)	246 (1559)				
Total	28700 (49716)	27471 (44317)	1230 (–14529 to 16988)	0.878	–7106 (–23590 to 9379)	0.396

NB: Not all totals add up due to rounding; [a]Standard parametric tests with validity tested using bootstrapping (bootstrapped results similar so not reported); [b]Adjusted for baseline CGAS, baseline %mBMI, age, sex and region

Table 5 Outcome measures at baseline, 6 and 12-month follow-up

Outcome measure	Specialist		Generic		Unadjusted[a]		Adjusted[ab]	
	N	Mean (SD)	n	Mean (SD)	Mean difference (95% CI)	p-value	Mean difference (95% CI)	p-value
Baseline								
%mBMI	191	82.70 (11.10)	105	83.60 (9.90)	−0.90 (−3.46 to 1.66)	0.489		
CGAS	174	43.22 (14.40)	99	47.86 (13.29)	−4.64 (−8.11 to −1.17)	**0.009**		
HoNOSCA	45	21.04 (8.43)	16	14.88 (5.77)	6.17 (1.60 to 10.74)	**0.009**		
6-months								
%mBMI	143	91.98 (8.51)	67	89.62 (12.89)	2.37 (−0.59 to 5.31)	0.116	2.58 (0.16 to 5.01)	**0.037**
CGAS	115	58.94 (17.17)	55	63.27 (17.05)	−4.33 (−9.88 to 1.21)	0.125	0.49 (−5.14 to 6.12)	0.864
HoNOSCA	17	9.47 (7.43)	16	11.88 (10.31)	−2.40 (−8.76 to 3.95)	0.446	−6.61 (−15.54 to 2.31)	0.140
12-months								
%mBMI	106	94.70 (10.61)	39	93.36 (9.46)	1.34 (−2.48 to 5.16)	0.489	0.09 (−3.54 to 3.73)	0.960
CGAS	97	68.39 (17.95)	38	71.58 (21.41)	−3.19 (−10.37 to 4.00)	0.382	−0.65 (−8.26 to 6.96)	0.866
HoNOSCA	12	7.42 (4.48)	7	13.57 (16.94)	−6.15 (−16.88 to 4.57)	0.243	−12.42 (−31.07 to 6.23)	0.171

[a]Standard parametric tests; [b]Adjusted for baseline CGAS, baseline %mBMI, age, sex and region; %mBMI percentage of median expected BMI for age and sex (higher percentage, better outcome), CGAS Children's Global Assessment Scale (scored between 1 and 100; higher score, better outcome), HoNOSCA Health of the Nation Outcome Score for Children and Adolescents (scored between 0 and 52; higher score, poorer outcome)

generic group, generating an incremental cost-effectiveness ratio of £10,932 (−£7106/− 0.65). This suggests that assessment in a generic service generates a unit improvement in CGAS score for an additional cost of approximately £11,000, compared to specialist services. The cost-effectiveness plane in Fig. 1 illustrates that the scatter points fall in all four quadrants, but the largest proportion are in the South-West quadrant where specialist services are cheaper (below the x-axis)

and less effective (left of the y-axis). At the 6-month follow-up, adjusted total costs per participant were lower in the specialist group and adjusted CGAS scores slightly higher (better outcomes), so specialist services dominated generic services (Fig. 2).

Cost-effectiveness acceptability curves (Fig. 3), are downward sloping, suggesting that the cost-effectiveness of specialist eating disorders services declines as willingness to pay for improvements in CGAS increase, but

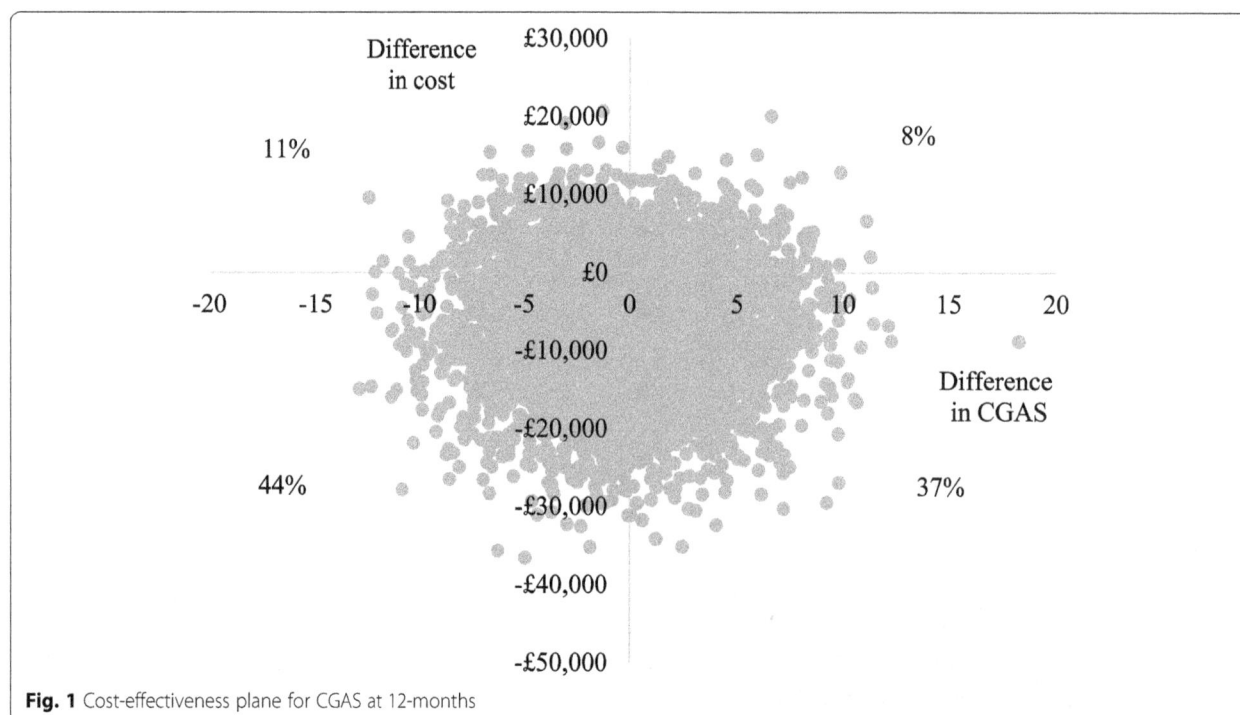

Fig. 1 Cost-effectiveness plane for CGAS at 12-months

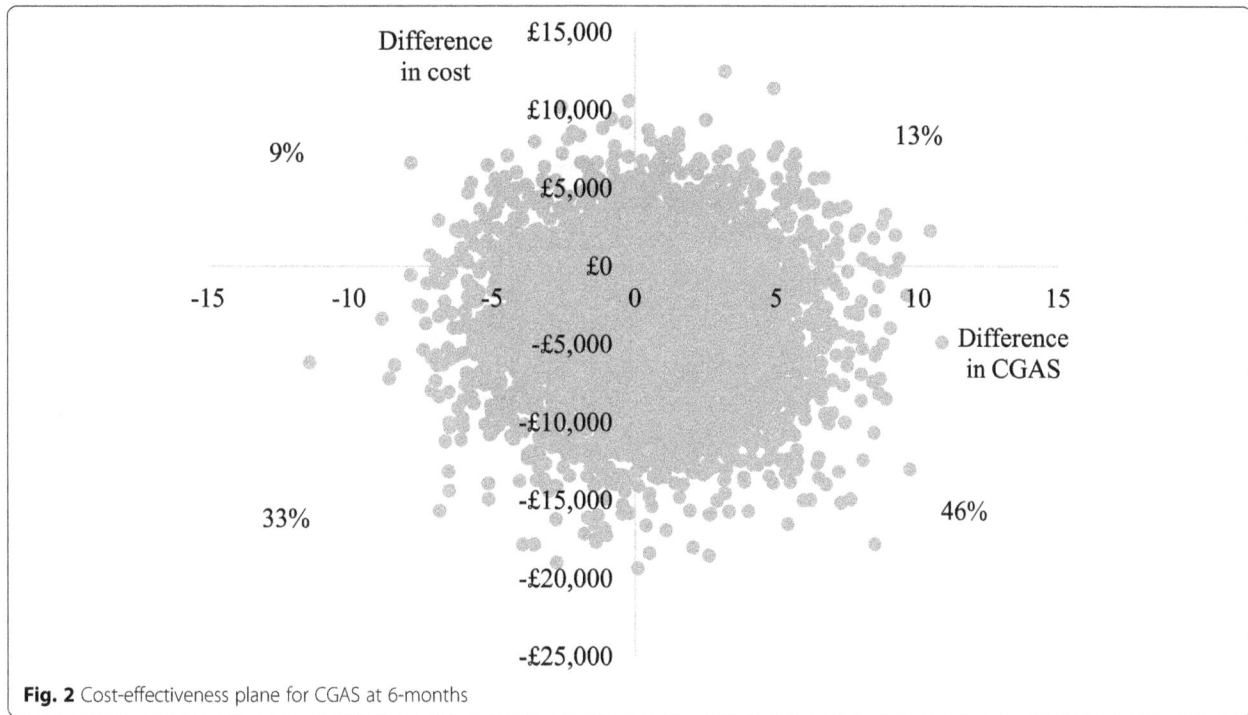

Fig. 2 Cost-effectiveness plane for CGAS at 6-months

does not fall below 50% over the willingness to pay range tested. This is due to the lower cost of the specialist group and the small differences in effects (i.e., at low levels of willingness to pay, society favours the cheaper option, but at higher levels of willingness to pay, society becomes increasingly indifferent between the two options). The curves illustrate that there is a higher probability of assessment in specialist services being cost-effective compared to generic services at both follow-ups, with probabilities at 12-months ranging from around 90% at zero willingness to pay for improvements in CGAS to 50% at willingness to pay of £30,000.

In terms of %mBMI, the secondary measure of effect, adjusted total costs per participant were lower and %mBMI scores were slightly higher (better outcome) in the specialist than the generic group at both the 6-

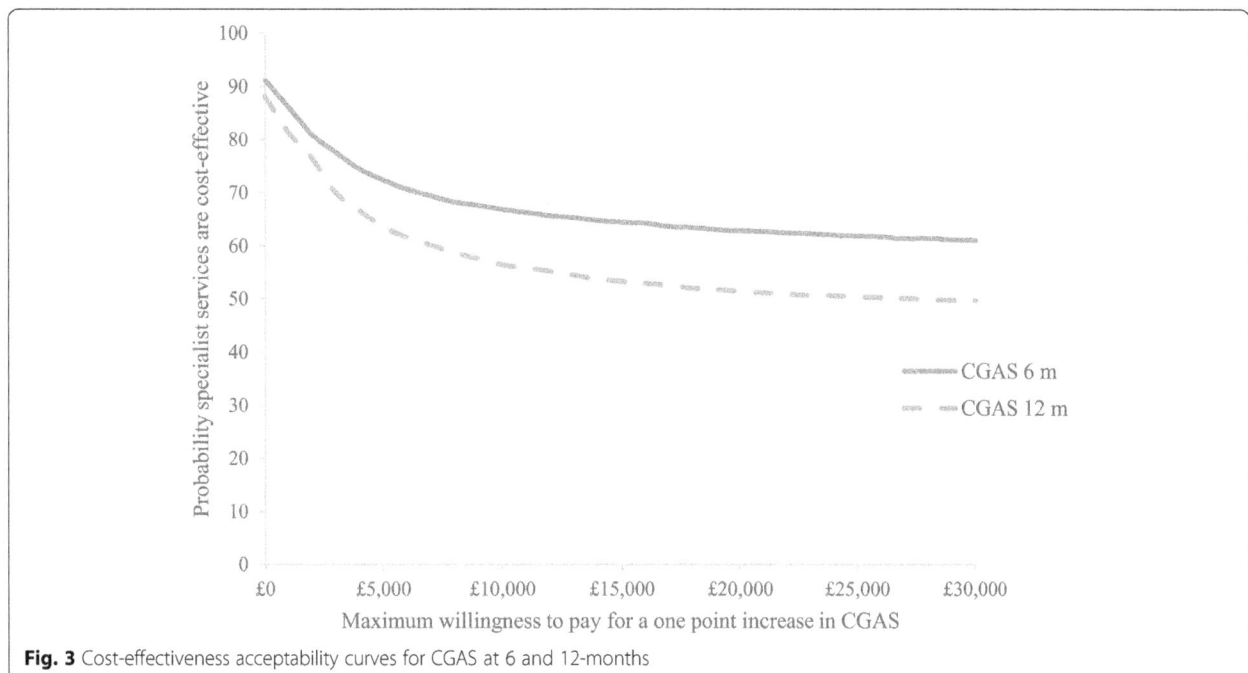

Fig. 3 Cost-effectiveness acceptability curves for CGAS at 6 and 12-months

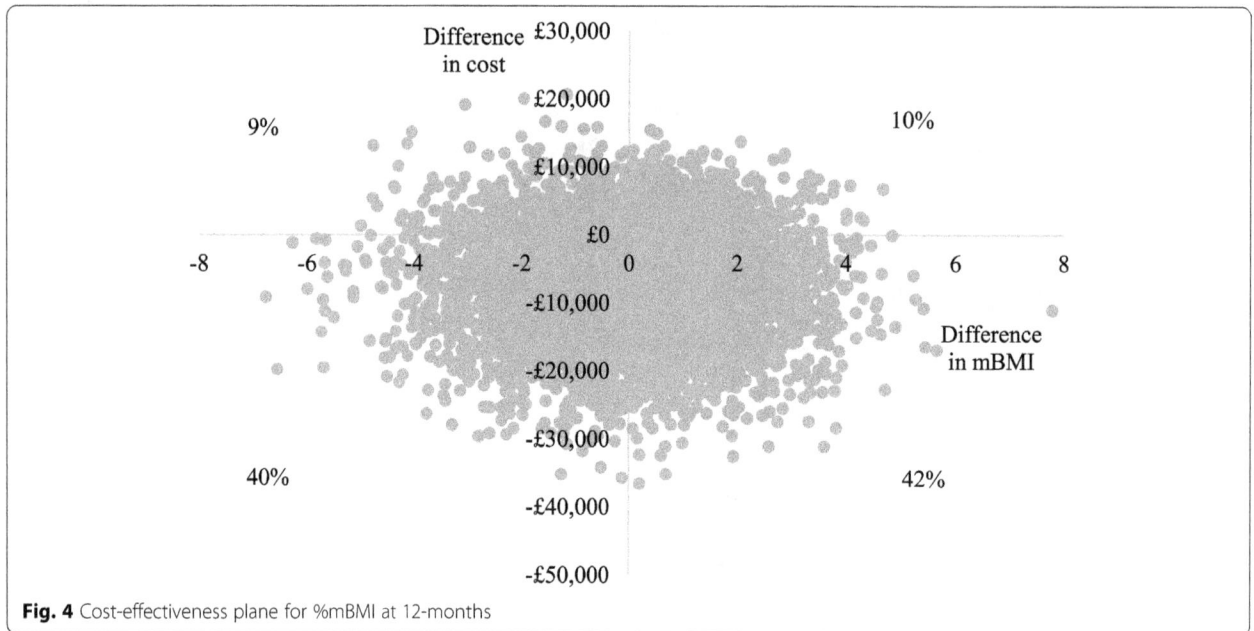

Fig. 4 Cost-effectiveness plane for %mBMI at 12-months

month and 12-month follow-ups, so specialist services dominated generic services (Figs. 4 and 5). Cost-effectiveness acceptability curves (Fig. 6) suggest there is a higher probability of initial assessment in specialist services being cost-effective compared to generic services at both follow-ups, with probabilities at 12-months ranging from 76% at zero willingness to pay to 56% at willingness to pay of £30,000.

Discussion

Overview of the results

The results presented suggest that for children and adolescents aged 8 to 17 with anorexia nervosa in the UK and Republic of Ireland, assessment in specialist eating disorders services has a similar or higher probability of being cost-effective than assessment in generic CAMHS. At 12-months follow-up, specialist eating disorders

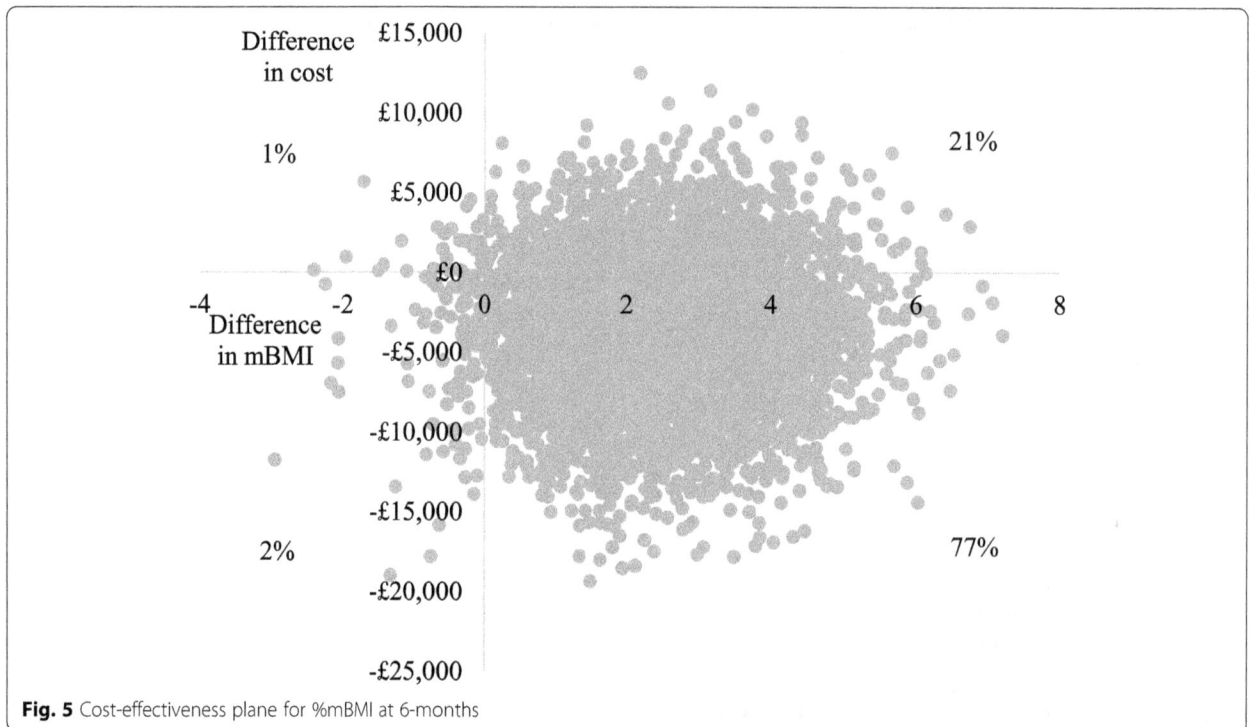

Fig. 5 Cost-effectiveness plane for %mBMI at 6-months

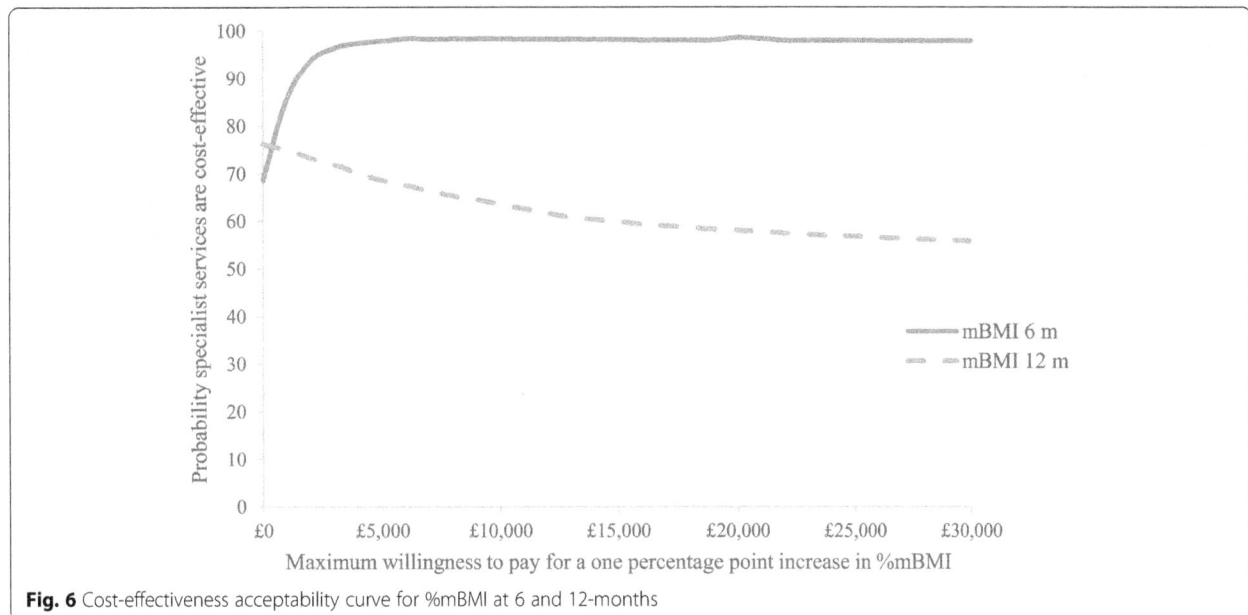

Fig. 6 Cost-effectiveness acceptability curve for %mBMI at 6 and 12-months

services had a higher probability of being cost-effective than generic CAMHS at low levels of willingness to pay for improvements in CGAS score and improvements in %mBMI; at higher levels of willingness to pay, the probability of either specialist or generic being cost-effective was around 50%. At 6-months follow-up, assessment in specialist eating disorders services had a higher probability of being cost-effective for the full range of willingness to pay values tested (£0 to £30,000). Without knowledge of the amount society is willing to pay for improvements in CGAS or %mBMI, no firm conclusions can be reached. However, we would hypothesise that it is unlikely that decision-makers would be willing to pay in excess of £30,000 for a one percentage point improvement in either measure, which is the minimum amount that would need to be spent for generic CAMHS to have a similar or higher probability of being cost-effective compared to specialist services.

Cost-effectiveness findings in favour of specialist services were due to similar outcomes in the two groups alongside lower costs in the specialist group, following adjustment for poorer baseline clinical status in the specialist group. Despite this poorer baseline status, children and adolescents assessed in specialist services achieved significantly better weight outcomes 6-months after assessment and similar outcomes at 12-months compare to those assessed in generic CAMHS, with a similar level of health service use, and thus similar costs.

These results are in line with previous evidence to support the cost-effectiveness of specialist services for children and adolescents with anorexia nervosa. One RCT carried out in the UK, concluded that specialist out-patient treatment has a higher probability of being cost-effective than inpatient or general outpatient treatment [9, 11]. In common with the CostED study, there were no differences in outcomes, however the specialist outpatient group had substantially lower costs than the comparison groups over two-year follow-up. Similar results were seen in a London-based study [34]. Whilst no significant differences in outcome were evident, admissions were significantly lower over one-year follow-up for children and adolescents assessed and treated in a specialist service (15% admitted) compared with those assessed and treated in a non-specialist service (40%).

From a pragmatic point of view, combining the CostED study results with previous evidence to support the cost-effectiveness of specialist community-based services [11] and to suggest that specialist services reduce admissions and costs [34], the evidence as a whole supports the provision of specialist eating disorders services, which is in line with recent guidance for and investment into the development of community eating disorders services for children and adolescents in England [22]. In addition, the CostED results should be considered alongside other factors of relevance to investment decisions, in particular the preferences of patients and carers. Existing evidence suggests a preference from these groups for specialist services [34–36], making the differential use of inpatient and outpatient services identified – with children and adolescents assessed in specialist services having greater contact with eating disorders facilities and less contact with general psychiatry services than those assessed in generic services – of particular importance.

Strengths and limitations

Anorexia nervosa is a relatively rare disorder, in comparison to other childhood mental health disorders, such as depression, making it difficult to recruit adequately powered samples for clinical trials. This surveillance study was able to gather case notifications from almost one hundred services across the UK and Republic of Ireland, which for a clinical trial would be prohibitively expensive. After accounting for duplicates and withdrawals, 298 cases were eligible for inclusion, a sample which is larger than RCTs in this population have been able to achieve to date [9, 37, 38]. However, it should be noted that this sample does not reflect the entire population of children and adolescents with an anorexia nervosa diagnosis for the first time in this age range, as only 50% of case notification cards were returned. Whilst a proportion of these would have been 'nil' returns (no case of anorexia nervosa to report), some will have been missing cases of anorexia nervosa meeting the study inclusion criteria.

In addition, the study benefits from being 'real world', reflecting actual clinical practice with standard clinical populations, broad inclusion criteria and limited exclusion criteria. However, the results were clearly affected by baseline differences in outcome scores between the two groups, which is a limitation of evaluations that do not randomly allocate participants, and may also reflect a level of participant self-selection, at least in those participants with access to both types of services. All analyses were therefore adjusted for baseline variables to minimise the impact of this limitation. Alternative approaches to the handling of observational data were considered, but small sample sizes, missing data, and imbalance in the size of the two groups precluded such approaches and thus the results should be interpreted within the context of the methodological limitations of the study.

At baseline, 63% of questionnaires were returned allowing cases to be assessed for eligibility for inclusion in the follow-up. Of those assessed as eligible, 74% of 6-month follow-up questionnaires and 63% of 12-month follow-up questionnaires were returned. Missing data was therefore a limitation which impacts upon the generalisability and interpretation of the results. However, imputation of missing data produced very similar results to complete case analyses, giving greater confidence in the results presented. In contrast, missing items in returned questionnaires were small in number, except for the HoNOSCA, suggesting that clinical services are not using this measure in routine practice. As a result, the HoNOSCA was removed as the pre-specified primary outcome measure and replaced with the CGAS, which had substantially higher response rates.

Some limitations arose directly from reliance on retrospective data contained within clinical records, rather than prospective collection from children and adolescents. In particular, availability of outcome data was limited to CGAS scores and %mBMI. These outcomes are too narrow to capture all impacts clinical services may have on the quality of life of children and adolescents with anorexia nervosa which suggests the need for clinical services to consider the consistent collection of measures of change, including measures relevant to eating disorders and broader measures of quality of life, to aid investigation of the effectiveness of services from both a clinical and a research point of view. Similarly, service use was limited to those health services for which data were likely to be available to all clinicians from clinical records, although this did capture the key services found in previous evaluations to account for the vast majority (over 90%) of the total costs in similar samples [11, 34]. Adjustment for confounding factors was also limited by the availability of data in clinical records, and thus it is possible that unobserved factors of importance were missed.

Whilst recruitment from across the UK and Republic of Ireland avoids biases inherent in studying clinical samples from a small number of services across a narrow range of geographical locations, bias in reporting and questionnaire completion is likely to be a problem. Specialist services have larger numbers of eating disorders cases than generic CAMHS, placing a greater questionnaire completion burden on clinicians, which may reduce their willingness to respond. However, those in specialist services are more likely to have an interest in the research, which may have a positive effect on their willingness to take part. Whilst the direction of any bias at the reporting stage is unknown, it is worth noting that a much larger proportion of the total number of services reporting at least one notification were generic CAMHS (over 60%), suggesting that these services were engaging with the study. However, biases in questionnaire completion at follow-up were evident, with completion rates being higher in the specialist group (77% at 6-months; 71% at 12-months follow-up) compared to generic CAMH S (69% at 6-months; 47% at 12-months follow-up).

The CostED study was also open to bias from loss to follow-up due to referral elsewhere or discharge – likely to be a particular problem as adolescents reach 18 years of age and move to university or to take up employment. Follow-up data were less likely to be available for participants who were doing well and had been discharged prior to follow-up, for participants who were doing badly and had been admitted to hospital or referred from generic CAMHS to specialist services, and for participants who had moved out of area. Although the small differences in outcomes between the groups may suggest that loss to follow-up due to discharge may also be similar, evidence that children and adolescents treated in generic services are supported for longer than those in specialist services [34] would suggest that loss of data due to discharge may have been greater for specialist services.

In terms of loss of data due to hospital admission, specialist services will generally remain in regular contact with their patients while they are in hospital and will also continue outpatient treatment following discharge. Although practice is variable, this is less likely to be the case in generic services, so data loss as a result of referral may have been greater in generic services. It is also worth noting that there was considerably greater loss to follow-up in generic services, particularly at 12-months (53% versus 29%), and if this indicates a greater proportion of participants doing badly who are admitted to hospital or referred to specialist community services, this would have biased the results in favour of generic CAMHS. This type of loss to follow-up may also explain the surprisingly low lengths of admissions in the CostED sample compared to other studies [34, 39].

A further bias may arise from the exclusion of children and adolescents admitted directly to inpatient facilities without any contact with community-based services, which may be more likely in areas where community-based specialist eating disorders services are not available. This potentially introduces a bias in favour of generic CAMHS since these children and adolescents will be receiving considerably more expensive care as inpatients than the cost of treating them in community-based generic services would have been. Finally, it should be noted that nationally applicable unit costs were applied to most services, which increases the generalisability of the results to the national picture but reduces variability and the local applicability of the results.

Conclusion

Assessment and diagnosis in a specialist eating disorders service for children and adolescents with anorexia nervosa may have a higher probability of being cost-effective than assessment and diagnosis in generic CAMHS, as specialist services were able to achieve larger gains in clinical effectiveness but without additional expenditure.

Appendix

Case notification definition

Please report any child/young person aged 8 to 17 years and 11 months inclusive, who meets the case notification definition criteria below for the first time in the last month. One bullet point criterion from each group below should be fulfilled.

Group A

- Restriction of food, low body weight, or
- Weight less than expected for age

Group B

- Fear of gaining weight, or
- Fear of becoming fat, or
- Behaviour that interferes with weight gain, for example excessive exercising, self-induced vomiting, use of laxatives and diuretics

Group C

- Body image disturbance, or
- Persistent lack of recognition of the seriousness of the current low body weight

Exclusions

- Patients who are not underweight
- Patients with bulimia nervosa, binge eating disorder, avoidant restrictive food intake disorder or other failure to thrive presentations

DSM5 analytic definition

The tighter DSM5 analytic definition used to check the validity of the broad 'two-symptom' definition, included the following symptoms:

1. "Restriction of energy intake relative to requirements" and
2. "Intense fear of gaining weight or of becoming fat" or "Persistent behaviour that interferes with weight gain, despite low weight" and
3. "Perception that body shape/size is larger than it is" or "Preoccupation with body weight and shape" or "Lack of recognition of the seriousness of the current low body weight"

Clinical symptoms contained in the CostED questionnaires to support DSM5 diagnosis

Clinical symptoms included in the baseline, 6 and 12-month follow-up questionnaires were used to support diagnosis of DSM5 anorexia nervosa and included the following features which required a response of yes, no, not known or not applicable: restriction of energy intake relative to requirements; intense fear of gaining weight or of becoming fat; persistent behaviour that interferes with weight gain, despite low weight; perception that body shape/size is larger than it is; preoccupation with body weight and shape; lack of recognition of the seriousness of the current low body weight; excessive exercise; self-induced vomiting (including frequency); laxative or diuretic abuse; and binge eating (including frequency). In addition, for females, clinicians were asked if the young person had reached menarche and, if yes, whether there was secondary amenorrhoea.

Abbreviations

BMI: Body Mass Index; %mBMI: Percentage of median expected body mass for age and sex; CAMHS: Child and Adolescent Mental Health Services; CAPS S: Child and Adolescent Psychiatry Surveillance System; CGAS: Children's Global Assessment Scale; CostED: Cost-effectiveness of models of care for young people with Eating Disorders; DSM5: Diagnostic and Statistical Manual of Mental Disorders Fifth Edition; HoNOSCA: Health of the Nation Outcome Score for Children and Adolescents; NHS: National Health Service; QALY: Quality Adjusted Life Year; UK: United Kingdom

Acknowledgements

We would like to thank all the clinicians who were kind enough to give up their time to provide the CostED study with CAPSS notifications and to complete questionnaires. We know your time is precious and in short supply and we are truly grateful. We would also like to thank the team at the Child and Adolescent Psychiatry Surveillance System, based at the Royal College of Psychiatrist's Centre for Care Quality and Improvement, for their support with the design and running of the surveillance aspect of this study, and all the members of our study steering committee for their invaluable advice.

Authors' contributions

SB led the study, managed the King's College London research staff, contributed to the design of the study and the data analysis, and drafted the manuscript. HP contributed to data collection, data entry, data cleaning, data analysis, and commented on and approved the manuscript. BB contributed to the design of the study, the data analysis, and commented on and approved the manuscript. TF contributed to the design of the study, provided expertise on CAPSS methodology, provided clinical expertise, and commented on and approved the manuscript. DN contributed to the design of the study, provided expertise on CAPSS methodology, provided clinical expertise, and commented on and approved the manuscript. MS contributed to the design of the study, provided clinical expertise, and commented on and approved the manuscript. SG contributed to the design of the study, provided clinical expertise, and commented on and approved the manuscript. GM contributed to the design of the study, managed the Northern Ireland research staff, and commented on and approved the manuscript. RS contributed to data collection, data entry, data cleaning and data analysis, and commented on and approved the manuscript. NL contributed to data collection, data entry and data management in Northern Ireland, and commented on and approved the manuscript. GK contributed to data collection, data entry and data management in Northern Ireland, and commented on and approved the manuscript. JK provided PPI expertise, advised on the design and supported the implementation of the Delphi survey and commented on and approved the manuscript. KJ provided clinical expertise and commented on and approved the manuscript. HS provided clinical expertise and commented on and approved the manuscript. IE contributed to the design of the study, provided clinical support to the research team, and commented on and approved the manuscript. The author(s) read and approved the final manuscript.

Authors' information

SB Professor of Health Economics
HP Trial Manager
BB Senior Lecturer in Health Economics
TF Professor of Child and Adolescent Psychiatry
DN Reader in Child and Adolescent Psychiatry
MS Consultant Child and Adolescent Psychiatrist
SG Professor of Adolescent Psychiatry
GM Professor of Social Work
RS Research Assistant
NL Research Fellow
GK Research Fellow
JK Policy Officer
KJ Consultant Child and Adolescent Psychiatrist
HS Consultant Forensic Child and Adolescent Psychiatrist
IE Professor of Family Psychology and Family Therapy

Funding

The study was funded by the NIHR Health Services and Delivery Research Programme (11/1023/17) and the HSCNI Public Health Agency Research and Development Division (COM/4716/12). The funding bodies had no role in the design of the study, the collection, analysis, and interpretation of data or in writing the manuscript. The views expressed are those of the authors and not necessarily those of the NHS, the NIHR or the Department of Health.

Availability of data and materials

As a result of the collection of confidential patient data without consent, and approval from the Health Research Authority (following advice from the Confidentiality Advisory Group) for data to be provided for the purposes of the specified activity only, the datasets generated and analysed during the current study cannot be made publicly available for other purposes. However, the CostED research group will consider requests for further analysis on a case by case basis, subject to appropriate ethical/HRA CAG approvals. All data enquiries should be submitted to the corresponding author for consideration in the first instance. Access to available anonymised data may be granted following review and if appropriate permissions are in place.

Competing interests

TF reports she is Chair of the Child and Adolescent Psychiatry Surveillance Service that was used to run part of the study, which is an unpaid position (other than travel expenses). KJ reports that he was principal investigator for the Aberdeen site for a Sunovion sponsored multisite trial on effectiveness of Lurasidone in paediatric schizophrenia. JK reports that Beat has contracts with some NHS Trusts and Clinical Commissioning Groups who provide and commission (respectively) community eating disorders services for children and young people. In these contracts Beat works with the local services to deliver awareness raising training for professionals and in some cases to offer peer coaching for carers. All other authors declare that they have no competing interests.

Author details

[1]Institute of Psychiatry, Psychology & Neuroscience at King's College London, PO24 David Goldberg Centre, De Crespigny Park, London SE5 8AF, UK. [2]Department of Psychiatry, University of Cambridge, Level 5 Clifford Allbutt Building, Cambridge Biomedical Campus, Hills Road, Cambridge CB2 0AH, UK. [3]Imperial College London, Division of Psychiatry, Department of Brain Sciences, Commonwealth Building, Du Cane Road, London W12 0NN, UK. [4]South London and Maudsley NHS Foundation Trust, Michael Rutter Centre for Children and Young People, De Crespigny Park, London SE5 8AZ, UK. [5]University of Liverpool, Mount Pleasant, Liverpool L69 3BX, UK. [6]University of Bristol, School for Policy Studies, 8 Priory Road, Bristol BS8 1TZ, UK. [7]Queen's University Belfast, School of Social Sciences, Education & Social Work, 6 College Park Ave, Belfast BT7 1PS, UK. [8]Queen's University Belfast, University Road, Belfast BT7 1NN, UK. [9]Beat, Unit 1 Chalk Hill House, 19 Rosary Road, Norwich, Norfolk NR1 1SZ, UK. [10]NHS Grampian and University of Aberdeen, CAMHS, City Hospital, Park Road, Aberdeen AB24 5AU, UK. [11]NHS Ayrshire and Arran, South CAMHS/NSAIU, CAMHS, Arrol Park Resource Centre, House 1, Doonfoot Road, Ayr KA7 2DW, UK. [12]South London and Maudsley NHS Foundation Trust, Maudsley Centre for Child and Adolescent Eating Disorders, Michael Rutter Centre for Children and Young People, De Crespigny Park, London SE5 8AZ, UK.

References

1. Arcelus J, Mitchell AJ, Wales J, Nielsen S. Mortality rates in patients with anorexia nervosa and other eating disorders. A meta-analysis of 36 studies. Arch Gen Psychiatry. 2011;68(7):724–31. https://doi.org/10.1001/archgenpsychiatry.2011.74.

2. Hoang U, Goldacre M, James A. Mortality following hospital discharge with a diagnosis of eating disorder: national record linkage study, England, 2001-2009. Int J Eat Disord. 2014;47(5):507–15. https://doi.org/10.1002/eat.22249.

3. Striegel-Moore RH, Leslie D, Petrill SA, Garvin V, Rosenheck RA. One-year use and cost of inpatient and outpatient services among female and male patients with an eating disorder: evidence from a national database of health insurance claims. Int J Eat Disord. 2000;27(4):381–9. https://doi.org/10.1002/(SICI)1098-108X(200005)27:4<381::AID-EAT2>3.0.CO;2-U.

4. Simon J, Schmidt U, Pilling S. The health service use and cost of eating disorders. Psychol Med. 2005;35(11):1543–51. https://doi.org/10.1017/S0033291705004708.

5. NHS Digital. Hospital episode statistics, admitted patient care - England, 2011-12: primary diagnosis, 4 characters table. Leeds: NHS Digital; 2012. https://digital.nhs.uk/data-and-information/publications/statistical/hospital-admitted-patient-care-activity/hospital-episode-statistics-admitted-patient-care-england-2011-12

6. NHS Digital. Hospital admitted patient care activity, 2015-16: diagnosis. Leeds: NHS Digital; 2016. https://digital.nhs.uk/data-and-information/publications/statistical/hospital-admitted-patient-care-activity/2015-16

7. Strober M, Freeman R, Morrell W. The long-term course of severe anorexia nervosa in adolescents: survival analysis of recovery, relapse, and outcome predictors over 10-15 years in a prospective study. Int J Eat Disord. 1997; 22(4):339–60. https://doi.org/10.1002/(SICI)1098-108X(199712)22:4<339::AID-EAT1>3.0.CO;2-N.

8. Lay B, Jennen-Steinmetz C, Reinhard I, Schmidt MH. Characteristics of inpatient weight gain in adolescent anorexia nervosa: relation to speed of relapse and re-admission. Eur Eat Disord Rev. 2002;10(1):22–40. https://doi.org/10.1002/erv.432.

9. Gowers SG, Clark A, Roberts C, Griffiths A, Edwards V, Bryan C, et al. Clinical effectiveness of treatments for anorexia nervosa in adolescents: randomised controlled trial. Br J Psychiatry. 2007;191(5):427–35. https://doi.org/10.1192/bjp.bp.107.036764.

10. House J, Schmidt U, Craig M, Landau S, Simic M, Nicholls D, et al. Comparison of specialist and nonspecialist care pathways for adolescents with anorexia nervosa and related eating disorders. Int J Eat Disord. 2012; 45(8):949–56. https://doi.org/10.1002/eat.22065.

11. Byford S, Barrett B, Roberts C, Clark A, Edwards V, Smethurst N, et al. Economic evaluation of a randomised controlled trial for anorexia nervosa in adolescents. Br J Psychiatry. 2007;191(5):436–40. https://doi.org/10.1192/bjp.bp.107.036806.

12. Le LK-D, Hay P, Mihalopoulos C. A systematic review of cost-effectiveness studies of prevention and treatment for eating disorders. Aust N Z J Psychiatry. 2018;52(4):328–38. https://doi.org/10.1177/0004867417739690.

13. Byford S, Petkova H, Stuart R, Nicholls D, Simic M, Ford T, et al. Alternative community-based models of care for young people with anorexia nervosa: the CostED national surveillance study. Health Serv Deliv Res. 2019;7(37):1–78.

14. Lynn RM, Viner RM, Nicholls DE. Ascertainment of early onset eating disorders: a pilot for developing a national child psychiatric surveillance system. Child Adolesc Ment Health. 2012;17(2):109–12. https://doi.org/10.1111/j.1475-3588.2011.00613.x.

15. American Psychiatric Association. Diagnostic and Statistical Manual of Mental Disorders DSM-5. 5th ed. Arlington: American Psychiatric Association; 2013.

16. Le Grange D, Doyle PM, Swanson SA, Ludwig K, Glunz C, Kreipe RE. Calculation of expected body weight in adolescents with eating disorders. Pediatrics. 2012;129(2):e438–46. https://doi.org/10.1542/peds.2011-1676.

17. Cole TJ, Freeman JV and Preece MA. Body mass index reference curves for the UK, 1990. Arch Dis Child. 1995;73:25–9.

18. Shaffer D, Gould MS, Brasic J, Ambrosini P, Fisher P, Bird H, et al. A children's global assessment scale (CGAS). Arch Gen Psychiatry. 1983;40(11):1228–31. https://doi.org/10.1001/archpsyc.1983.01790100074010.

19. Gowers SG, Harrington RC, Whitton A, Lelliott P, Beevor A, Wing J, et al. Brief scale for measuring the outcomes of emotional and behavioural disorders in children. Health of the nation outcome scales for children and adolescents (HoNOSCA). Br J Psychiatry. 1999;174(5):413–6. https://doi.org/10.1192/bjp.174.5.413.

20. National Institute for Health and Care Excellence. Guide to the methods of technology appraisal 2013. London, UK: National Institute for Health and Care Excellence; 2013. https://www.nice.org.uk/process/pmg9/resources/guide-to-the-methods-of-technology-appraisal-2013-pdf-2007975843781

21. Department of Health and Social Care. NHS reference costs 2015-2016. London, UK: Department of Health and Social Care; 2016. https://www.gov.uk/government/publications/nhs-reference-costs-2015-to-2016

22. NHS England. Access and waiting time standard for children and young people with an eating disorder: commissioning guide. London, UK: National Collaborating Centre for Mental Health; 2015. https://www.england.nhs.uk/wp-content/uploads/2015/07/cyp-eating-disorders-access-waiting-time-standard-comm-guid.pdf

23. Royal College of Psychiatrists' Section of Eating Disorders. Eating disorders in the UK: service distribution, service development and training. College Report CR170. London: Royal College of Psychiatrists; 2012.

24. Barber JA, Thompson SG. Analysis of cost data in randomized trials: an application of the non-parametric bootstrap. Stat Med. 2000;19(23):3219–36. https://doi.org/10.1002/1097-0258(20001215)19:23<3219::AID-SIM623>3.0.CO;2-P.

25. Efron B, Tibshirani RJ. An introduction to the bootstrap. London: Chapman & Hall; 1993. https://doi.org/10.1007/978-1-4899-4541-9.

26. Schafer JL. Multiple imputation: a primer. Stat Methods Med Res. 1999;8(1): 3–15. https://doi.org/10.1177/096228029900800102.

27. Morshed S, Tornetta P, Bhandari M. Analysis of observational studies: a guide to understanding statistical methods. J Bone Joint Surg. 2009; 91(Suppl 3):50–60. https://doi.org/10.2106/JBJS.H.01577.

28. Claxton K. The irrelevance of inference: a decision-making approach to the stochastic evaluation of health care technologies. J Health Econ. 1999;18(3): 341–64. https://doi.org/10.1016/S0167-6296(98)00039-3.

29. Stinnett AA, Mullahy J. Net health benefits: a new framework for the analysis of uncertainty in cost-effectiveness analysis. Med Decis Mak. 1998; 18(2_suppl):S68–80. https://doi.org/10.1177/0272989X98018002S09.

30. van Hout BA, Al MJ, Gordon GS, Rutten FF. Costs, effects and C/E-ratios alongside a clinical trial. Health Econ. 1994;3(5):309–19. https://doi.org/10.1002/hec.4730030505.

31. Fenwick E, Byford S. A guide to cost-effectiveness acceptability curves. Br J Psychiatry. 2005;187(2):106–8. https://doi.org/10.1192/bjp.187.2.106.

32. Smink FRE, van Hoeken D, Hoek HW. Epidemiology of eating disorders: incidence, prevalence and mortality rates. Curr Psychiatry Rep. 2012;14(4): 406–14. https://doi.org/10.1007/s11920-012-0282-y.

33. Gowers S, Levine W, Bailey-Rogers S, Shore A, Burhouse E. Use of a routine, self-report outcome measure (HoNOSCA-SR) in two adolescent mental health services. Br J Psychiatry. 2002;180(3):266–9. https://doi.org/10.1192/bjp.180.3.266.

34. Schmidt U, Sharpe H, Bartholdy S, Bonin E, Davies H, Easter A, et al. Treatment of anorexia nervosa: a multimethod investigation translating experimental neuroscience into clinical practice. Prog Grants Appl Res. 2017;5(16):1–207.

35. Mitrofan O, Petkova H, Janssens A, Kelly J, Edwards E, Nicholls D, et al. Care experiences of young people with eating disorders and their parents: a qualitative study. BJPsych Open. 2019;5:e6:108.

36. Escobar-Koch T, Banker JD, Crow S, Cullis J, Ringwood S, Smith G, et al. Service users' views of eating disorder services: an international comparison. Int J Eat Disord. 2010;43(6):549–59. https://doi.org/10.1002/eat.20741.

37. Herpertz-Dahlmann B, Schwarte R, Krei M, Egberts K, Warnke A, Wewetzer C, et al. Day-patient treatment after short inpatient care versus continued inpatient treatment in adolescents with anorexia nervosa (ANDI): a multicentre, randomised, open-label, non-inferiority trial. Lancet. 2014; 383(9924):1222–9. https://doi.org/10.1016/S0140-6736(13)62411-3.

38. Eisler I, Simic M, Hodsoll J, Asen E, Berelowitz M, Connan F, et al. A pragmatic randomised multi-centre trial of multifamily and single family therapy for adolescent anorexia nervosa. BMC Psychiatry. 2016;16(1):422. https://doi.org/10.1186/s12888-016-1129-6.

39. Goddard E, Hibbs R, Raenker S, Salerno L, Arcelus J, Boughton N, et al. A multi-centre cohort study of short term outcomes of hospital treatment for anorexia nervosa in the UK. BMC Psychiatry. 2013;13(1):287. https://doi.org/10.1186/1471-244X-13-287.

16

The Development and Psychometric Evaluation of FABIANA-checklist: a Scale to Assess Factors Influencing Treatment Initiation in Anorexia Nervosa

Laurence Reuter[1]* [iD], Denise Kästner[1], Justine Schmidt[1], Angelika Weigel[1], Ulrich Voderholzer[2,3,4], Marion Seidel[5], Bianca Schwennen[6], Helge Fehrs[7], Bernd Löwe[1†] and Antje Gumz[1†]

Abstract

Background: A long duration of untreated illness (DUI) is an unfavorable prognostic factor in anorexia nervosa (AN) and is associated with chronic illness progression. Although previous preventive measures aimed at reducing DUI and thus improving short- and long-term treatment outcomes have been partially successful, a better understanding of the factors involved in the sensitive phase prior to treatment initiation is needed. To date, there is no validated instrument available to assess these factors specifically for patients with AN. The FABIANA-project (Facilitators and barriers in anorexia nervosa treatment initiation) aims at identifying predictors of the DUI in order to target preventive measures better in the future. As part of this project, the FABIANA-checklist was developed, based on a multi-informant perspective and a multimodal bottom-up approach. The present study focusses on the process of item generation, item selection and psychometric validation of the checklist.

Methods: Based upon a previous qualitative study, an initial set of 73 items was generated for the most frequently mentioned facilitators and barriers of treatment initiation in AN. After a process of consensual rating and cognitive pre-testing, the resulting 25-item version of the FABIANA-checklist was provided to a sample of female patients (N = 75), aged ≥ 14 years with AN that underwent their first psychotherapeutic treatment in the last 12 months. After item analysis, dimensionality of the final version of the FABIANA-checklist was tested by Principal Component Analysis (PCA). We evaluated construct validity assuming correlations with related constructs, such as perceived social support (F-SozU), support in the health care system (PACIC-5A), illness perception and coping (BIPQ).

Results: We included 54 adult and 21 adolescent patients with AN, aged on average 21.4 years. Average BMI was 15.5 kg/m^2, age of onset was 19.2 years and average DUI was 2.25 years. After item analysis, 7 items were excluded. The PCA of the 18-item-FABIANA-checklist yielded six components explaining 62.64% of the total variance. Overall internal consistency was acceptable (Cronbach's α = .76) and construct validity was satisfactory for 14 out of 18 items. Two consistent components emerged: "primary care perceived as supportive and competent" (23.33%) and

*Correspondence: l.reuter@uke.de
†Shared last authorship: Bernd Löwe and Antje Gumz.
[1] Department of Psychosomatic Medicine and Psychotherapy, University Medical Center Hamburg-Eppendorf, Martinistr. 52, W37, 20246 Hamburg, Germany
Full list of author information is available at the end of the article

"emotional and practical support from relatives" (9.98%). With regard to the other components, the heterogeneity of the items led to unsatisfactory internal consistency, single.item loading and in part ambiguous interpretability.

Conclusions: The FABIANA-checklist is a valid instrument to assess factors involved in the process of treatment initiation of patients with AN. Psychometrics and dimensionality testing suggests that experienced emotional and practical support from the primary health care system and close relatives are main components. The results indicate that a differentiated assessment at item level is appropriate. In order to quantify the relative importance of the factors and to derive recommendations on early-intervention approaches, the predictive effect of the FABIANA-items on the DUI will be determined in a subsequent study which will further include the perspective of relatives and primary caregivers.

Plain English summary

Early treatment contributes to a more favorable illness course and an improved prognosis in patients with anorexia nervosa (AN). The current study presents the development of the FABIANA checklist, which aims to assess factors which influence duration of untreated illness. The FABIANA checklist was developed on the basis of interviews with patients, their relatives and primary care practitioners. It provides data from the first use of the checklist in a German sample of 75 patients with AN. The results of our study suggest that the FABIANA-checklist is a valid instrument to assess factors involved in the process of treatment initiation. Emotional and practical support from the primary health care system and close relatives were the most consistent components. A follow-up study will investigate the relationship between the FABIANA-items and the DUI in order to guide the conception of effective secondary prevention measures.

Keywords: Anorexia nervosa, Duration of untreated illness, Early intervention, Facilitators and barriers, Psychotherapy, Psychometrics, Construct validity

Background

Anorexia nervosa (AN) is a serious mental disorder often characterized by variable outcomes, high mortality rates and a high risk for a chronic course of the illness [1, 2]. Only a minority of patients are inwardly motivated to immediately seek specialized treatment [3–5], and it often takes several years for patients to receive appropriate therapy [6–8]. A recent review [6] including 14 studies found a mean duration of untreated illness (DUI) of 29.9 months (range = 6.4 to 39.9 months) in patients with AN. In children under 12 years of age, the DUI averaged 10 months, compared with 35 months in adolescents and adults.

Patients with AN have a better prognosis if evidence-based treatment [12] is provided timely and at early stages of illness [13, 14]. A delayed access to treatment has been associated with higher levels of psychological distress as well as with social and occupational impairment [15, 16]. Ambwani et al. [17] reported e.g. a positive association between disease duration and symptom severity at admission. Patients with a longer duration of illness (defined as > 3 years) had poorer long-term treatment outcomes and showed less improvement in their social or occupational adjustment one year after the end of treatment, compared with a group of patients with a recent onset (< 3 years). The importance of a rapid intervention in patients with AN is further supported by a

growing number of studies showing that the maladaptive behaviors in eating disorders become increasingly automated over time and, thus, more resistant to change [18–20].

Most studies divide the DUI into two phases [8–10]. The first phase describes the period between the initial manifestation of the disease and the patient's first contact with primary health care. This phase, which constitutes the larger part of DUI [4, 11], is characterized by a high degree of inner ambivalence of the patient with regard to the disease and the therapy. In a favorable case, the patient develops an acceptance of the illness and a motivation for treatment. The decision to seek help marks the transition to the second phase, which is mainly characterized by waiting for a referral to specialized treatment. Parents or relatives play an important role in the initial phase of the disease. Since they often live closely with young patients, they might address the AN at an early stage of the illness and accompany the patient to primary health care. The waiting time until referral to specialized care, on the other hand, depends more on the structural conditions and interdisciplinary cooperation within the respective health system.

Preventive interventions aiming at facilitating help-seeking behavior and optimizing pathways to specialized care lead to divergent outcomes [21–23]. In a previous study, members of our research group implemented a systemic public health intervention (psychenet), which aimed at facilitating the early recognition and treatment initiation in patients with AN [9, 24]. The implementation of a wide-range of preventive measures, such as disseminating information about AN, developing specialized treatment programs, establishing a multidisciplinary health network and setting up a specialized outpatient clinic, however, did not lead to a significant reduction of the DUI [21]. In the UK, the FREED-up program [10, 22] addresses the waiting time between the first contact with primary care and the start of a specialized treatment. Through person-centered contacts, referred patients receive information about their eating disorder and are given the opportunity to talk about fears and concerns regarding treatment. The aim is to build up motivation for a subsequent assessment and specialized AN-treatment [10, 22]. In the recently published FREED-up study [22], it has been shown that FREED participants had a significantly shorter DUI, faced shorter waiting times and had higher rates of treatment uptake in comparison to TAU. When FREED was optimally implemented (e.g. immediate specialist evidence-based assessment and treatment directly at help-seeking), which was the case for 56.5% of the total sample (N = 278), the reduction of DUI was pronounced, underlining the importance of well-interlinked care. However, the time span from the onset of the disease to the first contact with a specialist was not targeted by FREED. Moreover, a significant proportion of potential patients were not fully reached by the program, i.e. they dropped out of the program between referral from primary care and assessment. The authors attribute this to the ongoing ambivalence of many patients with AN regarding treatment initiation [22]. The results of this promising program suggest that the focus of interventions on service-related factors, might not be sufficient to address DUI in this highly ambivalent group of patients.

In order to target preventive measures better at the different phases in the process of treatment initiation, it is crucial to assess which factors are involved in the process of treatment initiation. Among the barriers involved in treatment initiation in patients with eating disorders (ED), Innes et al. [25] included patient-related factors such as stigma, unhelpful past treatment experiences, fear of change or low motivation. Service-related barriers are predominantly service availability, service restrictions and treatment costs [25]. The authors of this literature review, which included 11 studies, point out that the heterogeneity of the samples included (exclusively ED diagnosis or subclinical sample; female vs. mixed gender; adults vs. adults and adolescents; different ethnic background) and the methods applied (qualitative vs. quantitative methods, retrospective vs. prospective; dichotomous vs. dimensional assessment) do not allow

comparisons between the studies or a quantification of the barriers assessed. The diagnostic representation of the different types of ED including binge-eating disorder (BED), bulimia nervosa (BN) and AN was furthermore unbalanced, with an underrepresentation of patients with AN in the studies included.

According to the assessment of the barriers, five studies used a qualitative methodology with an open question about inhibiting or helpful factors in the process of treatment initiation. When checklists or rating scales were used, items were mainly derived from previous research on help-seeking behavior in patients with different mental health issues. The authors concluded that the "few instruments that have quantitatively assessed barriers have developed instruments without a clear justification for the items and importantly the instruments lacked psychometric rigor" (p. 18). None of the studies reported data on reliability or validity of the measures employed nor provided psychometrical support for the dimensionality of the applied factors or subscales [25].

Subsequent to the literature review, Innes et al. [26] provided psychometric data and analyzed the construct validity of the "Perceived Barriers to Psychological Treatment Scale" [27] for a sample (N = 708) of female patients aged > 14 years with disordered eating behavior. The sample included 53.81% of patients within the clinical range of ED, and about 20% of the clinical subgroup fulfilled the criteria for an AN. Factor analysis yielded a seven-factor solution including—sorted in descending order of importance—access to services, time constraints, stigma, lack of motivation, negative evaluation of treatment, emotional concerns, participation restrictions and access restriction. The overall score of perceived barriers was negatively correlated to general help-seeking intentions (r = − .28) and to intentions to seek help from a mental health professional (− .19). Although this questionnaire has good psychometric values, it registers general barriers to seeking psychological treatment. It does not register disorder-specific barriers (e.g. fear of gaining weight). This might be reflected by the low correlations with help-seeking behavior in the population of patients with disordered eating behavior.

In a more recent paper, Ali et al. [28, 29] assessed and quantified barriers to help-seeking among a clinical sample of patients with different types of ED. The 15 barriers, which had been extracted from a literature review [28] were systemized in the "Barriers toward seeking help for eating disorders questionnaire" (BATSH-ED). The BATSH-ED covers a broad range of barriers for help-seeking behavior and mainly refers to patient-related barriers, such as internal attitudes, experiences and beliefs regarding the ED. These include aspects such as denying the disease or not perceiving its severity, not wishing to be a burden for others, feeling ashamed about the ED or the fear of losing control. While these and other aspects, such as a lack of knowledge or information about eating disorders, are suitable for potential preventive measures, other aspects, such as "previous negative experiences" or "comorbidities" cannot be addressed by preventive measures. The few barriers related to the health system or the social environment are described by more general items, so that it seems rather difficult to derive concrete measures here as well.

In addition to the question whether the barriers of the BATSH-ED are suitable for deducing preventive measures, it also remains questionable as to what extent the measure, which was developed for ED in general, is suitable to specifically address AN-specific factors. The use of the BATSH-ED in a population with different eating disorders (N = 291) showed, despite the small size of the AN-subsample (N = 10), differences with regard to the importance of the barriers in treatment initiation in the ED-subgroups [29]. Patients with AN were more frequently embarrassed about their problems, were more afraid of treatment or saw treatment as a sign of weakness. A further limitation of the BATSH-ED is, that it includes only those barriers that were mentioned in the previous literature review. Aspects that might be relevant to patients but have not yet been researched are not addressed by the checklist. Furthermore, it does not take into account the factors that facilitate help seeking behavior, nor includes the perspective of primary caregivers and relatives.

In view of the limitations of the existing measures, the aim of the FABIANA-study (Facilitators and barriers in anorexia nervosa treatment initiation, [30]) was to develop, in a first step, a checklist to assess factors (facilitators and barriers) of treatment initiation in patients with AN using a multi-method and multi-informant approach.

To achieve a wide spectrum of factors involved in treatment initiation in patients with AN we used semi-structured interviews (N = 22) with patients, relatives and primary care physicians [31]. Using Grounded Theory we identified facilitators and barriers within the patient, the social environment, the health care system and society. Based upon the most prominent factors (see Additional file 1) of this study [31] the FABIANA-checklist was developed.

The present study reports on the process of item construction and item selection of the FABIANA-checklist and examines the psychometric properties and dimensionality of the checklist among a sample of German patients with AN. It further quantifies factors involved in AN treatment initiation as experienced by patients.

The long-term goal of the FABIANA study is to quantify the magnitude of the effects of the factors assessed with the FABIANA-checklist on the DUI (upcoming study) with the intention of giving recommendations to guide the conception of effective secondary prevention approaches.

Method

(1) The development of the FABIANA-Checklist

Instrument and item generation were based on a recommended procedure for mixed-method studies [32]. Details and data on item generation, item evaluation and item selection can be found in the Additional file 1.

Item generation

For item generation, we considered facilitators and barriers which had been mentioned in at 25% of the interviews (N = 22) of our previous qualitative study [31] and/or had more than 10 codings and had been considered as addressable through secondary prevention measures. The latter rating was provided after consensual discussion in the research team, consisting of one professor of psychosomatic medicine and psychotherapy, two post-doctoral clinical psychologists and one clinical psychologist. Two frequently named factors were excluded due to difficult modifiability, namely "(not) living, being or eating alone"; "good personal connections" to somebody working within medical services. Two further factors ("waiting time and availability of treatment"; "fit between individual patient and service setting") were considered to be too unspecific and exclusively related to primary prevention and, therefore, excluded.

Based upon prototypical quotes from our previous qualitative study [31], items were formulated for each of the selected 21 factors. It was ensured that the items represented all facets of each factor. As the content of some factors was more heterogeneous than others, the number of items per factor ranged from 1 to 7.

Item selection

The first set of 73 items was rated independently by the research team named above. Raters considered clinical relevance, addressability through secondary prevention measures and comprehensibility of each item and assigned a composite score from 1 to 3 points, with 1 = inappropriate item recommended for exclusion, 2 = potentially appropriate item requiring modifications to improve understandability, and 3 = very appropriate item recommended for inclusion in the checklist.

Interrater-reliability (Fleiss' Kappa for ordinal data) was moderate ($k = 0.45$; 95% CI [0.39, 0.53]). The agreement was substantial for item inclusion ($k=0.60$; 95% CI: [0.51, 0.70]), moderate for item exclusion ($k=0.47$; 96% CI [0.35, 0.54] and fair for potentially suitable items ($k=0.32$; 95% CI [0.23, 0.43]).

Items with a full agreement for inclusion (mean score of 3 points; $n=15$) were included in the checklist. Items with both a mean score < 2 points and single ratings ≤ 2 points ($n=20$) were excluded from the checklist. For the remaining items ($n=38$), group discussions were held in the research group until consensus regarding inclusion (n = 15) or exclusion (n = 13) was reached. Suggestions about alternative formulations were considered and it was ensured that each factor was represented by at least one item. If necessary, the wording of some items was revised. A total of 30 items was considered for the first version of the checklist, which subsequently underwent cognitive pre-testing.

Cognitive pre-tests

The 30-item FABIANA-checklist underwent cognitive pretesting in a sample of 9 adult female patients with AN (average age 22.8 years, $SD=5.6$, [18, 35]) recruited in a specialized inpatient unit for AN treatment (inpatients $n=8$, day-care $n=1$). The sample had an average BMI of 16.8 kg/m^2 ($SD=1.9$) and was predominantly diagnosed with a restrictive type of AN (N=8). Exclusion criteria were a participation in our previous qualitative study or insufficient German language skills. After informed consent, patients completed the FABIANA checklist, which took on average about five minutes ($M=04$:25).

Patients were asked to rate the extent each aspect applied to their personal experiences in the period from illness onset to the start of a specialized psychotherapeutic treatment on a 5-point Likert scale (1 = strongly disagree to 5 = strongly agree). After completing the checklist, personal interviews addressed the relevance ("How important was this aspect for initiating the psychotherapeutic treatment?"), comprehensibility ("How comprehensible is the item?") and the recallability ("How well do you remember the described aspect?") for each item and answers were rated on a 3-point scale, with 1 = not at all, 2 = partially and 3 = very much.

The interrater reliability (ICC with mixed effects model and absolute agreement) was good (ICC=0.89; 95% CI [0.85, 0.92]). With regard to the assessed relevance, the 30 items were normally distributed around the mean value of 1.96 ($SD=0.47$). Average comprehensibility ($M=2.88$, SD=0.17) and recallability ($M=2.95$, $SD=0.08$) were very high.

After discussion of the results in the research group, 5 items were excluded from the checklist. Decisive was a combination of low relevance (< 2 points), a similarity to other items of the same factor or an unspecific

formulation and thus the difficulty of deriving preventive measures. The resulting FABIANA-checklist with 25 items underwent psychometric validation.

(2) Psychometric analysis and validation of the FABIANA-checklist

The FABIANA-study has been registered (NCT03713541) and ethical approval was obtained prior to recruitment (PV5108).

Data collection

Data for the psychometric validation of the FABIANA-checklist was collected between July 2018 and June 2019 in 11 cooperating in- and outpatient centers specialized in the psychotherapeutic treatment for ED. Inclusion criteria were an age ≥ 14 years, female gender and typical or atypical AN diagnosis. We included patients who were either currently in their first AN treatment or who had initiated their first psychotherapeutic AN treatment within the last 12 months. Psychotherapeutic treatments were defined by a minimum duration of seven days in an inpatient setting or five consecutive sessions in an outpatient setting. We planned to include at least four participants for each item of the FABIANA-checklist [30, 33].

After obtaining written informed consent from the patients and their legal guardians, eligible patients completed the assessment battery, which consisted of sociodemographic data, the 25-item version of the FABIANA-checklist and the questionnaires used for construct validation. Clinical data such as the current treatment diagnosis, Body Mass Index (BMI, kg/m^2) and the date of treatment initiation were provided by the treating specialist. Patients subsequently participated in structured clinical interviews (SCID-5-CV, [34]) to validate the AN diagnosis and to assess AN subtypes and comorbidity.

Particular attention was paid to the assessment of illness and weight history. To ensure a higher recall accuracy anchor examples, as for example relevant events in the patients' life, were marked on a timeline at the respective age of the patient. The interviewer repeatedly referred to this timeline in order to support patients in recalling their symptoms at a given time point. Age of onset (AOO) was defined as the age (in years) of the patient at the moment when the criteria for AN were fully met for the first time. The DUI was defined as the difference between the date of illness onset and the date of first treatment initiation (in years).

For sample characteristics we considered descriptive data. To account for differences between adults and adolescents regarding DUI and AOO we used simple t-tests. All calculations were performed with SPSS 27.

Item analysis and dimensionality of the FABIANA-checklist

For item analysis, we considered descriptive data (*N, mean, standard deviation, range*), graphical distributions of the raw values (histogram, Q-Q plot), skewness, kurtosis and item difficulty. For item discrimination we used Pearson's correlation coefficient (r^{it}), i.e. the correlation between the single item and the global score. Internal consistency was evaluated by Cronbach's alpha. Before performing scale statistics, polarity of negatively poled items was reversed (see also annotations in Table 2 and 3). We used consensual group discussions to decide upon inclusion or exclusion of the items in the final version of the checklist. The aim was to obtain an economic and internally consistent scale (Cronbach's $\alpha > 0.70$) that captures a broad spectrum of factors involved in treatment initiation of patients with AN.

Dimensionality of the FABIANA-checklist was tested by Principal Component Analysis (PCA). Data suitability test included the Kaiser–Meyer–Olkin (KMO) criterion and Bartlett' test for sphericity. We considered components with eigenvalues ≥ 1 [35] and tested for varimax, quartimax and equamax rotation on data. We considered and reported factor loadings of > 0.30. In the case of cross-loadings on multiple components, we considered the loading that showed the best interpretability. For each component the explained variance, the eigenvalues and the internal validity (Cronbach's alpha) are given. At item level correlations between the item and the respective component (r^{it}) and changes in the internal validity of the component when the item is deleted are provided.

Construct validity of the FABIANA-checklist

We evaluated construct validity of FABIANA-checklist by testing hypotheses regarding correlations with related well-established constructs, namely to collaborative support from health care providers, perceived social support and illness-perception. All assumptions for construct validation were made for each item separately. Expected correlations are shown in Table 3.

We expected positive correlations between the FABIANA-items related to experienced support from health care members (e.g. general practitioners, gynecologist, psychiatrist) and the global score of the *Patient Assessment of Chronic Illness Care questionnaire*. The PACIC-5A [36] is a brief self-administrated instrument to assess whether the patients were provided with patient-centered collaborative care prior to their psychotherapy. The PACIC-5A relates to the chronic care model [39] and measures the extent to which professionals tried to induce behavioral changes in patients. The 5A approach is evidence-based, has achieved widespread acceptance and is considered the most appropriate and psychometrically robust instrument assessing patient experience

with chronic disease care [40]. The global score includes the assessment of present behavior, patient counselling, collaborative agreement with the patient about realistic goals, assisting the patient during her lifestyle changes, and frequent follow-ups.

We further assumed positive correlations between the FABIANA-items, which include concern or concrete support from relatives or the social environment with the total score of the *Social Support Questionnaire* (F-SozU [37]). The unidimensional short version of the F-SozU assesses general perceived social support. For comparability, patients were asked in the introduction to refer to the period between the onset of AN and the initiation of specialized psychotherapeutic treatment. The 14 items of the F-SozU are rated on a scale from $0 =$ did not apply to $4 =$ did fully apply. The total score results from the mean value of all items. The F-SozU shows good psychometric properties and a good internal consistency (Cronbach's $\alpha = 0.94$).

For the FABIANA-items relating to societal factors, as for example the influence of media or stigmatization, we assumed correlations with subscales of Brief illness perception Questionnaire. The *Brief Illness Perception Questionnaire* (BIPQ [38]) assesses patients' illness representations, including the degree of understanding of the illness, the perceived personal and treatment control, the experience of symptoms, concerns about the illness and emotional effects of the illness on a numeric rating scale (0–10). For construct validation, we considered positive correlations between the FABIANA-items (see Table 3) and personal control, treatment control and illness comprehensibility. In addition, we included the open-ended BIPQ item on subjective illness causes, in which patients are asked to record the three major causes of their AN. Since we were particularly interested in the influence of media, we assessed whether or not (dichotomous variable) answers regarding the influence of media were given in the open-ended item of the BIPQ.

Construct validity was tested with bivariate correlations. We report correlation coefficients and *p*-values for one-tailed testing ($\alpha < 0.10$). Correlation coefficients were interpreted based on Cohen's d with $d = {} < 0.30$ as a small, $d = 0.30–50$ medium and $d > 0.50$ as large [41].

Results

Sample characteristics

We recruited 75 female patients with AN of which 54 were adult and 21 were adolescent. Mean age was 21.4 years ($SD = 7.35$ [14.0, 61.0]). Most patients (89%) were diagnosed with typical AN and 77% presented the restrictive AN-subtype. The mean BMI was 15.5 kg/m^2 ($SD = 1.96$ [10.6, 23.0]). Most patients (77%) had at least

Table 1 Sample characteristics

	n = 75	Adults (n = 54)	Adolescents (n = 21)	F, p
Age; M in years, (SD, [range])	21.4 (7.35, [14, 61])	23.69 (4.47, [18, 61])	15.52 (1.17 [14, 17])	
Setting; n (%)				
Inpatient	70 (93.3)	51 (94.4)	19 (90.5)	
Outpatient	5 (6.7)	3 (5.6)	2 (9.5)	
Diagnosis – DSM V; n (%)				
Typical anorexia nervosa (F50.0)	67 (89.3)	47 (87.0)	20 (95.2)	
Atypical anorexia nervosa (F50.1)	8 (10.7)	7 (13.0)	1 (4.8)	
AN subtype; n (%)				
restrictive	58 (77.3)	40 (74.1)	18 (85.7)	
binge-purging	17 (22.7)	14 (25.9)	3 (14.3)	
DUI; M in years, (SD, [range])	2.25 (4.33, [.15, 19.6])	2.93 (4.94, [.15, 19.6])	.49 (.59, [− .17, 2.29])	5.083*
AOO; M in years, (SD, [range])	19.15 (5.18, [12, 41])	20.75 (5.26, [12, 41])	15.03 (1.07, [13, 17])	24.182***
BMI; M in kg/m² , (SD, [range])	15.5 (1.96, [10.6, 23.0] /)	15.5 (1.91, [10.6–21.1])	15.0 (2.12, [13.0, 23.3])	
Comorbid mental disorder; n (%)				
None	17 (22.6)	10 (18.5)	7 (33.3)	
One	42 (56.0)	23 (63.0)	8 (38.1)	
Two or more	16 (21.4)	10 (18.5)	6 (28.6)	
Comorbid personality disorder; n (%)				
None	70 (93.3)	49 (90.7)	21 (100)	
One	5 (6.7)	5 (9.3)	0 (0)	

DUI = Duration of untreated illness; AOO = Age of onset; F-values for simple t-tests comparing adults to adolescents, with * for $p < .05$ and *** for $p < .001$ (two-sided)

one comorbid mental disorder, diagnosed by SCID-5-CV interview [34]. Table 1 shows the sample characteristics.

In our sample we observed an average DUI of 2.25 years ($SD = 4.33$, [− 0.17, 19.59]. Note regarding negative DUI: one patient with atypical AN fully met the diagnostic criteria for AN after treatment initiation). DUI in adolescent patients ($M = 0.49$ years, $SD = 0.59$ [−0.17, 2.29]) was significantly shorter compared to adults ($M = 2.93$ years, $SD = 4.94$, [0.15, 19.59], $p = 0.027$). A treatment initiation within the first year after illness onset could be observed in 64% of patients, predominantly in the first three quartiles (Q1: 17.3%, Q2: 25.3%, Q3: 17.3%, and Q4: 4%). A DUI between one and three years was found in 17.4% of the patients, 13.3% had a DUI between 3 and 7 years and 5.3% had a DUI between 18 and 20 years. The average AOO was 19.15 years ($SD = 5.18$, [12, 41]). Adolescents had significantly lower AOO compared to adults (with $M = 15.03$; $SD = 1.07$ [13.0, 17.0] and $M = 20.75$, $SD = 5.26$, [12.0, 41.0]; $p = 0.000$).

Item analysis and dimensionality
Results from item analysis are shown in Table 2. For each item, the total range between the minimum and maximum value (1–5) was used. After consensual group discussion, 7 items were excluded. Reasons for exclusion were poorer item-total correlation values compared to another item of the same factor (item a: $r^{it} = 0.17$ vs.

item 2: $r^{it} = 0.42$, item b: $r^{it} = − 0.08$ vs. item 3: $r^{it} = 0.03$ and item d: $r^{it} = 0.13$ vs. item 8: $r^{it} = 0.50$). Item c, e, f and g showed r^{it} values around or below 0. As these factors were also judged to be less modifiable we opted for the exclusion of these items and the respective factors (e.g. the factor "somatic symptoms and/or exacerbation and personal breaking point reached"). Excluding these 7 items increased internal consistency of the checklist (Cronbach's alpha) from 0.70 to 0.77. The final version of the FABIANA-checklist included 17 of the factors extracted from the qualitative interviews [31], represented by 18 items.

PCA was performed after item selection. Sample size ($N = 75$) was adequate (KMO = 0.72) and Bartlett's test of sphericity indicated that data structure was appropriate for running PCA ($\chi^2 = 307.26$; $p < 0.001$). A scree-plot yielded empirical justification for retaining six factors with eigenvalues > 1, which accounted for 62.46% of the total variance. Among the tested rotations, the varimax-rotated solution was the most interpretable. Table 3 indicates results of the PCA. At the component level, the internal consistency for the first two factors was in an acceptable range (Cronbach's $\alpha = 0.67–0.79$). The first component explained 23.33% of the variance. The eight items included aspects of the health care system that patients experienced as supportive and helpful (e.g., trust in the treating physician, the treating physician's

Table 2 Item characteristics of the FABIANA-checklist

FABIANA-checklist (N = 18)	N	M	M¹	SD	Adults		Adolescents		p	Item analysis			25 items		18 items	
					M	SD	M	SD		SK	KT	DIF	r^tt	α	r^tt	α
1 People from my social environment have never addressed my anorexia, or have done so too late.[1]	75	3.1	2.9	1.17	3.0	1.18	3.4	1.12		.24	−.63	.47	.06	.71	.15	.77
2 There was at least one person in my social environment who understood at an early stage of the illness that I needed professional help (e.g. from a doctor, a psychotherapist or an counselling center)	75	3.6		1.51	3.7	1.51	3.3	1.53		−.63[3]	−1.16	.65	.42	.67	.34	.75
3 It helped me to look at or read articles regarding the successful treatment of anorexia or the recovery of other people with anorexia (e.g. books, reports, social media)	73	3.0		1.34	3.1	1.39	2.8	1.20		−.08	−1.12	.50	.03	.71	.09	.77
4 My social environment often expressed concern about my anorexia	75	4.2		1.02	4.1	1.01	4.3	1.06		−1.00[3]	.18	.79	.50	.68	.47	.75
5 At least one person from my social environment supported me practically in treatment initiation (e.g. arranged or accompanied me to medical appointments)	75	4.1		1.41	4.1	1.41	4.1	1.46		−1.31[3]	.18	.78	.24	.69	.18	.77
6 My environment has encouraged me to take up treatment	74	4.5		.98	4.5	.93	4.5	1.15		−2.20[3]	4.78	.86	.50	.68	.44	.75
7 My relatives or persons I relate to closely informed themselves on the subject of anorexia (e.g. read books, researched on the internet, visited a counseling center or a doctor[2])	75	2.7		1.59	3.3	1.40	4.1	1.11	*	−.35	−1.18	.63	.31	.69	.26	.76
8 I had a doctor[2] who arranged that I received appropriate treatment	75	3.2		1.46	3.2	1.44	3.2	1.55		−.09	−1.38	.55	.50	.67	.53	.74
9 I had a doctor[2] who recognized my anorexia at an early stage of the illness	75	2.3		1.40	2.2	1.42	2.4	1.36		.73[4]	−.77	.31	.47	.67	.55	.74
10 I had a doctor[2] who told me unambiguously that I had anorexia	75	3.1		1.63	3.1	1.61	3.0	1.72		−.13	−1.60	.51	.34	.68	.45	.75
11 I had a doctor[2] who dealt badly with my difficulties concerning food, body-shape or weight (e.g. did not take my complaints seriously or trivialized them).[1]	75	2.7	3.3	1.59	2.7	1.56	2.5	1.69		−.38	−1.44	.58	.33	.68	.28	.76
12 After my anorexia was recognized, I had regular appointments with a doctor[2]	74	3.3		1.43	3.2	1.40	3.8	1.45		−.33	−1.22	.58	.39	.68	.40	.75
13 I had a doctor[2] I trusted	75	3.4		1.48	3.3	1.43	3.4	1.63		−.39	−1.25	.59	.47	.67	.51	.74
14 I had a doctor[2] with high competence in the field of eating disorders	75	2.7		1.38	2.6	1.37	2.9	1.41		.18	−1.24	.41	.49	.67	.55	.74
15 I had a doctor who collaborated well with my other practitioners[2]	74	2.5		1.45	2.5	1.42	2.4	1.57		.60[4]	−.96	.36	.49	.67	.52	.74
16 It was difficult for me and/or my relatives or persons I relate to closely to find out whom I could consult best to get help.[1]	75	3.3	2.7	1.40	3.3	1.41	3.2	1.38		.33	−1.16	.42	.20	.70	.22	.76
17 I believed that undergoing psychotherapy was a sign of weakness.[1]	74	3.3		1.43	3.3	1.44	3.5	1.44		.28	−1.25	.42	.11	.70	.14	.77
18 By comparing with girls or women in the media (e.g. television, internet, social media) I considered a certain diet (e.g. a very restricted diet), a very slim figure or a very low weight to be normal so that I didn't feel the need for treatment.[1]	75	3.8	2.2	1.32	3.8	1.31	3.7	1.35		.68[4]	−.79	.30	.17	.70	.12	.77
Excluded items (N = 7)																
a My social environment did not understand my illness (e.g. "Just start eating again").[1]	74	3.7	2.3	1.03	3.7	.98	3.7	1.17		.45	−.58	.32	.17	.70		
b It helped me to exchange ideas with people who had already undergone psychotherapy	73	2.8		1.61	2.8	1.65	2.8	1.54		.12	−1.62	.45	−.08	.72		
c At least one person from my social environment has frequently blamed me for my anorexia nervosa.[1]	75	2.7	3.3	1.43	2.7	1.50	2.8	1.26		−.26	−1.24	.57	.02	.71		

Table 2 (continued)

FABIANA-checklist (N = 18)	N	M	M¹	SD	Adults		Adolescents		p	Item analysis			25 items		18 items	
					M	SD	M	SD		SK	KT	DIF	r^{it}	α	r^{it}	α
d	After my anorexia was diagnosed, I was in medical treatment for a long time without getting a clear recommendation for psychotherapy.[1]	73	1.8	4.2	1.09	1.7	.97	2.1	1.35		−1.55[3]	1.79	.81	.13	.70		
e	I was only ready for treatment as my (physical or mental) breaking point was reached	74	4.0		1.18	4.1	1.18	3.8	1.20		−1.07[3]	.30	.75	−.15	.72		
f	I was afraid that the treatment would not be compatible with other things important to me (e.g. school, job, children).[1]	75	4.4	1.6	1.06	4.4	1.14	4.3	.86		1.61[4]	1.72	.16	.08	.70		
g	Without my physical symptoms and complaints, I would not have undergone psychotherapy	73	4.2		1.11	4.1	1.22	4.4	.61		−1.44[3]	1.37	.80	−.01	.71		
Cronbach's alpha (scale)													.70		.77	

[1] Items were inverted for item analysis

[2] Patients are asked in the introduction of the questionnaire, to refer to the physicians they consulted before being referred to specialized care

[3] Left-skewed item

[4] Right-skewed items

N = number of participants who completed the item; M = mean value, M^1 = Mean value after item inversion, SD = standard deviation, p-values for simple t-tests comparing adults to adolescents, $*p < .05$, SK = skewness, KT = kurtosis, DIF = item difficulty (0–1), r^{it} = item-total correlation, α = Cronbach's alpha when item is deleted,

Table 3 Principal component analysis and construct validation of the FABIANA-checklist (18 items)

Components (Eigenvalue)	Items (Nr.)	Principal Components Analysis								Construct validity	
		1	2	3	4	5	6	r^{it}	α	Assumptions	r, p
1 Primary care perceived as supportive and competent (4.20)	I had a doctor[2] I trusted. (13)	.84						.61	.75	PACIC-5A	.59***
	I had a doctor[2] with a great competence in the field of eating disorders. (14)	.78						.59	.75	PACIC-5A	.42***
	I had a doctor[2] who cooperated well with my other practitioners. (15)	.61				.31		.50	.77	PACIC-5A	.29*
	After my anorexia was diagnosed, I had regular appointments with a doctor[2]. (12)	.51				.38		.41	.78	PACIC-5A	.42***
	I had a doctor[2] who arranged that I received appropriate treatment. (8)	.49	.35			.26		.51	.76	PACIC-5A	.24*
	I had a doctor[2] who recognized my anorexia at an early stage of the illness. (9)	.46	.27	.58				.54	.76	PACIC-5A	.32**
	I had a doctor[2] who dealt badly with my difficulties concerning food, body-shape or weight (e.g. did not take my complaints seriously or trivialized them).[1] (11)	.45			−.47			.35	.79	PACIC-5A	.35**
	I had a doctor[2] who told me unambiguously that I had anorexia. (10)	.43		.35			.33	.48	.77	PACIC-5A	.34**
2 Emotional and practical support from the social environment/ relatives (1.80)	My social environment encouraged me to take up treatment. (6)		.82					.60	.45	F-SozU	.21*
	My social environment often expressed concern about my anorexia. (4)	.25	.72					.43	.64	F-SozU	.43***
	At least one person from my social environment supported me practically in treatment initiation (e.g. arranged or accompanied me to medical appointments). (5)		.71					.46	.64	F-SozU	.14
3 Need and Searching for Orientation and Help (1.60)	It was difficult for me and/ or my relatives or persons I relate to closely to find out whom I could consult best to get help.[1] (16)			.75	.24			−.16		PACIC-5A	.14
	It helped me to look at or read articles regarding the successful treatment of anorexia or the recovery of other people with anorexia (e.g. in books, reports, social media). (3)	.36		−.57				−.16		BIPQ: Personal control[3] BIPQ: Treatment control[4] BIPQ: Comprehensibility[5]	−.26* .23* .09
4 Social environment recognizing AN and need for help (1.39)	People from my social environment have never addressed my anorexia, or have done so too late.[1] (1)				.76			.34	.20	F-SozU	.15
	There was at least one person in my social environment who understood at an early stage of the illness that I needed professional help. (2)				.43	.40	.32	.22	.40	F-SozU	.22*
	I believed that undergoing psychotherapy was a sign of weakness.[1] (17)	.36			.61	.28	.29	.22	.38	BIPQ: Personal control[3] BIPQ: Treatment control[4] BIPQ: Comprehensibility[5]	.14 .16 .20*

Table 3 (continued)

Components (Eigenvalue)	Items (Nr.)	Principal Components Analysis								Construct validity	
		1	2	3	4	5	6	r^{it}	α	Assumptions	r,p
5 Informed relatives (1.22)	My relatives or persons I relate to closely informed themselves on the subject of anorexia (e.g. read books, researched on the internet, visited a counselling center or a doctor²). (7)					.82				F-SozU	.05
6 Absence of negative media influence (1.05)	By comparing with girls or women in the media (e.g. television, internet, social media) I considered a certain diet (e.g. a very restricted diet), a very slim figure or a very low weight to be normal so that I didn't feel the need for treatment.¹ (18)						.85			BIPQ:Comprehensibility⁵ BIPQ: Causal representation "Media"⁶ (−)	.20* −.31**
Variance explained (%)		23.33	9.98	8.86	7.71	6.76	5.82				
Cronbach's alpha		.79	.67	−.38	.42						

¹ The polarity of item 1, 11, 16, 17 and 18 was inverted

² Patients are asked in the introduction of the questionnaire, to refer to the physicians they consulted before being referred to specialized care

³ BIPQ item 3 with 0 = absolutely no personal control and 10 = extreme personal control

⁴ BIPQ item 4 with 0 = perception that treatment is not helpful at all and 10 = perception of treatment as extremely helpful

⁵ BIPQ item 7 with 0 = no illness perception and 10 = very clear illness perception

⁶ BIPQ Item 9, open item asking for the tree major subjective causes for the illness

All illness causes related to influences of media were considered. r^{if} = item-factor correlation, α = Cronbach's alpha of the component if the item is deleted, (−) negative correlation expected, *p < .05, **p < .01; ***p < .001 (one-sided)

competence in the area of eating disorders or good cooperation between different physicians). The second component, explained 9.98% of the variance and included three items related to emotional and practical support from relatives. On the third component ("Need and searching for orientation and help"), inconsistencies in terms of factor loadings manifested in negative internal consistency. On the one hand, this component reflected the disorientation of the patients and their relatives, not knowing whom to consult for help, and on the other hand it included the patient's attempt to gather information about helpful treatment processes from books or social media. The fourth component (7.71%) included items showing that AN was taken seriously (not trivialized) by the patients or their social environment (e.g. AN was not addressed too late or at least one person of the environment understood the need for professional help). Internal consistency of this factor was however insufficient (Cronbach's $\alpha = 0.42$). Component four and five showed single-item loadings, relating on relatives who informed themselves about AN (6.76%) and the absence of negative media influence (5.82%).

Construct validity

As hypothesized, patients who reported supportive experiences relating to the health care system perceived more patient-centered, collaborative care prior to treatment initiation, which was reflected by significant correlations with the PACIC-5A total score with 8 out of 9 items of the FABIANA-checklist (with r varying from 0.24 to 0.59). The strongest correlations were found for the feeling of trust in the practitioner (item 13, $r = 0.59$, $p < 0.001$), perceived competence of the practitioner and regular contact after AN diagnosis (items 12 and 14, both $r = 0.42$, $p < 0.001$). Moderate correlations were found for the items describing early recognition of AN by the practitioner (item 9, $r = 0.32$, $p = 0.006$) and directly addressing the AN (item 10, $r = 0.34$, $p = 0.004$). Dealing well with patient's difficulties (not trivializing complaints) (item 11, $r = 0.35$, $p = 0.003$), arranging appropriate treatment (item 8, $r = 0.24$, $p = 0.029$) and cooperating with other practitioners (item 15, $r = 0.29$, $p = 0.012$) were, as expected, related to perceived care. The FABIANA-checklist item 16, indicating difficulties to find out whom to consider for appropriate help, did not correlate significantly with the PACIC-5A score ($r = 0.14$, $p = 0.134$).

Half of expected relations between items of the FABIANA-checklist that have proximity to the concept of social support and the total score of the F-SozU could be confirmed. The strongest correlation was found for the concerns expressed by the social environment (item 4, $r = 0.43$, $p < 0.001$). Early recognition of the need for treatment by significant others (item 2, $r = 0.22$, $p = 0.032$)

and encouragement of the patient to seek help (item 6, $r = 0.21$, $p = 0.041$) were significant at a lower level. The items regarding whether the relatives directly addressed AN (item 1, $r = 0.15$, $p = 0.100$), informed themselves about the AN in the media (item 7, $r = 0.5$, $p = 0.352$) or provided concrete practical support (item 5, $r = 0.15$, $p = 0.130$) were not significantly related to experienced social support.

The expected correlation between consuming media about successful treatments (item 3) and treatment control (BIPQ), i.e. the belief that treatment might be helpful, was confirmed ($r = 0.23$, $p = 0.028$). However, the consumption of media about successful treatments was, contrary to expectations, associated with less personal control ($r = -0.26$, $p = 0.015$) and showed no significant correlation with illness comprehensibility ($r = 0.09$, $p = 0.221$). Patients who did not perceive undergoing a psychotherapy as a weakness (item 17) had, as expected, a significantly better understanding of their illness ($r = 0.20$, $p = 0.049$, BIPQ), but we found no positive relation to personal control ($r = 0.14$, $p = 0.124$) or treatment control ($r = 0.16$, $p = 0.084$). Patients who reported a lower influence of their weight perception by media (item 18) had, as expected, a better understanding of illness ($r = 0.20$, $p = 0.042$) and named less often media influence as one of the causes of their illness ($r = -0.31$, $p = 0.004$). An overview on all assumptions on construct validity and corresponding correlations is given in Table 3.

Average scores of the FABIANA-items

Mean values for all FABIANA-items can be found in Table 2. The items with the highest average scores focused on practical and emotional support from the social environment, e.g. if relatives expressed concern about AN ($M = 4.2$, $SD = 1.02$), perceived the need for help ($M = 3.6$, $SD = 1.52$), informed themselves about AN ($M = 3.5$, $SD = 1.38$) encouraged the patient to seek treatment ($M = 4.5$, $SD = 0.98$), arranged medical appointments or accompanied the patients to medical consultations ($M = 4.1$, $SD = 1.41$). The average scores indicate, that the primary care provider was more likely not to recognize AN at an early stage ($M = 2.3$, $SD = 1.40$), and that cooperation with other providers was more likely to be less well organized ($M = 2.5$, $SD = 1.45$). Influenced by the media, patients tended to assume that low weight was "normal" or that they did not feel the need for help ($M = 3.8$, $SD = 1.28$). They were more likely to agree that, prior to treatment initiation they felt, that seeking therapy was a sign of weakness ($M = 3.4$, $SD = 1.43$). Differences between adult and adolescent patients were found only for item 7. Relatives of adolescent patients were more likely to inform themselves on the subject of

AN or to visit a counselling center ($M = 4.1$, $SD = 1.11$ vs, $M = 3.3$, $SD = 1.40$, $p = 0.012$).

Discussion

The current study reports on the development and psychometric evaluation of the FABIANA-checklist which aims at assessing factors involved in the process of treatment initiation in patients with AN. The development of the checklist was based on a multi-informant and mixed-method approach. The items of the checklist were derived from facilitators and barriers of treatment initiation that were most frequently named by patients with AN, their relatives and primary care providers in our previous qualitative study [31]. The process of item-selection included item ratings and consensual discussions in the research team, cognitive pre-tests and item-analysis.

Psychometric characteristics of the FABIANA-checklist were tested in a sample of 75 female patients with AN. After item analysis, PCA of the 18-item version of the checklist yielded six components. With Cronbach's α of 0.77, overall internal consistency was acceptable. The most consistent components regarded the support from the primary health care system and emotional and practical support from relatives or close others. Another yet less consistent component related to the supportive role of relatives in the early recognition of AN and their understanding of the need for treatment. With regard to the other components, the heterogeneity of the items led to unsatisfactory internal consistencies and single item loading. For 14 out of 18 items the expected proximity to well established measures of social support, health care system support, illness perception could be confirmed.

Perceived support from the primary health care system

The eight items of the first factor are related to the patients' contact with the health care system before being referred to a specialized treatment. They refer to the practitioners' competence in dealing with ED, early recognition of the disorder, taking the symptoms seriously and clear communication about the diagnosis. Regular appointments, referral to specialized treatment and the practitioner's good networking also loaded onto this component. All items of this component showed positive correlations with perceived patient-centered collaborative care, as measured by the PACIC-5A.

Studies show that the majority of patients with AN consult a medical doctor before being referred to specialized care [42, 43]. Often it is in primary care where AN is addressed for the first time and where possible treatment options are discussed [44]. However, previous studies indicate that about 40% of practitioners do not correctly identify AN and only 26–40% of patients with

AN-diagnosis are referred to specialized treatments by their practitioners [11, 45]. Patients with AN are particularly adept at hiding their weight and body shape from their medical doctor. Nevertheless, empirical evidence suggests that the majority of practitioners do not regularly screen for ED or believe to lack the necessary skills to intervene properly in ED [46] due to fear of patients' defensiveness or insecurity about which questions to ask. The authors hypothesized that medical doctors may be adopting a "watchful waiting" approach, which is frequent when it comes to diagnosing mental illness in primary care [47]. However, even if patients with AN are referred to specialized treatment, this does not guarantee that they will start or complete a psychotherapeutic treatment [48, 49]. Hay et al. [50] showed that the subsequent use of specialized psychiatric treatment was influenced by whether or not mental health issues were raised in primary care visits.

Previously developed checklists and reviews on treatment barriers usually include some factors related to the health system [6, 25, 28, 29, 51]. However, these factors mainly address general aspects, such as difficulties in accessing specialized care, long waiting times or high treatment costs. The FABIANA-checklist focusses more on the practitioner's specific approach to the disorder in the frame of a doctor-patient relationship and networking with colleagues. From the responses of the patients in our sample, there are indications that the early treatment of AN by the practitioner and pathways to specialized care may be further optimized. While patients quite often stated that they had a doctor they could trust, they less often agreed with the items related to their doctor's competence in dealing with ED, organizing cooperation with other treatment providers or dealing directly with their AN. The recognition and competent management of AN within the health care system therefore seems to be an important starting point for preventive measures. It is important to note that the FABIANA-checklist does not refer exclusively to contacts with general practitioners but to any contact with the medical care system that took place prior to referral for specialized treatment.

Support from the relatives and close others

The second factor refers to three items which describe the perceived support from relatives and close others. Correlations between the items and the F-SozU [37], a validated measure for social support, were all positive. The correlation with item 5 was however too small to be significant. While the F-SozU captures more general aspects of social support, item 5 refers to a quite specific assistance in initiating treatment, which was even further specified by presenting examples e.g. e close relatives "arranged doctor's appointments" or "accompanied me to medical appointments". It is possible that the correlation would have been larger without this further restriction through examples.

Social support is mentioned in the checklist on treatment barriers proposed by Ali et al. [29] and in existing systematic reviews on barriers to help-seeking behavior [51, 52]. While the BATSH-ED refers to a general lack of support or encouragement from others or to the inability of others to provide help, the FABIANA-checklist differentiates the relatives' concern for the patient, the encouragement of the patient to seek treatment and concrete practical support. Barriers and helpful factors are not necessarily comparable in their influence, even if they are endpoints on the same spectrum. For example, Cachelin et al. [52] reported that in 23–35% of patients with ED, encouragement from friends was a major facilitator for entering treatment. However, a lack of support was perceived by only 3% as a barrier.

In our sample patients agreed particularly often with factors of emotional and practical support. Moreover, the item on early detection of AN by relatives was on average more likely to be endorsed than the item referring to early detection of AN by practitioners. Although no causal conclusions can be drawn from our data, this indicates that close others play an important role in early detection and in supporting the patient on her way to specialized care.

Three items mainly loaded onto the fourth component, which, however, had insufficient internal consistency. One item refers to an inner attitude of the patient (perceiving the need of psychotherapy as a sign of weakness) and two items address the early recognition of AN and the need for help by close others. This component might be related to some extent to aspects of stigmatization and shame, which have been found to be potential barriers to treatment initiation in other studies [25, 28, 51]. On the one hand, it could be assumed that patients who consider therapeutic help as a sign of personal weakness, might feel more embarrassed and ashamed when personal problems occur and might be more afraid of being blamed by others. Thus, they might hide their problems from their relatives or close others, which in turn will present more difficulties in recognizing and addressing their need for help. On the other hand, dealing openly with weaknesses and disorders in the family (or in society) can make it easier for the patient to confide in others and to get the necessary support from close relatives. Interestingly, there was no general correlation between relatives addressing AN (item 1) and the total score of perceived social support. But the item was correlated with a single FSozU item, namely with the feeling of (the

patient) of being able to share happiness and sorrow with close others.

Further components

The other components were characterized by either negative internal consistency or single item loadings. These components describe similar topics, namely knowledge about AN and available treatments and the consideration of role models in the period prior to treatment uptake. Ali et al. [29] describe a lack of knowledge about the ED as a barrier to help-seeking behavior and mention a factor about knowledge about where to get help and about which treatments are available, which coincides with item 16 of the FABIANA-checklist. This item could not be validated with the PACIC-5A [36] as expected. It probably refers more to a general feeling of orientation, in the sense of knowing where to search for help, rather than to have perceived concrete support from the health system.

In addition to the patients' level of knowledge, the FABIANA-checklist also recorded whether any relatives had informed themselves about AN. In this item (7) differences between adolescent and adult patients emerged, with the relatives of adolescents searching more frequently for advice or information about AN. In contrast to our expectations this item was not correlated to general social support. It probably refers more to the support that relatives seek for themselves in literature or counselling in order to be able to in turn support patients.

Item 3 was retained in the checklist despite having an item-total correlation close to zero, because it represented an aspect that was not represented by any other item, namely the orientation towards other patients with successful therapy courses (as role models). This item, which did not correlate significantly with any other item of the checklist, complicated the interpretation of the PCA. Contrary to our expectation, it had a negative impact, contributed to a negative Cronbach's alpha on the third component and was neither associated with more personal control nor with more illness comprehensibility. We were not able to fully interpret the third component. This should be seen as an indication that this item needs be examined more closely and, if necessary, excluded from the checklist.

Patients with AN confirmed that comparing themselves to other girls or women in the (social) media had an impact on the fact that they considered their low weight or their dieting as normal and that they subsequently did not felt the need to seek treatment. Patients who were less influenced by the media had, as expected, a better understanding of their disease and were also less likely to perceive the media as a cause of their illness in the BIPQ [38].

Strengths and limitations

To the best of our knowledge, the FABIANA-checklist is the only checklist of factors involved in treatment initiation in patients with AN that underwent psychometric validation.

In contrast to a classic questionnaire, which is based on theoretical concepts, the FABIANA-checklist was created using a mixed-method and a multi-informant (patients, their relatives and practitioners) approach, and is thus summarizing aspects that were considered relevant to the agents involved in treatment initiation. The use of a bottom-up approach (based on qualitative interviews) ensures the external validity of our checklist. Through the inclusion of the most frequently mentioned categories it is ensured that the factors listed in the checklist address a broad group of patients with AN. Even though it was important to us to collect a broad range of factors, we were unable to include all aspects mentioned in the interviews. For reasons of parsimony and applicability of the checklist, we had to exclude factors that were mentioned by only a few patients or that were very similar to other factors, even if they covered slightly different aspects. Moreover, even if we had a large qualitative sample, it is possible that aspects were not covered or were underrepresented in our sample.

Another strength is the process of item selection, which was guided by consensual rating discussions within the research group and a focus on items that are potentially modifiable by secondary prevention measures.

The sample of our study is representative of female patients with AN. The decision to include only female patients with AN was based on the fact, that women are by far the most frequently affected patient group. In addition, it is possible that other factors are involved in men's treatment uptake [53]. However, in order to study gender specific barriers and facilitators, we would have had to collect a much larger sample, which would have demanded a lot of time and resources. In addition, since the preliminary study was based exclusively on interviews with female patients, we assume that the factors contained in the checklist can only be transferred to a limited extent to a male target group.

As the survey was conducted at 11 sites, the sample is fairly representative of patients with AN undergoing specialized treatment in Germany. Since the large majority of patients was recruited at inpatient units, these patients are overrepresented in the sample. With an average BMI of 15.5 kg/m^2 and a comorbidity rate of 77%, the analyzed population is comparable to other studies [6, 54]. We found a mean DUI of 2.25 years for female patients with AN. The DUI is slightly below the mean DUI for patients with AN from seven countries described by Austin et al. [6] in their recent systematic review (2.42 years), and similar to another German sample from the Hamburg metropolitan area [44]. In the subgroup of adolescent patients, DUI was a little less than 6 months and thus significantly shorter than in adults. Mean AOO was around 19 years, with 15.5 years for adolescent patients and 20.7 years for adults. The shorter DUI found in adolescent patients has been demonstrated in other studies [6, 42, 47] and can be attributed to significantly lower dispersion in the subsample of adolescents. Moreover, other studies suggest, that adolescents are more likely living with their relatives, who support the recognition and help-seeking process.

With regard to the sample size, it can be said that approximately 3 participants per item is acceptable but in the lower range of the recommendations for PCAs. It is therefore possible that the PCA was underpowered.

Finally, the FABIANA-checklist explicitly refers to the time that preceded the first psychotherapeutic treatment, it will not allow conclusions on correlates of treatment-seeking in general. Moreover, retrospective memory creates distortions, i.e. some factors are experienced as more significant or less significant than they were at the given time. The literature provides no sufficient evidence on the optimal recall period to minimize the impact of memory effects (e.g., recall biases) for self-reported utilization of healthcare services [55]. However, it is recommended to use periods of three or six months when frequently used services are surveyed while salient visits and rarely used medical care services seem to be accurately reported over a longer period [55]. We assume the commencement of a psychotherapeutic treatment to be a salient and rare event, justifying the use of a 12-month-period for our study purposes.

Conclusion

The FABIANA-checklist is a psychometrically evaluated instrument, which specifically refers to factors involved in treatment initiation in patients with AN. The 18-item version has an acceptable internal consistency and due to the bottom-up approach a high external validity. The present study provided initial data on the expression of these factors in a population of patients who were currently or recently undergoing their first specialized AN treatment. As the focus of the FABIANA-checklist has been laid on modifiable factors, it offers a good starting point for the overall aim of the FABIANA-project, i.e. deriving preventive measures. To quantify the relative importance of the factors assessed by the FABIANA-checklist and to derive recommendations on early-intervention approaches, the effect of these factors on the DUI will be determined in our upcoming study. Furthermore, we plan to investigate differences between the perspectives of patients, their close relatives and primary caregivers on factors involved in the process of treatment initiation.

Abbreviations

AN: Anorexia nervosa; AOO: Age of onset; BATSH-ED: Barriers toward seeking help for eating disorders questionnaire; BED: Binge eating disorder; BIPQ: Brief illness perception questionnaire; BN: Bulimia nervosa; DUI: Duration of untreated illness; ED: Eating disorder; FABIANA: Facilitators and barriers in anorexia nervosa treatment initiation; FREED: First episode and rapid early intervention in eating disorders; F-SozU: Social Support Questionnaire (Fragebogen der sozialen Unterstützung); PACIC-5A: Patient assessment of chronic illness care questionnaire.

Acknowledgements

We would like to thank all our interview partners and our cooperating partners who were involved in the recruitment of study participants. Alphabetically ordered, these are: Asklepios Clinic Nord-Ochsenzoll (Hamburg), Asklepios Clinic West Hamburg (Hamburg), Clinic Lüneburger Heide (Bad Bevensen), Dipl. Psych. Kaufmann, A.L. (Flensburg), MediClin Seepark Clinic (Bad Bodenteich), Schön Clinic Bad Arolsen (Bad Arolsen), Schön Clinic Bad Bramstedt (Bad Bramstedt), Schön Clinic Hamburg Eilbek (Hamburg), Schön Clinic Roseneck (Prien am Chiemsee), Training Center for Behavior Therapy Falkenried (VTFAW, Hamburg), University Hospital Hamburg-Eppendorf (Hamburg), University Hospital Heidelberg (Heidelberg), University Clinic Regensburg (Regensburg).

Authors' contributions

The study's principal investigators, BL and AG, designed the study assisted by DK and AW. Funding was obtained by BL (FABIANA-sub-study 1) and AG (FABIANA-sub-study 2 and 3). UV, MS, BS, HF were involved in the recruitment of patients. DK, JS and LR conducted data collection. JS, LR, AW and AG analyzed the data. LR and JS wrote the first draft of the manuscript. All other authors provided substantial input to the first draft. All authors read and approved the final manuscript.

Competing interests

The authors declare that they have no competing interests.

Author details

[1]Department of Psychosomatic Medicine and Psychotherapy, University Medical Center Hamburg-Eppendorf, Martinistr. 52, W37, 20246 Hamburg, Germany. [2]Department of Psychiatry and Psychotherapy, University Hospital, LMU Munich, Munich, Germany. [3]Schön Clinic Roseneck, Prien am Chiemsee, Germany. [4]Department of Psychiatry and Psychotherapy, University Hospital of Freiburg, Freiburg, Germany. [5]Schön Clinic for Psychosomatic Medicine and Psychotherapy, Bad Arolsen, Germany. [6]Medclin Seepark Clinic for Acute Psychosomatic Care, Bad Bodenteich, Germany. [7]Department of Psychosomatic Medicine and Psychotherapy, Asklepios Westklinikum Hamburg, Hamburg, Germany.

References

1. Fichter MM, Quadflieg N, Crosby RD, Koch S. Long-term outcome of anorexia nervosa: Results from a large clinical longitudinal study. Int J Eat Disord. 2017. https://doi.org/10.1002/eat.22736.
2. Steinhausen HC. The outcome of anorexia nervosa in the 20th century. Am J Psychiatry. 2002;159(Suppl 8):1284–93. https://doi.org/10.1176/appi.ajp.159.8.1284.
3. Forrest LN, Smith AR, Swanson SA. Characteristics of seeking treatment among U.S. adolescents with eating disorders. Int J Eat Disord. 2017;50(Suppl 7):826–33. https://doi.org/10.1002/eat.22702.
4. Hart LM, Granillo MT, Jorm AF, Paxton SJ. Unmet need for treatment in the eating disorders: a systematic review of eating disorder specific treatment seeking among community cases. Clin Psychol Rev. 2011;31(Suppl 5):727–35. https://doi.org/10.1016/j.cpr.2011.03.004
5. Solmi F, Hotopf M, Hatch SL, Treasure J, Micali N. Eating disorders in a multi-ethnic inner-city UK sample: prevalence, comorbidity and service use. Soc Psychiatry Psychiatr Epidemiol. 2016;51:369–81. https://doi.org/10.1007/s00127-015-1146-7.
6. Austin A, Flynn M, Richards K, Hodsoll J, Duarte TA, Robinson P, Kelly J, Schmidt U. Duration of untreated eating disorder and relationship to outcomes: A systematic review of the literature. Eur Eat Disord Rev. 2020. https://doi.org/10.1002/erv.2745.
7. Weigel A, Rossi M, Wendt H, Neubauer K, von Rad K, Daubmann A, Romer G, Löwe B, Gumz A. Duration of untreated illness and predictors of late treatment initiation in anorexia nervosa. J Public Health (Germany). 2014;24:427–36. https://doi.org/10.1007/s10389-014-0642-7.
8. Schlegl S, Hupe K, Hessler JB, Diedrich A, Huber T, Rauh E, Aita S, Gärtner T, Voderholzer U. Wege in die Versorgung und Behandlungslatenzen bei stationären Patienten mit Anorexia und Bulimia nervosa. Psychiatr Prax. 2019;46(Suppl 6):342–8. https://doi.org/10.1055/a-0922-5651.
9. Gumz A, Uhlenbusch N, Weigel A, Wegscheider K, Romer G, Löwe B. Decreasing the duration of untreated illness for individuals with anorexia nervosa: study protocol of the evaluation of a systemic public health intervention at community level. BMC Psychiatry. 2014;14(1):1–8. https://doi.org/10.1186/s12888-014-0300-1.
10. Brown A, McClelland J, Boysen E, Mountford V, Glennon D, Schmidt U. The FREED project (first episode and rapid early intervention in eating disorders): service model, feasibility and acceptability. Early Interv Psychiatry. 2018;12(2):250–7. https://doi.org/10.1111/eip.12382.
11. Volpe U, Monteleone AM, Ricca V, Corsi E, Favaro A, Santonastaso P, de Giorgi S, Renna C, Abbate Daga G, Amianto F, Balestrieri M, Luxardi GL, Clerici M, Alamia A, Segura-Garcia C, Rania M, Monteleone P, Maj M. Pathways to specialist care for eating disorders: An Italian multicentre study. Eur Eat Disord Rev. 2019;27(Suppl 3):274–82. https://doi.org/10.1002/erv.2669.
12. Zipfel S, Wild B, Grob G, Friederich HC, Teufel M, Schellberg D, Giel KE, de Zwaan M, Dinkel A, Herpertz S, Burgmer M, Löwe B, Tagay S, von Wietersheim J, Zeeck A, Schade-Brittinger C, Schauenburg H, Herzog W. Focal psychodynamic therapy, cognitive behaviour therapy, and optimised treatment as usual in outpatients with anorexia nervosa (ANTOP study): Randomised controlled trial. Lancet. 2014;383(Suppl 9912):127–37. https://doi.org/10.1016/S0140-6736(13)61746-8.
13. Allen KL, Mountford V, Brown A, Richards K, Grant N, Austin A, Glennon D, Schmidt U. First episode rapid early intervention for eating disorders (FREED): From research to routine clinical practice. Early Interv Psychiatry. 2020;14(Suppl 5):625–30. https://doi.org/10.1111/eip.12941.
14. Zipfel S, Giel KE, Bulik CM, Hay P, Schmidt U. Anorexia nervosa: Aetiology, assessment, and treatment. Lancet Psychiatry. 2015;2(Suppl 12):1099–111. https://doi.org/10.1016/S2215-0366(15)00356-9.
15. Davidsen AH, Hoyt WT, Poulsen S, Waaddegaard M, Lau M. Eating disorder severity and functional impairment: moderating effects of illness duration in a clinical sample. Eat Weight Disord. 2017;22(Suppl 3):499–507. https://doi.org/10.1007/s40519-016-0319-z.
16. De Vos JA, Radstaak M, Bohlmeijer ET, Westerhof GJ. Having an eating disorder and still being able to flourish? Examination of pathological symptoms and well-being as two continua of mental health in a clinical sample. Front Psychol. 2018;9:2145. https://doi.org/10.3389/fpsyg.2018.02145.
17. Ambwani S, Cardi V, Albano G, Cao L, Crosby RD, Macdonald P, Schmidt U, Treasure JA. multicenter audit of outpatient care for adult anorexia nervosa: Symptom trajectory, service use, and evidence in support of "early stage" versus "severe and enduring" classification. Int J Eat Disord. 2020;53(8):1337–48. https://doi.org/10.1002/eat.23246.
18. Werthmann J, Simic M, Konstantellou A, Mansfield P, Mercado D, van Ens W, Schmidt U. Same, same but different: Attention bias for food cues in adults and adolescents with anorexia nervosa. Int J Eat Disord. 2019;52(Suppl 6):681–90. https://doi.org/10.1002/eat.23064

19. Shott ME, Filoteo JV, Bhatnagar KAC, Peak NJ, Hagman JO, Rockwell R, Kaye WH, Frank GKW. Cognitive Set-Shifting in Anorexia Nervosa. Eur Eat Disord Rev. 2012;20(Suppl 5):343–9. https://doi.org/10.1002/erv.2172.

20. Steinglass JE, Walsh BT. Neurobiological model of the persistence of anorexia nervosa. J Eat Disord. 2016. https://doi.org/10.1186/s40337-016-0106-2.

21. Gumz A, Weigel A, Wegscheider K, Romer G, Löwe B. The psychenet public health intervention for anorexia nervosa: a pre-post-evaluation study in a female patient sample. Prim Health Care Res Dev. 2018;19(Suppl 1):42–52. https://doi.org/10.1017/S1463423617000524.

22. Flynn M, Austin A, Lang K, Allen K, Bassi R, Brady G, Brown A, Connan F, Franklin-Smith M, Glennon D, Grant N, Jones WR, Kali K, Koskina A, Mahony K, Mountford V, Nunes N, Schelhase M, Serpell L, Schmidt U. Assessing the impact of First Episode Rapid Early Intervention for Eating Disorders on duration of untreated eating disorder: a multi-centre quasi-experimental study. Eur Eat Disord Rev. 2020. https://doi.org/10.1002/erv.2797.

23. Schmidt U, Adan R, Böhm I, Campbell IC, Dingemans A, Ehrlich S, Elzak-kers I, Favaro A, Giel K, Harrison A, Himmerich H, Hoek HW, Herpertz-Dahlmann B, Kas MJ, Seitz J, Smeets P, Sternheim L, Tenconi E, van Elburg A, van Furth E, Zipfel S. Eating disorders: the big issue. Lancet Psychiatry. 2016;3(Suppl 4):313–5. https://doi.org/10.1016/S2215-0366(16)00081-X.

24. Weigel A, Gumz A, Kästner D, Romer G, Wegschneider K, Löwe B. Präven-tion und Versorgung von Essstörungen: Das Gesundheitsnetz Mager-sucht und Bulimie. Psychiatr Prax. 2015;42(Suppl 1):30–4. https://doi.org/10.1055/s-0034-1387651.

25. Innes NT, Clough BA, Casey LM. Assessing treatment barriers in eating disorders: a systematic review. Eat Disord. 2017;25(Suppl 1):1–21. https://doi.org/10.1080/10640266.2016.1207455.

26. Innes NT, Clough BA, Day JJ, Casey LM. Can the Perceived Barriers to Psychological Treatment Scale be used to investigate treatment barriers among females with disordered and non-disordered eating behaviours? Psychiatry Res. 2018;259:68–76. https://doi.org/10.1016/j.psychres.2017.09.070.

27. Mohr DC, Ho J, Duffecy J, Baron KG, Lehman KA, Jin L, Reifler D. Perceived barriers to psychological treatments and their relationship to depression. J Clin Psychol. 2010;66(Suppl 4):394–409. https://doi.org/10.1002/jclp.20659.

28. Ali K, Farrer L, Fassnacht DB, Gulliver A, Bauer S, Griffiths KM. Perceived barriers and facilitators towards help-seeking for eating disorders: a systematic review. Int J Eat Disord. 2017;50(Suppl 1):9–21. https://doi.org/10.1002/eat.22598.

29. Ali K, Fassnacht DB, Farrer L, Rieger E, Feldhege J, Moessner M, Griffiths KM, Bauer S. What prevents young adults from seeking help? Barriers toward help-seeking for eating disorder symptomatology. Int J Eat Disord. 2020;53(Suppl 6):894–906. https://doi.org/10.1002/eat.23266.

30. Kästner D, Buchholz I, Weigel A, Brunner R, Voderholzer U, Gumz A, Löwe B. Facilitators and barriers in anorexia nervosa treatment initiation (FABIANA): study protocol for a mixed-methods and multicentre study. BJPsych open. 2019;5(6):1–9. https://doi.org/10.1192/bjo.2019.77.

31. Kästner D, Weigel A, Buchholz I, Voderholzer U, Löwe B, Gumz A. Facilita-tors and barriers in anorexia nervosa treatment initiation: a qualitative study on the perspectives of patients, carers and professionals. J Eat Disord. 2021. https://doi.org/10.1186/s40337-021-00381-0.

32. Pentzek M, Wollny A, Herber OR, Porst R, Icks A, Abholz H-H, Wilm S. Item-konstruktion in sequenziellen Mixed-methods-Studien: Methodenbe-schreibung anhand eines Beispielprojekts. ZFA. 2012;88(Suppl 12):520–7. https://doi.org/10.3238/zfa.2012.0520-0527.

33. Tabachnik BG, Fidell LS. Using multivariate statistics. 3rd ed. Northridge: Harper Collins; 1996.

34. Beesdo-Baum K, Zaudig M, Wittchen HU, editors. SCID-5-CV Strukturiertes Klinisches Interview für DSM-5-Störungen–Klinische Version. Göttingen: Hogrefe; 2019.

35. Guttman L. Some necessary conditions for common-factor analysis. Psychometrika. 1954;19(2):149–61. https://doi.org/10.1007/BF02289162.

36. Rosemann T, Laux G, Droesemeyer S, Gensichen J, Szecsenyi J. Evaluation of a culturally adapted German version of the Patient Assessment of Chronic Illness Care (PACIC 5A) questionnaire in a sample of osteoarthritis patients. J Eval Clin Pract. 2007;13(Suppl 5):806–13. https://doi.org/10.1111/j.1365-2753.2007.00786.x.

37. Fydrich T, Sommer G, Brähler E. F-SozU: Fragebogen zur Sozialen Unter-stützung. [F-SozU: Questionnaire on social support.]. Göttingen: Hogrefe; 2007.

38. Broadbent E, Petrie KJ, Main J, Weinman J. The brief illness perception questionnaire. J Psychosom Res. 2006;60(Suppl 6):631–7. https://doi.org/10.1016/j.jpsychores.2005.10.020.

39. Wagner EH, Austin BT, Davis C, Hindmarsh M, Schaefer J, Bonomi A. Improving chronic illness care: translating evidence into action. Health Aff. 2001;20(Suppl 6):64–78. https://doi.org/10.1377/hlthaff.20.6.64.

40. Vrijhoef HJ, Berbee R, Wagner EH, Steuten LM. Quality of integrated chronic care measured by patient survey: identification, selection and application of most appropriate instruments. Health Expect. 2009;12(Suppl 4):417–29. https://doi.org/10.1111/j.1369-7625.2009.00557.x.

41. Cohen J. Statistical power analysis for the behavioral sciences. New York, NY: Routledge Academic; 1988.

42. Bühren K, Herpertz-Dahlmann B, Dempfle A, Becker K, Egberts KM, Ehrlich S, Föcker M. First sociodemographic, pretreatment and clinical data from a German web-based registry for child and adolescent anorexia nervosa. Z Kinder Jugendpsychiatr. 2017;45(5):393–400. https://doi.org/10.1024/1422-4917/a000544.

43. Cadwallader JS, Godart N, Chastang J, Falissard B, Huas C. Detecting eating disorder patients in a general practice setting: a systematic review of heterogeneous data on clinical outcomes and care trajec-tories. Eat Weight Disord. 2016;21:365–81. https://doi.org/10.1007/s40519-016-0273-9.

44. Neubauer K, Weigel A, Daubmann A, Wendt H, Rossi M, Löwe B, Gumz A. Paths to first treatment and duration of untreated illness in anorexia nervosa: Are there differences according to age of onset? Eur Eat Disord Rev. 2014;22(Suppl 4):292–8. https://doi.org/10.1002/erv.2300.

45. Higgins A, Cahn S. Detection of anorexia nervosa in primary care. Eat Disord. 2018;26(Suppl 3):213–28. https://doi.org/10.1080/10640266.2017.1397419.

46. Linville D, Brown T, O'Neil M. Medical providers' self perceived knowledge and skills for working with eating disorders: a national survey. Eat Disord. 2012;20:1–13. https://doi.org/10.1080/10640266.2012.635557.

47. Currin L, Waller G, Schmidt U. Primary care physicians' knowledge of and attitudes toward the eating disorders: do they affect clinical actions? Int J Eat Disord. 2009;42(Suppl 5):453–8. https://doi.org/10.1002/eat.20636.

48. House J, Schmidt U, Landau S, Simic M, Nicholls D, Hugo P, Berelowitz M, Eisler I. Comparison of specialist and nonspecialist care pathways for adolescents with anorexia nervosa and related eating disorders. Int J Eat Disord. 2012;45(Suppl 8):949–56. https://doi.org/10.1002/eat.22065.

49. Waller G, Schmidt U, Treasure J, Murray K, Aleyna J, Emanuelli F, Crockett J, Yeomans M. Problems across care pathways in specialist adult eating disorder services. Psychiatr Bull. 2009;33(Suppl 1):26–9. https://doi.org/10.1192/pb.bp.107.018325.

50. Hay P, Ghabrial B, Mannan H, Conti J, Gonzalez-Chica D, Stocks N, Heriseanu A, Touyz S. General practitioner and mental healthcare use in a community sample of people with diagnostic threshold symptoms of bulimia nervosa, binge-eating disorder, and other eating disorders. Int J Eat Disord. 2020;53(1):61–8. https://doi.org/10.1002/eat.23174.

51. Regan P, Cachelin FM, Minnick AM. Initial treatment seeking from profes-sional health care providers for eating disorders: A review and synthesis of potential barriers to and facilitators of "first contact." Int J Eat Disord. 2017;50(Suppl 3):190–209. https://doi.org/10.1002/eat.22683.

52. Cachelin FM, Striegel-Moore RH. Help seeking and barriers to treatment in a community sample of Mexican American and European American women with eating disorders. Int J Eat Disord. 2006;39(2):154–61. https://doi.org/10.1002/eat.20213.

53. Richardson C, Paslakis G. Men's experiences of eating disorder treatment: a qualitative systematic review of men-only studies. J Psychiatr Ment Health Nurs. 2021;28(2):237–50. https://doi.org/10.1111/jpm.12670.

54. Salbach-Andrae H, Lenz K, Simmendinger N, Klinkowski N, Lehmkuhl U, Pfeiffer E. Psychiatric comorbidities among female adolescents with anorexia nervosa. Child psychiatry Hum Dev. 2008;39(Suppl 3):261–72. https://doi.org/10.1007/s10578-007-0086-1.

55. Bhandari A, Wagner T. Self-reported utilization of health care ser-vices: improving measurement and accuracy. Med Care Res Rev. 2006;63(2):217–35. https://doi.org/10.1177/1077558705285298.

A Pilot Trial of Repetitive Transcranial Magnetic Stimulation of the Dorsomedial Prefrontal Cortex in Anorexia Nervosa: Resting fMRI Correlates of Response

D. Blake Woodside[1,2,3,4*] (iD), Katharine Dunlop[5], Charlene Sathi[6], Eileen Lam[6], Brigitte McDonald[6] and Jonathan Downar[2,3,6,7]

Abstract

Background: Patients with anorexia nervosa (AN) face severe and chronic illness with high mortality rates, despite our best currently available conventional treatments. Repetitive transcranial magnetic stimulation (rTMS) has shown increasing efficacy in treatment-refractory cases across a variety of psychiatric disorders comorbid with AN, including major depression, Obsessive Compulsive Disorder (OCD), and Post traumatic Stress Disorder (PTSD). However, to date few studies have examined the effects of a course of rTMS on AN pathology itself.

Methods: Nineteen patients with AN underwent a 20–30 session open-label course of dorsomedial prefrontal rTMS for comorbid Major Depressive Disorder (MDD) ± PTSD. Resting-state functional MRI was acquired at baseline in 16/19 patients.

Results: Following treatment, significant improvements were seen in core AN pathology on the EDE global scale, and to a lesser extent on the shape and weight concerns subscales. Significant improvements in comorbid anxiety, and to a lesser extent depression, also ensued. The greatest improvements were seen in patients with lower baseline functional connectivity from the dorsomedial prefrontal cortex (DMPFC) target to regions in the right frontal pole and left angular gyrus.

Conclusions: Despite the limited size of this preliminary, open-label study, the results suggest that rTMS is safe in AN, and may be useful in addressing some core domains of AN pathology. Other targets may also be worth studying in this population, in future sham-controlled trials with larger sample sizes.

Keywords: Anorexia nervosa, R-TMS, fMRI, Anorexia, Treatment, Neuromodulation

* Correspondence: b.woodside@utoronto.ca
[2] Program for Eating Disorders, University Health Network, Toronto, Canada
Centre for Mental Health, University Health Network, Toronto, Canada
Full list of author information is available at the end of the article

Plain English summary

Anorexia nervosa is a serious illness that is difficult to treat. New treatments are urgently needed. This paper describes a preliminary study of a potential new treatment for Anorexia Nervosa, transcranial magnetic stimulation. In this treatment a magnetic field is generated and applied from outside the skull to affect specific areas of the brain thought to be involved in Anorexia nervosa. The results of this preliminary trial, conducted with 19 subjects over 6 weeks, showed some improvements in the way people with Anorexia nervosa think about weight, shape and their eating. The benefits were associated with areas of the brain involved in decision making and in regulating emotions. These changes did not appear to be related to improvements in other conditions, such as depression.

Keywords: Anorexia nervosa, R-TMS, fMRI, Anorexia, Treatment, Neuromodulation

Introduction

Anorexia Nervosa (AN) is a serious medical condition with a chronic, treatment-resistant course as well as substantial rates of mortality. While perhaps half of those affected will eventually respond to conventional treatments, many do not, and either develop a chronic intractable course or die from their condition. The evidence base for conventional treatments is weak, and the development of new treatments for AN has been slow, with few truly innovative new treatments over the last several decades. Given the severity of the condition, it is urgent that new approaches to treatment be examined.

Repetitive transcranial magnetic stimulation (rTMS) is an emerging neuromodulation treatment currently approved in major depression and obsessive-compulsive disorder, and used investigationally in a variety of other psychiatric conditions. The most common target of stimulation in most conditions is the dorsolateral prefrontal cortex. However, as the technology has matured, new stimulatory targets have become available, including the dorsomedial prefrontal cortex (DMPFC) [1]. In addition, the emergence of functional imaging, such as functional magnetic resonance imaging (fMRI) has allowed for visualization of changes in brain activity in response to various treatments, and clinical improvement can be correlated to changes in such activity over the course of treatment.

Our group has recently examined the use of neuronavigated DMPFC-rTMS supplemented by fMRI in a number of conditions relevant to eating disorders. DMPFC-rTMS has achieved significant symptom improvement in Bulimia Nervosa (BN, [11]), Obsessive-Compulsive Disorder [10], and Post-Traumatic Stress Disorder (PTSD, [20]). In the first two studies, we were able to correlate changes in key symptoms to alterations in relevant brain circuitry function seen on resting-state fMRI. However, to date, no studies have reported clinical or neuroimaging findings during DMPFC-rTMS for AN.

To date, there is an extremely small literature on the use of rTMS in AN. All of this literature involves stimulation of the dorsolateral prefrontal cortex (DLPFC). Van den Eynde et al. [19] reported on 10 subjects who received a single session of DLPFC rTMS and noted some subjective reductions in feeling 'fat' or 'full', and some reduction in anxiety. McClelland et al. [14] reported on two cases of severe AN who received approximately 20 sessions of DLPFC rTMS, noting some improvements in EDE symptoms and mood, persisting out to 1 month post treatment. One patient reported decreases in the frequency of bingeing and vomiting. This team then reported on the results of a single session, double blind DLPFC protocol on 49 AN subjects [15] showing non-significant improvements in some AN symptoms amongst those who received active treatment. Finally, Choudhary et al. [6] reported on a single individual with severe AN who received 21 sessions of DLPFC rTMS, and while the authors reported that the patient improved across a wide variety of domains, no quantitative data were presented aside from BMI scores.

The current study extends some of the above findings using a new target for stimulation, the dorsomedial prefrontal cortex (DMPFC), in an open-label sample of 19 patients with AN. We report the effects of this intervention on AN psychopathology, as well as associated changes in brain activity on resting-state fMRI that may correlate with any changes in AN psychopathology..

Methods
Demographic and psychometric data
Between May 2012 and July 2017, 19 female patients with AN (ages 21–56, mean 31.2 ± SD 9.8; BMI 14.5–18.5, mean 16.4 ± SD 1.3) underwent a course of DMPFC-rTMS at the UHN Magnetic Resonance Imaging (MRI)-Guided rTMS Clinic, in each case for an indications other than the AN per se (i.e., comorbid major depression and/or PTSD). The diagnosis of AN was based on a full clinical interview conducted by a Canadian Royal College-certified psychiatrist (authors DBW, JD)

according to the Diagnostic and Statistical Manual fourth edition (DSM-IV) criteria.

rTMS treatment parameters

All patients underwent an initial course of 20 sessions of bilateral DMPFC-rTMS, administered once daily on weekdays over 4 weeks; extension to 30 sessions was offered to those showing partial clinical improvement (mean course length, 22.6 sessions). Stimulation followed the same procedures we have reported previously for DMPFC-rTMS in MDD [1]. To summarize, treatment sessions employed a MagPro R30 stimulator and Cool-DB80 coil positioned laterally to the midline at 25% of the nasion-inion distance, with stimulation of the left then right hemisphere accomplished by orienting the coil handle to the right then to left during the two runs of stimulation on each daily session. All subjects received at least 20 sessions of 10 Hz stimulation.

Outcome measures

Clinical and psychometric data was collected at the initiation and conclusion of treatment. Subjects were administered the Eating Disorders Examination (EDE 16.0D, [7]), the Beck Depression Inventory (BDI, [3]), the Hamilton Depression Inventory (HAM-D, [13]), the Beck Anxiety Inventory (BAI, [2]) and the Difficulties with Emotional Regulation Scale (DERS, [12]). The EDE and HAM-D were administered by trained assessors. Significance testing for changes from pre- to post-treatment was performed via paired t-tests on each measure.

fMRI acquisition and analysis

For 16 participants, a baseline (pre-treatment) structural and resting-state functional fMRI was available to investigate resting-state functional connectivity correlates to Global EDE improvement. Subjects underwent scanning the week prior to rTMS treatment in a 3 T GE Signa HDx scanner equipped with an 8-channel phased-array head coil. A T1-weighted anatomical (TE(time to echo) = 12 ms; TI = 300 ms; flip-angle = 20 degrees; 116 sagittal slices; slice thickness = 1.5 mm, no gap, 256 × 256 matrix, FOV(field of view) = 240 mm) and a 10-min eyes-open resting-state functional MRI scan (TE = 30 ms; TR = 2000 ms; flip-angle = 85 degrees; 5 mm thick axial slices, no gap, 64 × 64 matrix, FOV = 220 mm, 300 volumes) were collected.

Resting-state fMRI data was preprocessed using the Conn functional connectivity toolbox (version 16b, http://www.nitrc.org/projects/conn/) under Matlab version 8.5.0 and implementing functions from SPM12 (Statistical Parametric Mapping, Wellcome Trust Centre for Neuroimaging, London, UK; http://www.fil.ion.ucl.ac.uk/spm). The following preprocessing steps were taken:

removal of the first 5 volumes to account for image stabilization; functional realignment, unwarping and centering; slice-timing correction; structural centering, segmentation and normalization; ART-based (Artifact detection tool) motion-parameter scrubbing, functional smoothing (6 mm FWHM:full width at half maximum); aCompCor-based (anatomical component correction) removal of physiological noise [4]; linear regression of de-meaned confounding motion effects; band-pass filtering (0.008–0.09 Hz), and linear de-trending.

Analysis focused on two regions of interest (ROI), as utilized in our previous studies [10, 18]. Briefly, a bilateral DMPFC and dorsal anterior cingulate cortex (dACC) ROI were defined a priori from a parcellation atlas by Craddock et al. [8]. These ROIs were selected based on their proximity to the stimulation target and for consistency with our previous fMRI studies of DMPFC-rTMS. The time series of each ROI was used as a regressor to generate statistical parametric maps at the individual-level. The resultant statistical parametric maps were subsequently used in a higher-level mixed-effects general linear model (GLM). For both GLMs, ROI resting-state functional connectivity was correlated with de-meaned global-EDE percent improvement from pre- to the first follow-up visit at 0–4 weeks post treatment, with age and Body Mass index (BMI) included as covariates. If the first follow-up data was unavailable, end-of-treatment data was used ($n = 4$). Group-level analyses were thresholded at false-discovery rate corrected cluster-$p < 0.05$ and a height threshold of $p < 0.001$.

Results

Clinical measures

Results are presented in Table 1. Average BMI at treatment was 16.4, and declined slightly to 16.3 at the end

Table 1 Pschometric measures of effect for DMPFC-rTMS in AN

Variable	Pre-treatment	Post-treatment	p-value
EDE global	**4.12**	**3.35**	**.010****
EDE restraint	3.65	3.21	.095
EDE eating concerns	3.92	3.52	.054
EDE shape concerns	4.64	3.63	*.042* *
EDE weight concerns	4.23	3.35	*.024* *
BDI	36.16	30.24	*.041* *
HAM-D	15.50	14.28	.066
BAI	23.43	12.87	*<.001* *
DERS	115.33	117.00	.594
Age at start of treatment	21–56, mean 31.2 ± SD 9.8		
Body Mass Index	14.5–18.5, mean 16.4 ± SD 1.3		

Significant improvements were seen in the EDE global score and the BAI, after Bonferroni correction for multiple comparisons (** = $p < 0.05$, corrected). Considering uncorrected p-values in an exploratory fashion, the EDE subscales for shape and weight concerns as well as the BDI showed significant improvement (* = $p < 0.05$, uncorrected) of treatment. The EDE global scale showed significant improvement from pre- to post-treatment ($p < 0.010$) even after Bonferroni correction for the 5 clinical scales examined. Exploratory analyses of the EDE subscales, using an uncorrected threshold of $p < 0.05$, showed significant improvements in shape concerns ($p = 0.042$) and weight concerns ($p = 0.024$), and a trend toward improvement in eating concerns ($p = 0.054$). There was also a significant improvement in anxiety as measured on the BAI ($p < 0.001$), which remained significant after Bonferroni correction across the 5 scales examined. The BDI also showed improvement ($p = 0.041$), and the HAMD a trend toward improvement ($p = 0.066$), although these did not survive correction for multiple comparisons.

fMRI results

dACC resting-state connectivity
Baseline resting-state functional connectivity to the dACC ROI did not significantly correlate with global EDE score improvement for any area of the brain.

DMPFC resting-state connectivity
Baseline resting-state functional connectivity to the DMPFC ROI revealed two significant clusters that negatively correlated with percent global EDE score improvement. Lower pre-treatment resting-state functional connectivity from the DMPFC to the right frontal pole and left angular gyrus significantly correlated with symptomatic improvement (Table 2; Fig. 1). Mean parameter estimates extracted from each cluster also significantly correlated with percent EDE improvement (Frontal pole/ EDE improvement $r = -0.63$, $p = 0.009$; Angular gyrus/ EDE improvement $r = -0.64$; $p = 0.008$).

Discussion
This study is the first examining the use of DMPFC-rTMS in AN, and only the second study that we are aware of that has provided subjects with a full course of treatment (i.e., ≥ 20 sessions). It is the first study of rTMS in AN with associated functional imaging.

Regarding clinical outcomes, the psychometric findings showing some modest reductions in core AN psychopathology are of interest, especially as the improvements in these core domains of pathology were seen over a rapid timeframe of 4–6 weeks, and there was no

adjunctive eating disorder treatment (psychotherapy or medication adjustments) being received by subjects. The lack of change in weight over the 4–6 week course is not unexpected, given the short duration of the treatment. The accompanying improvements in mood and anxiety are consistent with observations we have previously reported in other studies of DMPFC-rTMS in eating disorders [10, 11, 20], and suggestive of a transdiagnostic mechanism of effect for DMPFC-rTMS, as proposed elsewhere [9].

The neuroimaging findings offer some suggestion that patients who show EDE improvement may have distinctive patterns of network connectivity centering on the stimulation site. For example, the frontal polar region identified in the present study (Fig. 1) has been previously shown in healthy controls to be functionally coactive with the 'salience network', a network of regions that includes the DMPFC and which plays a major role in cognitive control and impulse control [16]. In the present study, patients lacking this connectivity (perhaps in reflection of a lesser capacity for cognitive control over perseverance or negative self-referential thinking) showed the greatest EDE improvement in DMPFC-rTMS. Notably, in healthy controls, DMPFC-rTMS has been shown to enhance the capacity for impulse control on the delay discounting task [5]. The possibility that DMPFC-rTMS may be particularly well suited to a subpopulation of AN patients with comorbid impulsivity or emotional dysregulation bears further investigation in future studies.

A number of limitations to the present study bear acknowledgement. First, this preliminary study had a small sample size, which may have led to underpowering to detect therapeutic effects, and may also have made it difficult to identify or characterize DMPFC-rTMS responsive subgroups of patients, as above. Second, the study used an open-label design, precluding assessment of the contribution of non-specific/placebo effects in the therapeutic response. Mitigating this point, the patients in this question were presenting for treatment of major depression or PTSD, without expectation of changes in core AN pathology as assessed on the EDE. Nonetheless, follow-up studies to this preliminary pilot work should employ a randomized, sham-controlled design. Finally, as this was primarily a clinical sample, only baseline and

Table 2 Regions showing significant correlation between baseline DMPFC resting-state functional connectivity and subsequent improvement in EDE global score

MNI			# Voxels	cluster p-FDR	Hemi	Region
x	y	z				
18	64	16	100	0.048	R	Frontal Pole
−46	−62	44	90	0.048	L	Sup. Lat. Occipital Cortex, Angular Gyrus

Abbreviations: *Hemi* Hemisphere; *FDR* False Discovery Rate; *L* Left; *Lat* Lateral; *MNI* Montreal Neurological Institute; *R* Right; *Sup* Superior

A Pilot Trial of Repetitive Transcranial Magnetic Stimulation of the Dorsomedial Prefrontal Cortex in Anorexia...

197

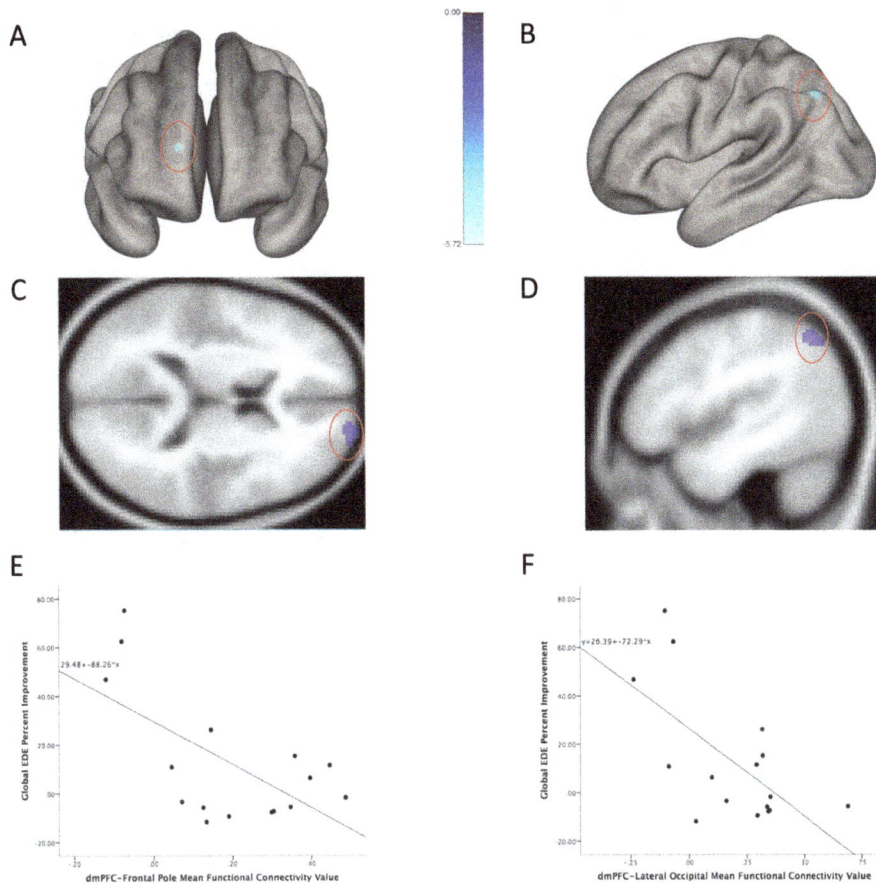

Fig. 1 Brain regions where baseline functional connectivity to DMPFC predicted subsequent improvement in EDE global score. For regions in the right frontal pole (**a**, **c**) and left angular gyrus (**b**, **d**), lower baseline connectivity to the DMPFC predicted greater subsequent improvement following the course of DMPFC-RTMS (**e**, **f**)

not follow-up MRIs were available; this precluded the assessment of changes in DMPFC connectivity that might illuminate the mechanisms of therapeutic effect. As we have previously reported that changes in DMPF C-striatal-thalamic connectivity are associated with improvement in MDD, BN, and OCD symptoms [10, 11, 18], it would be interesting to determine whether similar changes accompany improvement in core AN pathology on the EDE.

Conclusions

This preliminary case series suggests that DMPFC-rTMS may yield improvements in some elements of AN pathology. Given that previous work suggesting that DMPF C-rTMS enhances impulse control [5], further investigation may clarify whether the treatment is best suited to a subgroup of AN patients with deficits in salience network integrity and impulsivity of thought and behavior. It may also be worth investigating whether a more recently developed rTMS target in the right orbitofrontal cortex, originally showing benefits in OCD [17], might address different elements of AN pathology, such as

obsessionality, rigidity, or perseveration. Targeting the neural substrates of AN pathology non-invasively with rTMS may eventually provide an important adjuvant to conventional treatments, in cases where such treatments have failed to achieve meaningful improvement.

Abbreviations

AN: Anorexia Nervosa; rTMS: Repetitive transcranial magnetic stimulation; OCD: Obsessive Compulsive Disorder; PTSD: Post Traumatic Stress Disorder; MDD: Major Depressive Disorder; DMPFC: Dorsomedial Prefrontal Cortex; rMRI: Functional magnetic resonance imaging; BN: Bulimia Nervosa; DLPF C: Dorsolateral Prefrontal Cortex; MRI: Magnetic resonance imaging; DSM: Diagnostic and Statistical Manual; EDE: Eating Disorders Examination; BDI: Beck Depression Inventory; HAM: Hamilton Depression Inventory; BAI: Beck Anxiety Inventory; DERS: Difficulties with Emotional Regulation Scale; ROI: Region of interest; TE: Time to echo; SPM: Statistical Parametric Mapping; ART: Artifact Detection Tool; FWHM: Full width half medium; aComp-Cor: Anatomical Component Correction; dACC: Dorsal anterior cingulate cortex; GLM: General Linear Model; BMI: Body Mass Index

Authors' contributions

Authors' contributions: DBW and JD conceptualized and designed the study, and were the leads in implementing the study and writing the paper. KD performed the analysis of the imaging data. EL and BM coordinated the study and assisted in recruitment. CS performed a literature review on rTMS in AN, All authors have read and approved the manuscript.

Competing interests
The authors declare that they have no competing interests.

Author details
[1]Program for Eating Disorders, University Health Network, Toronto, Canada. [2]Centre for Mental Health, University Health Network, Toronto, Canada. [3]Department of Psychiatry, Faculty of Medicine, University of Toronto, Toronto, Canada. [4]Institute of Medical Science, University of Toronto, Toronto, Canada. [5]Feil Family Brain and Mind Research Institute, Weill Cornell Medicine, New York, USA. [6]MRI-Guided rTMS Clinic, University Health Network, Toronto, Canada. [7]Krembil Research Institute, University Health Network, Toronto, Canada.

References

1. Bakker N, Shahab S, Giacobbe P, Blumberger DM, Daskalakis ZJ, Kennedy SH, et al. rTMS of the dorsomedial prefrontal cortex for major depression: safety, tolerability, effectiveness, and outcome predictors for 10 Hz versus intermittent theta-burst stimulation. Brain Stimul. 2015;8(2):208–15. https://doi.org/10.1016/j.brs.2014.11.002.

2. Beck AT, Epstein N, Brown G, Steer RA. An inventory for measuring clinical anxiety: psychometric properties. J Consult Clin Psychol. 1988;56(6):893–7. https://doi.org/10.1037/0022-006X.56.6.893.

3. Beck AT, Ward CH, Mendelson M, Mock J, Erbaugh J. An inventory for measuring depression. Arch Gen Psychiatry. 1961;4(6):561–71. https://doi.org/10.1001/archpsyc.1961.01710120031004.

4. Behzadi Y, Restom K, Liau J, Liu TT. A component based noise correction method (CompCor) for BOLD and perfusion based fMRI. Neuroimage. 2007;37(1):90–101. https://doi.org/10.1016/j.neuroimage.2007.04.042.

5. Cho SS, Koshimori Y, Aminian K, Obeso I, Rusjan P, Lang AE, et al. Investing in the future: stimulation of the medial prefrontal cortex reduces discounting of delayed rewards. Neuropsychopharmacology. 2015;40(3):546–53. https://doi.org/10.1038/npp.2014.211.

6. Choudhary P, Roy P, Kumar Kar S. Improvement of weight and attitude towards eating behaviour with high frequency rTMS augmentation in anorexia nervosa. Asian J Psychiatr. 2017;28:160. https://doi.org/10.1016/j.ajp.2017.05.010.

7. Fairburn CG, Cooper Z, O'Connor M. The eating disorder examination. In: Fairburn CG, editor. Cognitive Behaviour Therapy and Eating Disorders. 16th ed. New York: Guilford Press; 2008. p. 270–308.

8. Craddock RC, James GA, Holtzheimer PE, Hu XP, Mayberg HS. A whole brain fMRI atlas generated via spatially constrained spectral clustering. Hum Brain Map. 2012;33(8):1914–28. https://doi.org/10.1002/hbm.21333.

9. Downar J, Blumberger DM, Daskalakis ZJ. The neural crossroads of psychiatric illness: an emerging target for brain stimulation. Trends Cogn Sci. 2016;20(2):107–20. https://doi.org/10.1016/j.tics.2015.10.007.

10. Dunlop K, Woodside B, Lam E, Olmsted M, Colton P, Giacobbe P, et al. Increases in frontostriatal connectivity are associated with response to dorsomedial repetitive transcranial magnetic stimulation in refractory binge/purge behaviors. Neuroimage Clin. 2015;8:611–8. https://doi.org/10.1016/j.nicl.2015.06.008.

11. Dunlop K, Woodside B, Olmsted M, Colton P, Giacobbe P, Downar J. Reductions in Cortico-striatal Hyperconnectivity accompany successful treatment of obsessive-compulsive disorder with Dorsomedial prefrontal rTMS. Neuropsychopharmacology. 2016;41(5):1395–403. https://doi.org/10.1038/npp.2015.292.

12. Gratz KL, Roemer L. Multidimensional assessment of emotion regulation and Dysregulation: development, factor structure, and initial validation of the difficulties in emotion regulation scale. J Psychopathol Behav Assess. 2004;26(1):41–54. https://doi.org/10.1023/B:JOBA.0000007455.08539.94.

13. Hamilton M. A rating scale for depression. J Neurol Neurosurg Psychiatry. 1960;23(1):56–62. https://doi.org/10.1136/jnnp.23.1.56.

14. McClelland J, Bozhilova N, Nestler S, Campbell IC, Jacob S, Johnson-Sabine E, et al. Improvements in symptoms following neuronavigated repetitive transcranial magnetic stimulation (rTMS) in severe and enduring anorexia nervosa: findings from two case studies. Eur Eat Disord Rev. 2013;21(6):500–6. https://doi.org/10.1002/erv.2266

15. McClelland J, Kekic M, Bozhilova N, Nestler S, Dew T, Van den Eynde F, et al. A randomised controlled trial of Neuronavigated repetitive Transcranial magnetic stimulation (rTMS) in anorexia nervosa. PLoS One. 2016;11(3):e0148606. https://doi.org/10.1371/journal.pone.0148606.

16. Moayedi M, Salomons TV, Dunlop KAM, Downar J, Davis KD. Connectivity-based parcellation of the human frontal polar cortex. Brain Struct Funct. 2015;220(5):2603–16. https://doi.org/10.1007/s00429-014-0809-6.

17. Nauczyciel C, Drapier D. Repetitive transcranial magnetic stimulation in the treatment of obsessive-compulsive disorder. Rev Neurol. 2012;168(8–9):655–61. https://doi.org/10.1016/j.neurol.2012.05.006.

18. Salomons TV, Dunlop K, Kennedy SH, Flint A, Geraci J, Giacobbe P, et al. Resting-state cortico-thalamic-striatal connectivity predicts response to dorsomedial prefrontal rTMS in major depressive disorder. Neuropsychopharmacology. 2014;39(2):488–98. https://doi.org/10.1038/npp.2013.222.

19. Van den Eynde F, Guillaume S, Broadbent H, Campbell IC, Schmidt U. Repetitive transcranial magnetic stimulation in anorexia nervosa: a pilot study. Eur Psychiatry. 2013;28(2):98–101. https://doi.org/10.1016/j.eurpsy.2011.06.002.

20. Woodside DB, Colton P, Lam E, Dunlop K, Rzeszutek J, Downar J. Dorsomedial prefrontal cortex repetitive transcranial magnetic stimulation treatment of posttraumatic stress disorder in eating disorders: an open-label case series. Int J Eat Disord. 2017;50(10):1231–4. https://doi.org/10.1002/eat.22764.

18

The Role of Personality Traits, Sociocultural Factors and Body Dissatisfaction in Anorexia Readiness Syndrome in Women

Karolina Rymarczyk ⓘ

Abstract

Background: The mass media promote certain standards of physical attractiveness. The media coverage, in interaction with body dissatisfaction and personality traits, may intensify specified behaviors in women, that should help them to obtain an ideal body image, e.g., excessive concentration on body image, weight control, increase in physical activity. The intensification of these behaviors can develop anorexia readiness syndrome (ARS) in women. The paper presents a study on the role of the Five-Factor Model personality traits (neuroticism, extraversion, agreeableness, conscientiousness, and intellect/openness), sociocultural factors (internalization, sociocultural pressure, information seeking), and body dissatisfaction in anorexia readiness syndrome.

Methods: The study involved 1533 Polish women aged 18–36 ($M = 22.51$, $SD = 2.41$). The participants completed the online version of the set of questionnaires. The link to the study was shared in social media groups. Personality dimensions were measured with the BFI, sociocultural factors were evaluated by means of the SATAQ-3, the degree of body dissatisfaction was assessed with the BIQ, while ARS was measured using five self-reported items referring to specific behaviors from TIAE.

Results: Hierarchical multiple regression analysis revealed internalization, sociocultural pressure, and body dissatisfaction as significant predictors of ARS. While neuroticism was correlated with ARS, it lost its predictive value after entering body dissatisfaction in the regression model.

Conclusions: The factors associated with ARS were (1) neuroticism among personality traits, (2) internalization and pressure from sociocultural norms among sociocultural attitudes, and (3) body dissatisfaction. The key finding is the absence of statistical significance for neuroticism in predicting ARS after including body dissatisfaction. In future research, the group of men and patients with anorexia nervosa can be included, and the age range can be extended to include younger people. The catalog of potential ARS predictors may be expanded, which can help to explain the role of neuroticism in ARS.

Keywords: Neuroticism, Big five dimensions, Sociocultural factors, Body dissatisfaction, Anorexia readiness syndrome

Correspondence: k.rymarczyk@uksw.edu.pl
Institute of Psychology, Cardinal Stefan Wyszyński University in Warsaw,
Warsaw, Poland

Plain English summary

Mass culture conveys a lot of information that women should use to fit the specific canon of beauty regarding the female body. Media body image standards can be absorbed by many women who may feel the pressure of having to conform to these standards. Adopting and adhering to the sociocultural ideals of beauty contributes to the development of body dissatisfaction as well as anorexia readiness syndrome (ARS) that can even lead to eating disorders under certain non-favorable circumstances in the long term. The aim of the study was to examine the contributing factors of ARS – thoughts, emotions and behaviors that may lead to diagnosable anorexia nervosa (AN). The study involved 1533 Polish women from a nonclinical population. Based on a review of the literature, possible determinants of ARS were selected: personality traits, sociocultural factors and degree of body dissatisfaction. Analyses confirmed that internalization and pressure from sociocultural norms (two sociocultural factors), and body dissatisfaction may help predict ARS. Neuroticism (personality trait) was also related to ARS. Knowledge of which factors may contribute to ARS may help in understanding how AN develops and what treatments may help prevent the illness from developing. In future research, it is also worth conducting the study on a group of patients with eating disorders and a group of men. Research on a more diverse group will help to understand the determinants of ARS.

Keywords: Neuroticism, Big five dimensions, Sociocultural factors, Body dissatisfaction, Anorexia readiness syndrome

Background

Mass media promote specified norms of attractiveness and the ideal female body and women can engage in certain behaviors, which in their opinion could help them to achieve this ideal body [1]. Such behaviors may be attributable to comparing oneself to unrealistic ideals while depreciating one's attractiveness, and include: a greater interest in nutrition, calorie counting, dieting, weight control methods, increased physical activity, excessive focus on body image, emotional lability related to eating and body perception, the desire to control one's body dimensions and weight, high competitiveness and perfectionism, as well as the need for control (cf. [2–4]). The above symptoms were classified by Ziółkowska [4] as elements of anorexia readiness syndrome (ARS) defined as "a set of indicators in the cognitive, emotional, and behavioral spheres of functioning giving rise to suspicion of abnormality in meeting one's nutritional needs and in one's attitude to one's body" (p. 37).

Substantial research on ARS has been devoted to the extent of this phenomenon among adolescent and adult people. Factors that may lead to body dissatisfaction and, in the long term, to eating disorders, include sociocultural factors (cf. [2, 5, 6]) and personality traits (cf. [4, 7, 8]). However, in previous investigations those factors were examined separately. The present study focused on sociocultural factors and personality traits jointly in order to determine significant ARS predictors.

Personality determinants of ARS

One of the personality models used in body image research is the Five-Factor Model [9], which consists of neuroticism, extraversion, agreeableness, conscientiousness, and intellect/openness to experience [9–11]. Research into the Big Five [9] has revealed that various personality traits have been significant in explaining body dissatisfaction, and especially neuroticism was relevant [12, 13] that: (1) was associated with perceiving one's own body as larger than it is objectively over time [8]; (2) predicted body image dissatisfaction in men and women [12]; (3) predicted investment in body image and self-consciousness of appearance [14]; (4) was linked to actual-ideal weight discrepancy [15]; (5) was useful in explaining emotions related to depression caused by ideal self-discrepancies [16]; (6) was associated with eating disorders and low self-esteem [17]; (7) was a significant risk factor for eating disorder symptoms [18].

The trait of neuroticism (vs. emotional stability) comprises emotional instability, oversensitivity, the tendency to experience negative emotions, adjustment and resilience to stress [9]. Due to the tendency to experience negative emotions and dissatisfaction, neuroticism may be linked to negative body image (cf. [15]). Therefore, it would be worthwhile to examine the role of neuroticism in the development of ARS before the onset of a major eating disorder. Indeed, neuroticism appears to be a trait of special importance to disturbed body image, and ultimately to eating disorders (cf. [7, 12, 18]).

Sociocultural factors as determinants of ARS

Body image perception in women is determined by various factors, that could labeled as sociocultural factors, and include: the assimilation of media influence and the internalization of the media body ideal [13, 19], the family environment [4, 20, 21], peer pressure among youth [22, 23], and cultural influence [24].

Thompson and collaborators [25], who termed sociocultural factors attitudes, distinguished: (1) internalization; (2) pressures from sociocultural norms; (3) seeking information about body image. The attitudes adopted by people are affected by the mass media, which promote certain norms of physical attractiveness (cf. [25, 26]). In conjunction with some physical characteristics (e.g., BMI) and psychological factors (e.g., ideal self-discrepancies, personality traits), media plays an important role in one's body image (cf. [1, 27]).

The internalization of the thin ideal contributes to postponing the satisfaction of basic needs (e.g., food) and lowers the awareness of one's own body in women [1]. The body ideal present in culture may affect body perception leading to objectification [28] and an instrumental attitude (using the body for attaining certain goals and benefits). According to the study of Młożniak and Schier [29], objectified body perceptions tend to be more severe in those who described their bodies as, e.g., a machine, instrument, or object [29].

The study of Izydorczyk and Rybicka-Klimczyk [1] showed that the mass media constitute an important source of information about beauty ideals for women. The subjects experienced pressure from sociocultural norms in connection to the female body image standards promoted by the media and internalized them to a significant extent. In their paper on ARS, Chytra-Gędek and Kobierecka [5] found that the key assessment criterion for women was being slim, which was associated with good looks, popularity, as well as being successful and attractive to men. Based on the responses given in the study, in the group of examined women, 6.5% of them were found to exhibit ARS (mostly in the dimension of attributing high value to body slimness) [5].

Sociocultural factors play a role not only in eliciting body dissatisfaction, but also in the development of eating disorders [6, 30–32], which may follow from persistent dissatisfaction with one's looks, a critical evaluation of one's appearance, and vulnerability to external influence (e.g., the mass media). Therefore, these factors should be examined in terms of their predictive value for ARS.

Body dissatisfaction as a determinant of ARS

Body image may be defined as an internalized belief about one's appearance [33], including convictions about how one is perceived by others and the associated emotions (cf. [34]). The cognitive dimension of body image consists of individuals' thoughts, beliefs, and cognitive patterns about their appearance. A negative perception may imply a lack of acceptance leading to adverse emotional states, excessive weight control, a tendency for perfectionism, and internalization of attractiveness standards [4, 5, 35, 36]. The cognitive sources of distorted body image are also investigated by neuroscience. Its affective element may be associated with changes in the prefrontal cortex, insula, and amygdala, with the perception component being linked to changes in the parietal lobe (cf. [37]).

Body dissatisfaction and negative emotional states often result from comparisons with the ideal [38–40] that is frequently and conspicuously presented in the mass media [41, 42]. Abnormal body image perceptions may be also attributable to depressive symptoms or major depression [43]. Rzeszutek and Schier [43] reported that young adults with depressive symptoms tended to be more critical of their bodies. Body dissatisfaction may result from discrepancies between real perceptions of one's body and of the body presented in the media and entails a higher risk of eating disorders [39]. Hagman et al. [44] showed that patients with anorexia nervosa (AN) had a higher level of body dissatisfaction than healthy women and overestimated their body size more.

Therefore, if body dissatisfaction is associated with the risk of developing eating disorders, it seems reasonable to explore its role in predicting ARS.

Present study

The present study explored possible determinants of ARS among the variables described above, identified in the literature as the most important predictors of ARS. One can expect that (a) personality traits and especially neuroticism (cf. [18]), (b) sociocultural factors, and especially internalization and pressure (cf. [3]), and (c) body dissatisfaction (cf. [2]) are positively related to ARS. Moreover, a question has been asked which of these variables will significantly increase the prediction of ARS. According to the Five-Factor Theory, in the first step personality traits (basic tendencies) were included in the analysis and in the next steps sociocultural factors and body dissatisfaction (characteristic adaptations) were added [45].

Considering that the image of the human body in the mass media, which has major implications for the way women perceive their own bodies [41, 42, 46], and numerous findings pointing to the significant role of neuroticism in body image perception, hierarchical multiple regression analysis was conducted to find out whether the aforementioned categories of variables can be used to predict ARS.

Methods

Participants

The study encompassed 1533 Polish women aged 18 to 36 years ($M = 22.51$, $SD = 2.41$), and was administered online using the University Online Survey System. The participants were recruited from groups in social media where the link to the study was shared. There were student groups and groups related to women's activity. Participants' anonymity was fully ensured, and the study did not include personal questions. The inclusion criterion was age - 18 years or more.

Among the participants, 52% had secondary education, 47.1% had higher education, with the remaining 0.9% having primary or vocational education. As many as 79.6% of the women were city dwellers, while 20.4% lived in rural areas. The medium BMI level was 22.10 (13.63–51.27). Most of the examined women (n = 1079) were of a normal weight (18.5–24.9), 203 women were underweight (below 18.5), and 169 women were pre-obese (25.0–29.9). In the BMI group of obesity, 58 women were obesity class I (30.0–34.9), 14 women were obesity class II (35.0–39.9), and only 6 women were obesity class III (above 40). Women also completed the Photographic Figure Rating Scale to assess the most closely resembled their own bodies (real) and the body that they would like to possess (ideal). To assess the direction of the real-ideal discrepancy, we used the Modified Contour Drawing Figure Rating Scale [47], which included nine line-drawings of women's bodies with covered faces. The real-ideal discrepancy showed that 1203 women would like to be thinner, 114 women would like to be fatter, and in 216 women there were no differences. Although the group of women who would like to be thinner was large, most of the women were still of a normal weight (BMI 18.5–24.9).

Measures

Measurement of personality traits

Personality traits were measured using the *Big Five Inventory* (BFI) [10], which consists of 44 items describing various behaviors. BFI evaluates five personality dimensions: extraversion, agreeableness, conscientiousness, neuroticism, and openness/intellect [11] using a five-point scale ranging from 1 (*strongly disagree*) to 5 (*strongly agree*). The Cronbach's alpha of the constituent trait scales ranged from 0.70 to 0.84.

Measurement of sociocultural factors

Sociocultural factors were measured using the *Sociocultural Attitudes Towards Appearance Questionnaire*-3 (SATAQ-3) [25]. The Polish version of the questionnaire prepared by Izydorczyk and Rybicka-Klimczyk [1, 26] consists of 24 items forming three scales (as opposed to four scales in the original): (1) internalization evaluating the degree of comparing oneself to and assimilating sociocultural norms concerning attractive body image standards, and especially those promoted by the mass media (nine items, e.g., "I wish I looked like the models in music videos"); (2) pressure from sociocultural norms assessing the strength of that pressure exerted by the mass media (seven items, e.g., "I've felt pressure from TV or magazines to lose weight"); (3) seeking information about body image measuring the frequency of seeking that information in the mass media (eight items, e.g., "TV commercials are an important source of information about fashion and "being

attractive"). Responses were given on a five-point scale ranging from 1 (*definitely disagree*) to 5 (*definitely agree*), with the Cronbach's alpha of the various scales being between 0.80 and 0.91. Since the scales revealed significant intercorrelations of more than 0.54, the overall score was used in the study (STQ). The overall score was supported by the scree plot on all 24 items which clearly shows a single factor that explains 42.44% of the variance of all variables while the second explains only 8.58%. The correlations of individual scales with the overall score exceeded 0.80. A parallel analysis was run on four scales and indicates a one-factor solution (first two eigenvalues from sample correlation matrix: 2.146, 0.908; first two average eigenvalues from parallel analysis: 1.056, 1.016).

Measurement of body dissatisfaction

The degree of body dissatisfaction was measured using the *Body Image Questionnaire* (BIQ-40) developed by Głębocka [39] containing 40 items grouped into four subscales (1) the cognition-emotions subscale evaluates one's opinions about one's appearance as well as the emotions experienced in relation to it (16 items, e.g., "I think my hips are too big"); (2) the behavior subscale consists of items referring to a healthy lifestyle (five items with reversed response scale, e.g., "I enjoy active leisure"); (3) the criticism from others subscale measures the subjective degree of acceptance of the woman by the people around her (six items, e.g., "I often hear critical comments about my looks"); (4) the pretty-ugly stereotype measures the degree of internalization of the prevalent standards of beauty (13 items, e.g., "Slim women are more attractive to men").

The overall score indicates the degree of dissatisfaction with one's body image. Using the overall score was supported by the scree plot on items which clearly shows a single factor that explains 32.09% of the variance of all variables while the second explains only 9.82%. A parallel analysis was run on three scales and indicates a one-factor solution (first two eigenvalues from sample correlation matrix: 2.171, 0.459; first two average eigenvalues from parallel analysis: 1.041, 1.001). Responses were given on a five-point scale from 1 (*definitely disagree*) to 5 (*definitely agree*) with the reliability for the overall score being Cronbach's alpha = 0.95, and that for the constituent subscales ranging from 0.81 to 0.95.

Measurement of ARS

ARS was measured using behavioral indicators from the questionnaire for *Testing Individual Approach to Eating* (TIAE) [4]. Five items were selected due to their specific content: (1) "I've fasted, dieted, restricted food"; (2) "I've taken purgatives"; (3) "I'm angry when I eat too much"; (4) "I've taken weight-loss drugs/appetite suppressants; (5) "I'm trying to cut down on fat and carbohydrates".

Categorical confirmatory factor analysis, in which the selected items formed a latent factor, fitted the data well: $df = 5$; $\chi^2 = 53.3$; CFI = 0.976; RMSEA = 0.079 [0.061–0.099]. Responses were given on a binary scale from 0 (*no*) to 1 (*yes*). The total score is the sum of five behavioral items selected from the categorical confirmatory factor analysis. The factor loadings of the items ranged from 0.53 to 0.86. Cronbach's alpha for the five selected items was 0.66.

Statistical analyses

There were no missing data for the self-report questionnaires because the answer to each question was required. In the first step, correlation analysis was conducted to compare associations between the studied variables: personality traits, sociocultural factors, body dissatisfaction, and ARS. Subsequently, hierarchical multiple regression was performed because we wanted to see how including subsequent variables changes the ARS prediction in the model [48]. The regression model was verified in three steps: after entering each variable, it was checked whether the percentage of explained variance increased. In this way, four variables were entered in three steps (called "blocks" in SPSS software): (1) personality traits; (2) sociocultural factors; and (3) body dissatisfaction. In each step we introduced variables assumed to be related to ARS based on theoretical reasoning and additional separate analysis. The variables had been included in this specific order based on Five-Factor Theory from basic tendencies (personality traits) by characteristic adaptations (sociocultural factors) to self-concept (body dissatisfaction) ([45], p. 192). It is especially important taking into account that personality traits are rather stable and hardly change while the other factors are much more prone to changing in the interventions.

After introducing each set of variables, it was checked whether the resulting model explained more variance and which variables were significant in predicting ARS. In particular, it was investigated whether neuroticism, which was significantly associated with body dissatisfaction, would maintain its significance after the introduction of other variables associated with body image.

Results

Descriptive statistics

Descriptive statistics for the scales used in the study are given in Table 1.

Table 2 presents descriptive statistics (*M* and *SD*), intercorrelations, and correlations between personality traits, sociocultural factors, body dissatisfaction, and ARS.

Considering the Big Five dimensions, it should be noted that neuroticism was most strongly correlated with body dissatisfaction ($r = 0.43$) and ARS ($r = 0.35$). In turn, the overall score calculated for the SATAQ-3 (STQ) was more closely associated with body dissatisfaction ($r = 0.52$) and ARS ($r = 0.57$) than any of its constituent scales, although the correlation between internalization and ARS was of a similar level ($r = 0.55$). A strong correlation was also found between ARS and body dissatisfaction ($r = 0.62$). Interestingly, there was no relationship between the Big Five openness and internalization ($r = 0.00$).

These correlations indicate that neuroticism is associated with the degree of body dissatisfaction, internalization, and ARS. In women, the tendency to adopt abnormal attitudes to eating and body image under stress was found to be strongly predicted by the degree of body dissatisfaction, and even more so by the opinions and emotions about one's appearance as well as the degree of internalization, that is, comparing oneself to and assimilating sociocultural norms concerning ideal body standards, especially those promoted by the mass media.

Regression analysis

The next step involved analysis of the hierarchical multiple regression model containing significant predictors of the dependent variable. The assumptions for the correlation and the linear regression were verified before conducting the analyses. The normal distribution has been confirmed based on values of skewness and kurtosis. Skewness and kurtosis statistics revealed that the results had a normal distribution, as they were in the standard deviation range of <– 1; + 1>. All predictor variables and the outcome variable were quantitative. The assumptions of multicollinearity (Variance inflation factor, VIF = 1.5605) and independent errors (Durbin-Watson test, DW = 1.726) were also satisfied. All the predictor variables were not correlated very highly (correlations of above 0.80 or 0.90) [48].

In order to predict ARS, four variables were introduced in three blocks: (1) personality traits, (2) sociocultural factors, and (3) body dissatisfaction. First, a linear regression analysis of personality traits showed that only neuroticism significantly predicted ARS (neuroticism: $\beta = 0.19$, $p < 0.01$; extraversion: $\beta = – 0.004$, $p > 0.01$; intellect/openness: $\beta = 0.06$, $p > 0.01$; agreeableness: $\beta = – 0.03$, $p > 0.01$; conscientiousness: $\beta = – 0.02$, $p > 0.01$). Thus, neuroticism was entered in hierarchical multiple regression analysis in the first block. The second block included two variables: internalization and pressure from sociocultural norms (sociocultural attitudes to body image) because in the separate regression, the third sociocultural factor (information seeking) was an insignificant predictor of ARS. The variable entered in the third block was body dissatisfaction, which was associated with emotions related to one's appearance. Three models with a good fit to the data were obtained, with

Table 1 Descriptive statistics of the questionnaires used in the study

		Min	Max	Mean	Standard deviation	Skewness	Kurtosis
BFI-44	Extraversion	1.13	5.00	2.93	0.78	− 0.03	− 0.63
	Agreeableness	1.00	5.00	3.46	0.59	− 0.20	0.01
	Conscientiousness	1.33	5.00	3.47	0.67	− 0.18	− 0.25
	Neuroticism	1.25	5.00	3.47	0.76	− 0.27	− 0.34
	Openness	1.40	5.00	3.71	0.63	− 0.33	− 0.09
SATAQ-3	Internalization	1.00	4.89	3.12	0.82	− 0.28	− 0.81
	Pressure from sociocultural norms	1.00	5.00	3.16	1.08	− 0.31	− 0.89
	Information seeking	1.00	5.00	2.53	0.83	0.17	− 0.47
BIQ-40	Cognition-emotions	1.00	5.00	2.80	1.04	0.17	− 1.08
	Behaviors	1.00	5.00	2.80	0.90	0.08	− 0.61
	Criticism from others	1.00	4.83	1.96	0.74	1.06	1.00
	Pretty-ugly stereotype	1.00	5.00	3.61	0.65	− 0.32	0.37
	Overall score	4.56	18.54	11.16	2.43	0.29	− 0.27
TIAE	ARS	0.00	1.00	0.46	0.19	0.15	− 0.51

analysis of variance being statistically significant for each of them (Table 3).

Model 1 with one predictor (neuroticism) explained as little as 4% of the variance in ARS. Model 2 with three predictors (neuroticism, internalization, and pressure from sociocultural norms) explained 19% of the variance.

Finally, Model 3, containing four predictors (neuroticism, internalization, pressure from sociocultural norms, and body dissatisfaction), explained 27% of the variance (Table 4).

As can be seen, Model 3 with four predictors explained the largest percentage of the variance. It is worth

Table 2 Descriptive statistics, intercorrelations, and correlations between the scales

	BFI-44					SATAQ-3				BIQ-40					TIAE
	E	A	C	N	O	IN	PSN	IS	STQ	BD	C-E	BEH	CRI	P-U	ARS
E	−														
A	0.25**	−													
C	0.16**	0.18**	−												
N	− 0.37**	− 0.32**	− 0.29**	−											
O	0.31**	0.14**	0.16**	− 0.12**	−										
IN	− 0.11**	− 0.10**	− 0.18**	0.29**	0.00	−									
PSN	− 0.09**	− 0.07**	− 0.13**	0.28**	− 0.04	0.60**	−								
IS	− 0.04	− 0.05	− 0.07**	0.17**	− 0.07*	0.61**	0.54**	−							
STQ	− 0.10**	− 0.09**	− 0.15**	0.29**	− 0.04	0.85**	0.87**	0.83**	−						
BID	− 0.28**	− 0.18**	− 0.31**	0.43**	− 0.17**	0.48**	0.50**	0.33**	0.52**	−					
C-E	− 0.16**	− 0.10**	− 0.20**	0.35**	− 0.08**	0.52**	0.55**	0.33**	0.55**	0.87**	−				
BEH	− 0.29**	− 0.15**	− 0.31**	0.27**	− 0.25**	0.12**	0.14**	0.07**	0.14**	0.60**	0.27**	−			
CRI	− 0.23**	− 0.16**	− 0.23**	0.35**	− 0.12**	0.29**	0.27**	0.21**	0.30**	0.74**	0.58**	0.25**	−		
P-U	− 0.11**	− 0.14**	− 0.13**	0.27**	− 0.02	0.46**	0.49**	0.37**	0.52**	0.68**	0.60**	0.12**	0.35**	−	
ARS	− 0.15**	− 0.16**	− 0.12**	0.35**	0.03	0.55**	0.50**	0.41**	0.57**	0.62**	0.72**	0.04	0.46**	0.58**	−
M	2.93	3.46	3.47	3.47	3.71	3.12	3.16	2.53	8.81	11.16	2.80	2.80	1.96	3.61	0.46
SD	0.78	0.59	0.67	0.76	0.63	0.82	1.08	0.83	2.32	2.43	1.04	0.90	0.74	0.65	0.19

Notes: **statistical significance at $p < 0.01$; * statistical significance at $p < 0.05$; $n = 1533$
BFI-44: *E* Extraversion, *A* Agreeableness, *C* Conscientiousness, *N* Neuroticism, *O* Openness; SATAQ-3: *IN* Internalization, *PSN* Pressure from sociocultural norms, *IS* Information seeking, *STQ* overall SATAQ-3 score; BIQ-40: *BD* Body dissatisfaction, overall score, *C-E* cognition-emotion, *BEH* behavior, *CRI* criticism from others, *P-U* pretty-ugly stereotype; TIAE: *ARS* anorexia readiness syndrome, *M* mean, *SD* standard deviation

Table 3 Summary of hierarchical multiple regression analysis

Model	Corrected R^2	Standard error	R^2 change	F	df1	df2	Significance
1	0.04	1.38	0.04	61.86	1	1531	0.000
2	0.19	1.27	0.15	143.47	2	1529	0.000
3	0.27	1.20	0.08	168.41	1	1528	0.000

Notes: Model 1: neuroticism; Model 2: internalization, pressure from sociocultural norms; Model 3: body dissatisfaction

noting that after the introduction of the variable "body dissatisfaction" neuroticism lost statistical significance: $\beta = -0.03$; $p > 0.01$.

As far as the research question is concerned, analysis showed that the only personality trait significant to body image, i.e., neuroticism was not retained in the hierarchical multiple regression model after entering other variables, equally relevant to body image. Thus, the final set of predictors significantly explaining ARS comprised internalization, pressure from sociocultural norms, and body dissatisfaction.

Discussion

The obtained results confirmed the adopted hypotheses about correlations between the Big Five factors, internationalization, pressure from sociocultural norms, body dissatisfaction, and ARS. Hierarchical multiple regression analysis revealed three variables that significantly predicted ARS, i.e., internalization, pressure from sociocultural norms, and body dissatisfaction.

Among the Big Five factors, only neuroticism exhibited the highest significant correlation with body dissatisfaction, which is consistent with the findings of Swami et al. [15], where neuroticism was significantly positively associated with body image in women (the higher scores on the scale indicate greater actual-ideal weight discrepancy) and significantly negatively associated with body appreciation (the higher scores on the scale reflect more positive body appreciation). In the study on male subjects, Benford and Swami [49] found a positive

correlation between neuroticism and drive for muscularity; while body appreciation was negatively related to neuroticism and positively to extraversion.

The presented study also analyzed sociocultural factors using the SATAQ-3. It was found that the higher the degree of internalization, the higher the extent of anorectic behaviors. A similar correlation, albeit somewhat weaker, was obtained for pressure from sociocultural norms. Thus, internalization was shown to be a significant predictor of ARS. Internalizing the beauty standards promoted by the mass media, women engage in behaviors aimed at attaining the ideal, such as the tendency to give in to mass culture, excessive concentration on the body image, comparing oneself to paragons of beauty, and emotional lability related to body image. However, when such behaviors intensify, women do not necessarily come closer to the ideal, but rather expose themselves to the risk of eating disorders (cf. [4]), which may be associated with sociocultural factors, as indicated by Murnen i Smolak [31] in a meta-analysis or relations between distorted body image and disordered eating. Anorectic behaviors may be also affected by one's opinion of, and emotions elicited by, one's appearance, as well as general body dissatisfaction, as shown by the high correlation identified in this study.

Hierarchical multiple regression analysis revealed three variables that significantly predicted ARS, i.e., internalization, pressure from sociocultural norms, and body dissatisfaction. Initially, the model also included neuroticism, but in the third step, after entering body dissatisfaction,

Table 4 Regression coefficients in the hierarchical multiple regression model

Model		b	Standard error	Beta	t	Significance
1	Constant	0.40	0.17	–	2.40	0.02
	Neuroticism	0.37	0.05	0.20	7.87	0.00
2	Constant	– 0.92	0.17	–	– 5.32	0.00
	Neuroticism	0.12	0.05	0.07	2.75	0.01
	Internalization	0.38	0.05	0.22	7.58	0.00
	Pressure from sociocultural norms	0.31	0.04	0.24	8.20	0.00
3	Constant	– 1.74	0.18	–	– 9.84	0.00
	Neuroticism	– 0.06	0.05	– 0.03	– 1.38	0.17
	Internalization	0.24	0.05	0.14	5.00	0.00
	Pressure from sociocultural norms	0.17	0.04	0.13	4.67	0.00
	Body dissatisfaction	0.21	0.01	0.36	13.00	0.00

neuroticism lost its statistical significance despite it being correlated with body dissatisfaction. In a similar study, Swami et al. [13] found that body dissatisfaction was significantly negatively correlated with extraversion, emotional stability, and openness, but regression analysis showed that the Big Five dimensions explained only a small proportion of the variance in body dissatisfaction. The authors suggested that the internalization of media influence may be the dominant predictor of body dissatisfaction, even more so than personality traits. Swami et al. [13] also showed that openness was not significantly associated with internalization-general (– 0.08), as in this article (0.00). Openness, as a personality trait, describes ideas, creativity, curiosity, and aesthetics [45]. Internalization is assimilating sociocultural norms (concerning attractive body image standards) [25], which is rarely considered as openness and following ideas, but rather as a demand associated with the achievement of certain aims (attractive body image). In psychopathology, internalizing disorders have been predicted by neuroticism and low conscientiousness [10]. Martin et al. [50] also reported that body dissatisfaction was significantly associated with neuroticism and with thin-ideal internalization (internalization of societal ideals of attractiveness). In turn, Reshadat et al. [51], who explored the relationship between personality traits and self-efficacy in weight control with unhealthy eating behaviors and attitudes, reported a significant negative correlation between such behaviors and neuroticism and psychoticism. As a result, neuroticism and psychoticism may be used to predict unhealthy eating behaviors. Finally, in the mentioned study of MacNeill et al. [12] disordered eating patterns were predicted by high neuroticism and extraversion as well as low conscientiousness in women, but not in men. Body image dissatisfaction was predicted by neuroticism in women and by neuroticism and low conscientiousness in men. The significant predictor of body image dissatisfaction was also BMI in both groups [12]. Those findings were partially confirmed in the present study, albeit only with neuroticism in models no. 1 and 2, which contained neuroticism, but not in model 3, from which that trait was eliminated. Thus, it should be considered whether the role of the general neurotic tendency is not in fact overestimated. According to model no. 3, internalization, pressure from sociocultural norms, and body dissatisfaction have greater explanatory power for ARS. Under the circumstances, neuroticism in particular and personality, in general, are no longer significantly associated with body image perceptions.

Limitations

The main limitations of the study are: (1) the focus on only women; (2) a cross-sectional design; (3) one country study. Future studies need some extensions to overcome these limitations. Future research could include not only women but also men. The study could be conducted on healthy people and patients diagnosed with eating disorders. A cross-cultural study could also provide substantial relations between personality, social factors, and body dissatisfaction in different groups. Future research could also include longitudinal studies and its results could verify the preventive and screening role of ARS.

Conclusions

The study examined the importance of personality traits, sociocultural attitudes, and body dissatisfaction on ARS in women. The factors most closely associated with ARS were (1) neuroticism among personality traits, (2) internalization and pressure from sociocultural norms among sociocultural factors, and (3) body dissatisfaction. The key finding is the absence of statistical significance for neuroticism in predicting ARS, even though that trait was strongly correlated with body image. The significant variables predicting ARS were internalization, pressure from sociocultural norms, and body dissatisfaction.

Implications

The knowledge of the predictors of ARS can be useful for the prevention of anorexia nervosa. The results in this article emphasize the important role of internalization and pressure from sociocultural norms and body dissatisfaction in the prediction of ARS. Neuroticism lost its role in predicting ARS after introducing these factors and this can be seen as an outcome that makes the prevention possible. Neuroticism is a stable, consistent, and enduring personality characteristic, determined biologically and therefore not changeable while sociocultural factors and body dissatisfaction could be changed. Thus, decreasing neuroticism in prevention or intervention can be impossible but increasing internalization and pressure from sociocultural norms or body dissatisfaction can be feasible. If those results will be confirmed in subsequent studies, anorexic behaviors (ARS symptoms) can be screened and preventively assessed in order to counteract the development of anorexia nervosa in the long term by focusing on changing these factors.

Abbreviations

ARS: Anorexia readiness syndrome; BFI: Big Five Inventory; BMI: Body Mass Index; BIQ-40: Body Image Questionnaire; SATAQ-3: Sociocultural Attitudes Towards Appearance Questionnaire-3; TIAE: Testing Individual Approach to Eating

Acknowledgements

The author would like to thank Professor Jan Cieciuch for the inspiration for writing this article, his valuable comments and remarks in refining the text and statistical support.

Author's contributions

The author(s) read and approved the final manuscript.

Declarations

Ethics approval and consent to participate
All procedures performed in studies involving human participants were in accordance with the ethical standards of the institutional and/or national research committee and with the 1964 Helsinki declaration and its later amendments or comparable ethical standards. Written informed consent for participation was not required for this study in accordance with the national legislation and the institutional requirements.

Competing interests
The author declare that the research was conducted in the absence of any commercial or financial relationships that could be construed as a potential conflict of interest.

References

1. Izydorczyk B, Rybicka-Klimczyk A. Środki masowego przekazu i ich rola w kształtowaniu wizerunku ciała u zróżnicowanych wiekiem życia kobiet polskich (analiza badań własnych) [Mass media and its influence on body image development among Polish women in different age (authors' own research)]. Probl Med Rodz. 2009;11:20–32.
2. Brytek-Matera A, Rybicka-Klimczyk A. Ocena nasilenia objawów syndromu gotowości anorektycznej u młodych kobiet - badania pilotażowe [assessment of anorexia readiness syndrome escalating symptoms in young women – a pilot study]. Stud Psychol UKSW. 2012;12:23–36.
3. Brytek-Matera A, Rybicka-Klimczyk A. Evaluation of body image among females with anorexia readiness syndrome. Arch Psychiatry Psychother. 2011;3:11–9.
4. Ziółkowska B. Uwarunkowania ekspresji syndromu gotowości anorektycznej [determinants of anorexia readiness Syndrom (ARS) expression]. Sborník Pr Filoz Fak Brněnské Univ Ann Psychol. 2000;48:35–55.
5. Chytra-Gędek W, Kobierecka A. Gotowość anorektyczna u dziewcząt i młodych kobiet [Anorexic readiness in girls and young women]. Psychiatria. 2008;5:7–12.
6. Pilecki MW, Salapa K, Józefik B. Socio-cultural context of eating disorders in Poland. J Eat Disord. 2016;4. https://doi.org/10.1186/s40337-016-0093-3(1):11.
7. Farstad SM, McGeown LM, von Ranson KM. Eating disorders and personality, 2004-2016: a systematic review and meta-analysis. Clin Psychol Rev. 2016;46: 91–105 https://doi.org/10.1016/j.cpr.2016.04.005.
8. Hartmann C, Siegrist M. A longitudinal study of the relationships between the big five personality traits and body size perception. Body Image. 2015; 14:67–71 https://doi.org/10.1016/j.bodyim.2015.03.011.
9. Costa PT Jr, McCrae RR. Revised NEO personality inventory (NEO–PI–R) and NEO five-factor inventory (NEO–FFI) professional manual. Odessa: Psychological Assessment Resources; 1992.
10. John OP, Srivastava S, John OP. The big-five trait taxonomy: history, measurement, and theoretical perspectives. In: Pervin LA, John OP, editors. Handb personal theory res. New York: Guilford Press; 1999. p. 102–38.
11. Strus W, Cieciuch J. Poza Wielką Piątkę - przegląd nowych modeli struktury osobowości [beyond the big five – review of new models of personality structure]. Pol Forum Psychol. 2014;19:17–49 https://doi.org/10.14656/PFP2 0140102.
12. MacNeill LP, Best LA, Davis LL. The role of personality in body image dissatisfaction and disordered eating: discrepancies between men and women. J Eat Disord. 2017;5. https://doi.org/10.1186/s40337-017-0177-8(1):44.
13. Swami V, Taylor R, Carvalho C. Body dissatisfaction assessed by the photographic figure rating scale is associated with sociocultural, personality, and media influences. Scand J Psychol. 2011;52(1):57–63. https://doi.org/1 0.1111/j.1467-9450.2010.00836.x.
14. da Silva Mendes JC, Figueiras MJ, Moss T. Influence of personality traits in self-evaluative salience, motivational salience and self-consciousness of appearance. Psychol Community Heal. 2016;5(2):187–97. https://doi.org/10. 5964/pch.v5i2.168.
15. Swami V, Tran US, Brooks LH, Kanaan L, Luesse EM, Nader IW, et al. Body image and personality: associations between the big five personality factors, actual-ideal weight discrepancy, and body appreciation. Scand J Psychol. 2013;54(2):146–51. https://doi.org/10.1111/sjop.12014.
16. Wasylkiw L, Fabrigar LR, Rainboth S, Reid A, Steen C. Neuroticism and the architecture of the self: exploring neuroticism as a moderator of the impact of ideal self-discrepancies on emotion. J Pers. 2010;78(2):471–92. https://doi.org/10.1111/j.1467-6494.2010.00623.x.
17. Gual P, Pérez-Gaspar M, Martínez-González MA, Lahortiga F, de Irala-Estévez J, Cervera-Enguix S. Self-esteem, personality, and eating disorders: baseline assessment of prospective population-based cohort. Int J Eat Disord. 2002; 31(3):261–73. https://doi.org/10.1002/eat.10040.
18. Miller JL, Schmidt LA, Vaillancourt T, McDougall P, Laliberte M. Neuroticism and introversion: a risky combination for disordered eating among a non-clinical sample of undergraduate women. Eat Behav. 2006;7(1):69–78. https://doi.org/10.1016/j.eatbeh.2005.07.003.
19. Cafri G, Yamamiya Y, Brannick M, Thompson JK. The influence of sociocultural factors on body image: a meta-analysis. Clin Psychol Sci Pract. 2005;12(4):421–33. https://doi.org/10.1093/clipsy/bpi053.
20. Amianto F, Martini M, Spalatro A, Abbate Daga G, Fassino S. Body image development within the family: attachment dynamics and parental attitudes in cross-sectional and longitudinal studies. Acta Psychopathol. 2017;3 https://doi.org/10.4172/2469-6676.100122.
21. Kluck AS. Family influence on disordered eating: the role of body image dissatisfaction. Body Image. 2010;7(1):8–14. https://doi.org/10.1016/j.bodyim.2009.09.009.
22. Ata RN, Ludden AB, Lally MM. The effects of gender and family, friend, and media influences on eating behaviors and body image during adolescence. J Youth Adolesc. 2007;36(8):1024–37. https://doi.org/10.1007/s10964-006-9159-x.
23. Hutchinson DM, Rapee RM. Do friends share similar body image and eating problems? The role of social networks and peer influences in early adolescence. Behav Res Ther. 2007;45(7):1557–77. https://doi.org/10.1016/j.brat.2006.11.007.
24. Markey CN. Culture and the development of eating disorders: a tripartite model. J Treat Prev. 2004;12(2):139–56. https://doi.org/10.1080/106402604 90445041.
25. Thompson JK, Van Den Berg P, Roehrig M, Guarda AS, Heinberg LJ. The sociocultural attitudes towards appearance Scale-3 (SATAQ-3): development and validation. Int J Eat Disord. 2004;35(3):293–304. https://doi.org/10.1002/eat.10257.
26. Izydorczyk B. Postawy i zachowania wobec własnego ciała w zaburzeniach odżywiania [attitudes and behaviors towards one's own body in eating disorders]. Warszawa: Wydawnictwo Naukowe PWN; 2014.
27. Izydorczyk B, Rybicka-Klimczyk A. Poznawcze aspekty obrazu ciała u kobiet a zaburzenia odżywiania [cognitive aspects of women's body image and eating disorders]. Endokrynol Pol. 2009;60(4):287–94.
28. Fredrickson BL, Roberts TA. Objectification theory: toward understanding Women's lived experiences and mental health risks. Psychol Women Q. 1997;21(2):173–206. https://doi.org/10.1111/j.1471-6402.1997.tb00108.x.
29. Młoźniak E, Schier K. The body as an object - a sociocultural perspective: the study of young adults' narratives. Sociol Res Online. 2016;21. https://doi.org/10.5153/sro.3865(1):17–34.
30. Loeber S, Burgmer R, Wyssen A, Leins J, Rustemeier M, Munsch S, et al. Short-term effects of media exposure to the thin ideal in female inpatients with an eating disorder compared to female inpatients with a mood or anxiety disorder or women with no psychiatric disorder. Int J Eat Disord. 2016;49(7):708–15. https://doi.org/10.1002/eat.22524.
31. Murnen SK, Smolak L. The cash effect: shaping the research conversation on body image and eating disorders. Body Image. 2019;31:288–93 https://doi.org/10.1016/j.bodyim.2019.01.001.
32. Suisman JL, Thompson JK, Keel PK, Burt SA, Neale M, Boker S, et al. Genetic and environmental influences on thin-ideal internalization across puberty and preadolescent, adolescent, and young adult development. Int J Eat Disord. 2014;47(7):773–83. https://doi.org/10.1002/eat.22321.
33. Thompson JK. Introduction: body image, eating disorders, and obesity-an emerging synthesis. In: Thompson JK, editor. Body image, Eat Disord Obes

An Integr Guid Assess Treat: American Psychological Association; 2001. p. 1–20. https://doi.org/10.1037/10502-001.

34. Izydorczyk B, Rybicka-Klimczyk A. Diagnoza psychologiczna poznawczych i emocjonalnych aspektów obrazu ciała u dziewcząt i młodych kobiet polskich [psychological diagnosis of cognitive and emotional aspects of body image in polish adolescents and young women]. Probl Med Rodz. 2008;10:24–35.

35. Perloff RM. Social media effects on young Women's body image concerns: theoretical perspectives and an agenda for research. Sex Roles. 2014;71(11-12):363–77. https://doi.org/10.1007/s11199-014-0384-6.

36. Rasińska R, Nowakowska I, Głowacka-Rębała A. Postrzeganie własnego ciała przez młodzież akademicką [Students' perception of their own body]. Zdr i Dobrostan. 2013;3:113–24.

37. Dakanalis A, Gaudio S, Serino S, Clerici M, Carrà G, Riva G. Body-image distortion in anorexia nervosa. Nat Rev Dis Prim. 2016;2 https://doi.org/10.1038/nrdp.2016.26.

38. Bąk W. E. Tory Higginsa teoria rozbieżności ja [E. tory Higgins's theory of the "self" descrepancy]. Przegląd Psychol. 2002;45:39–55.

39. Głębocka A. Niezadowolenie z wyglądu a rozpaczliwa kontrola wagi [dissatisfaction with appearance and desperate weight control]. Kraków: IMPULS; 2009.

40. Thompson JK. Assessing body image disturbance: measures, methodology, and implementation. In: Thompson JK, editor. Body image, Eat Disord Obes An Integr Guid Assess Treat: Am Psychol Assoc; 2001. p. 49–81. https://doi.org/10.1037/10502-003.

41. Femiak J, Rymarczyk P. Ciało jako temat narracji kultury masowej i narracji wewnętrznej [body as a theme of mass culture narration and internal narration]. Rozpr Nauk Akad Wych Fiz we Wrocławiu. 2015;9:28–33.

42. Romanowska-Tołłoczko A. Wizerunek kobiety w reklamie a percepcja i ocena własnego wyglądu przez dorastające dziewczęta [an effect of women's image in advertising on self-esteem and perception of appearance amongst adolescent girls]. Rozpr Nauk Akad Wych Fiz we Wrocławiu. 2015;49:34–41.

43. Rzeszutek M, Schier K. Tak bolesne, że aż obce? - Związek pomiędzy depresją a obrazem ciała u młodych dorosłych [so painful, that alien? – the link between depresssion and body image in young adults]. Psychoterapia. 2008;4:5–16.

44. Hagman J, Gardner RM, Brown DL, Gralla J, Fier JM, Frank GK. Body size overestimation and its association with body mass index, body dissatisfaction, and drive for thinness in anorexia nervosa. Eat Weight Disord Stud Anorexia Bulim Obes. 2015;20(4):449–55. https://doi.org/10.1007/s40519-015-0193-0.

45. McCrae RR, Costa PT Jr. Personality in adulthood: a five-factor theory perspective. 2nd ed. New York: Guilford Press; 2003. https://doi.org/10.4324/9780203428412.

46. Myers PN, Biocca FA. The elastic body image: the effect of television advertising and programming on body image distortions in young women. J Commun. 1992;42(3):108–33. https://doi.org/10.1111/j.1460-2466.1992.tb00802.x.

47. Swami V, Frederick DA, Aavik T, Alcalay L, Allik J, Anderson D, et al. The attractive female body weight and female body dissatisfaction in 26 countries across 10 world regions: results of the international body project I. Personal Soc Psychol Bull. 2010;36(3):309–25. https://doi.org/10.1177/0146167209359702.

48. Field A. Discovering statistics using SPSS. Los Angeles: SAGE Publications; 2009.

49. Benford K, Swami V. Body image and personality among British men: associations between the big five personality domains, drive for muscularity, and body appreciation. Body Image. 2014;11(4):454–7. https://doi.org/10.1016/j.bodyim.2014.07.004.

50. Martin SJ, Racine SE. Personality traits and appearance-ideal internalization: differential associations with body dissatisfaction and compulsive exercise. Eat Behav. 2017;27:39–44 https://doi.org/10.1016/j.eatbeh.2017.11.001.

51. Reshadat S, Zakiei A, Hatamin P, Bagheri A, Rostami S, Komasi S. A study of the correlation of personality traits (neuroticism and psychoticism) and self-efficacy in weight control with unhealthy eating behaviors and attitudes. Ann Med Health Sci Res. 2017;7:32–8.

19

Efficacy of Post-inpatient Aftercare Treatments for Anorexia Nervosa

Katrin E. Giel[1,2]*[iD], Simone C. Behrens[1,2], Kathrin Schag[1,2], Peter Martus[3], Stephan Herpertz[4], Tobias Hofmann[5], Eva-Maria Skoda[6], Ulrich Voderholzer[7,8,9], Jörn von Wietersheim[10], Beate Wild[11], Almut Zeeck[12], Ulrike Schmidt[13], Stephan Zipfel[1,2] and Florian Junne[1,2,14]

Abstract

Background: Early relapse after inpatient treatment is a serious problem in the management of anorexia nervosa (AN). Specialized aftercare interventions have the potential to bridge the gap between inpatient and outpatient care, to prevent relapse and to improve the long-term outcome for patients with AN.

Methods: Following the guidelines of the PRISMA statement, we conducted a systematic review, synthesizing the evidence from randomized-controlled trials (RCTs) investigating the efficacy of post-inpatient aftercare treatments for AN.

Results: Our search resulted in seven RCTs and three registered ongoing trials. Pharmacotherapy and low-threshold guided self-help have limited uptake and high dropout. Novel mobile guided self-help approaches seem promising due to high patient satisfaction, but their efficacy has yet to be investigated in larger trials. Cognitive-behavior psychotherapy may be beneficial in delaying relapse, but evidence is based on a single study.

Conclusion: Only a limited number of RCTs investigating aftercare interventions for patients with AN is available. There is no clear evidence favoring any one specific approach for post-inpatient aftercare in adult patients with AN. The field faces many challenges which generally affect intervention research in AN. A specific issue is how to increase uptake of and reduce dropout from aftercare interventions. This calls for better tailoring of interventions to patient needs and the integration of patient perspectives into treatment. Intensified research and care efforts are needed to address the problem of recurrent relapse after intensive inpatient treatment for AN and to eventually improve prognosis for this eating disorder.

Plain English summary

Patients with a severe form of anorexia nervosa (AN) are often treated as inpatients. Many of them benefit from this acute treatment. Unfortunately, a significant number of patients experience relapse after discharge. This problem could be addressed by specific treatments directly following inpatient therapy, so called aftercare interventions, which are tailored to patients' needs in this treatment period. This review looks at studies which have investigated

---

*Correspondence: katrin.giel@med.uni-tuebingen.de
[1] Department of Psychosomatic Medicine and Psychotherapy, Medical University Hospital Tübingen, Eberhard Karls University, Osianderstr. 5, 72076 Tübingen, Germany
Full list of author information is available at the end of the article

the efficacy of aftercare interventions for patients with AN directly after inpatient treatment. We included any studies which compared a novel aftercare intervention to a control treatment and where patients were randomly assigned to either of these treatments, as this procedure is considered to reduce bias. We found seven studies that investigated different aftercare intervention approaches, including medication, guided self-help and psychotherapy, and three ongoing studies. Based on the very limited evidence so far, no clear recommendations can be made favoring a specific approach for post-inpatient aftercare in adult patients with AN. The review shows that it should be a priority to increase uptake of aftercare interventions and to reduce dropout rates. This could be achieved by a better tailoring of interventions to patient needs and the integration of patient perspectives in intervention design. More studies are needed to find interventions which allow patients with AN to maintain treatment gains after intensive inpatient treatment.

Keywords: Aftercare, Anorexia nervosa, Eating disorder, Efficacy, Randomized-controlled trials, Relapse, Treatment, Therapy

Introduction

Anorexia nervosa (AN) is a severe mental disorder which often has a long-lasting and fluctuating course [1]. Up to 70% of patients with a severe course do not overcome the eating disorder (ED) in the long-term, and around 5% of patients die in long-term observation periods, yielding the highest mortality rate among all mental disorders [2–4]. A specific challenge in AN treatment, affecting all treatment settings and stages, is treatment adherence, with treatment discontinuation rates as high as 30–40% [5, 6]. To a certain extent this might reflect the ambivalence many patients experience towards weight gain and recovery [1, 7].

International treatment guidelines for EDs concur in their recommendation that psychotherapy is the first-line treatment for patients with AN, preferably in outpatient settings [8, 9]. There is currently no empirical evidence for the superiority of one specific psychotherapy approach in the treatment of adults with AN [8, 10]. For severely affected patients it is recommended that they are treated in specialized inpatient or day-hospital settings [8, 9]. However, these intensive acute treatments are not thought to replace outpatient therapy, but rather to enable it. Treasure et al. [11], concluded that continuous care which is matched to the stage of the illness may improve treatment outcomes. In line with this idea, treatment guidelines and recent suggestions for optimizing care pathways highlight the need for attending to the transition between different treatment settings in AN care [8, 12]. Related to this, the importance of ensuring post-inpatient care to prevent relapse and re-hospitalization has also been highlighted [12–14].

Regarding the implementation of these recommendations, evidence shows that inpatient treatment for AN is effective for many severely ill patients as they achieve weight gain and improvements in ED symptoms at least in the short-term [6, 10, 15]. Unfortunately, a considerable proportion of patients with AN experience deterioration or relapse in the first months after termination of inpatient treatment [16, 17]. This contributes to the unfavorable prognosis of AN [18] and also indicates that the post-discharge stage and transition from acute inpatient treatment to less intensive settings is a critical phase of transition which is currently not sufficiently addressed and managed in AN care. Accordingly, recent reviews and treatment guidelines point out that discharge from inpatient treatment often results in discontinuity of care and so far, empirical evidence about how to link intensive treatments with outpatient psychotherapy is scarce [1, 10, 13, 14, 17].

In addition to ensuring continuity of care, a post-inpatient intervention should ideally entail an approach that is tailored to the patient's illness stage and needs, i.e. provide a specialized maintenance or aftercare treatment [13, 16]. Typical components of interventions focusing on maintenance and relapse prevention comprise an assessment of the stage of illness and symptom profile, recovery and relapse history, psychoeducation on relapse processes, strengthening treatment motivation, identification and monitoring of high-risk situations for relapse, identification of coping strategies to prevent and manage relapse as well as strengthening of individual resources [19]. These key components of maintenance treatment have been most widely implemented and researched in the context of addictive behaviors [19]. However, they might also be effective in relation to the maintenance of behaviour change in other mental disorders, but with disorder-specific adaptations, i.e. to target maintenance mechanisms which have been identified for the specific core symptoms of the disorder in question. This could generally be achieved by a range of approaches, including pharmacological interventions.

As mentioned above, guidelines suggest that there is currently not enough evidence regarding which types of interventions can reduce the risk of relapse after successful inpatient treatment of AN [13]. Two further aspects might add to the difficulties of developing and investigating aftercare interventions in AN: Many adult patients with AN do not leave specialized inpatient or day-hospital treatment in a weight-recovered or fully remitted state, but are still underweight and at least partially fulfill diagnostic criteria for AN or another ED at the point of discharge [6]. This situation poses specific challenges for the treatment goals and components of effective aftercare, in terms of balancing a focus on maintaining gains achieved during inpatient care versus initiating further improvement and weight gain. When it comes to evaluating outcomes and efficacy of any aftercare interventions, a further challenge is the lack of any consensus definitions of relapse or recovery in AN [17, 20].

To summarize, early relapse after inpatient treatment is a common and serious problem in the management of adult patients with AN [16, 17] which contributes to the often lengthy course of this ED [18]. There are challenges in the development and evaluation of specialized, targeted aftercare interventions for AN. In order to summarize existing knowledge on which treatments might help patients with AN to maintain benefits after inpatient or day-hospital treatment, we conducted a systematic review synthesizing current evidence from randomized controlled treatment trials (RCTs). We decided to include only studies with a RCT design as this is considered the gold standard for efficacy research. The present review complements recent reviews which focused on identifying established core strategies of existing and emerging treatments for acute AN [21, 22], but did not focus on the transition between different treatment settings.

The aims of this systematic review are (1) to identify aftercare treatments following inpatient or day-hospital treatment for patients with AN, (2) to analyze their efficacy and (3) to explore how recovery processes and outcomes are operationalized in the different studies.

Method

A systematic literature research was performed following the PRISMA guidelines [23].

Search strategy

PubMed, PsychInfo, and Web of Science were searched for combinations including "eating disorders or anorexia nervosa", "relapse or maintenance" and "therapy, intervention, treatment or program". We did not use any limits in our search. We further searched the International Clinical Trials Registry Platform (ICTRP), German Clinical Trials Register (DRKS), ISRCTN registry, Clinicaltrials.gov and the Cochrane Controlled Trial Register for completed and ongoing trials. Search results were included into the analyses until 31.12.2020.

Eligibility criteria

After duplicates were removed, all records were screened and two raters (KEG and SCB) independently evaluated eligibility of the remaining studies. Disagreement was resolved through discussion and by integrating a further rater. Eligibility criteria were based on the PICOS taxonomy (participants, intervention, comparator, outcome, study design) according to the PRISMA statement [23]. Studies were considered eligible for the review if they met the following criteria:

(1) *Participants*: Examination of adult patients who had been diagnosed with AN or atypical AN at admission to acute treatment (inpatient / day-hospital treatment); (2) *Intervention*: treatment delivered after inpatient or day-hospital treatment and aiming at maintenance or the prevention of relapse; (3) *Comparator*: control group receiving either no treatment or treatment-as-usual (TAU); (4) *Outcome*: any measure indicative of AN psychopathology, e.g. Body Mass Index (BMI), Eating Disorder Examination (EDE) scores, percentage of relapse; (5) *Study design*: randomized controlled trial.

Case reports, narrative opinions or mere program descriptions were excluded as well as publications which did not undergo peer review.

Risk of bias assessment

Following the Cochrane Handbook for Systematic Reviews of Interventions [24], we used the RoB 2 tool (https://doi.org/10.1136/bmj.l4898) to assess risk of bias for the primary outcomes of the included studies. Risk of bias assessment was performed by one rater (SCB). The RoB 2 tool assesses risk of bias in five domains (randomization process, deviations from intended interventions, missing outcome data, measurement of the outcome and selection of the reported result). The tool defines an algorithm to categorize risk of bias for each domain as well as the overall study in "low", "some concerns" and "high".

Results
Study selection

Our systematic database search yielded 4822 results of published studies (see Fig. 1). After the screening process, 29 articles were included into the full-text assessment for eligibility. Of the 29 full-texts, 22 publications did not fulfill one or more of the inclusion criteria, leading to seven publications which were finally included into the in-depth analyses and summary. Agreement between raters was 87%. All included studies reported on aftercare interventions for adult patients with AN, while two trials reported data from mixed samples which also included adolescent patients [25, 26]. All included RCTs had a two-arm design. A total of 543 patients were included in

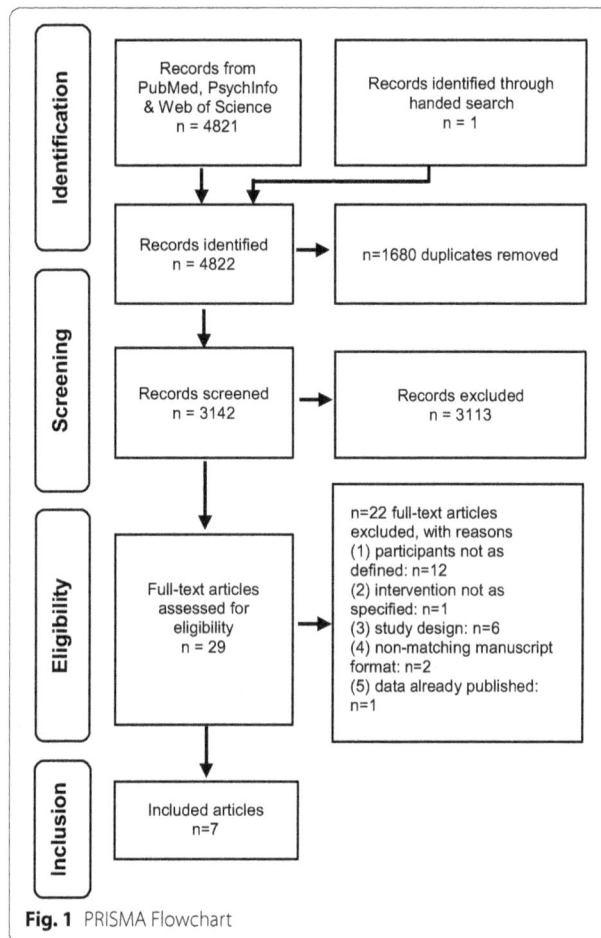

Fig. 1 PRISMA Flowchart

these RCTs. Different interventions were used, including pharmacological agents, guided self-help approaches and psychotherapy. Table 1 gives an overview on core aspects and outcomes of each trial. As Table 2 shows, risk of bias within or across studies was moderate with the exception of one study with high risk of bias which was predominantly due to high dropout rates [27]. The calculated effect sizes for the trials ranged between -0.024 and 1.0 (Table 3). Additionally, our search on trial registration platforms yielded three ongoing registered RCTs [28–30].

RCTs reporting on pharmacological interventions

Two studies investigated the efficacy of fluoxetine versus placebo administration over one year following inpatient treatment for AN to prevent relapse [31, 32]. The rationale for testing pharmacological agents for relapse prevention in AN was that pharmacotherapy, which is largely ineffective in the treatment of acute AN [31–33], might unfold its effects in weight-restored patients [31], and that it might contribute to recovery by targeting common comorbidities such as depression [32].

In one of these trials [31], patients had to be weight restored at trial entry (minimum BMI of 19 kg/m^2) and fluoxetine intake was adjunctive to individual cognitive-behavioral therapy (CBT) [34]. In the other trial, only patients suffering from the restrictive subtype of AN were included and an adjunctive outpatient psychotherapy was optional and taken up by some trial participants [32].

One of the trials determined *prevention of relapse* as primary outcome [32], and relapse was defined as dropout from the trial. Trial participation was terminated based on patient, physician or carer evaluation in case of a deteriorating clinical course of a patient, e.g. in terms of severe weight loss or severe ED symptom reoccurrence [32]. The second trial chose *time to relapse* as primary outcome [31], and relapse was defined based on several criteria reflecting severe deterioration of AN symptoms or comorbidities (see Table 1). In case of a relapse, trial participation was terminated [31].

The earlier and smaller trial reports limited intervention uptake with one third of eligible patients agreeing to participate, and a substantial dropout from the trial, especially in the placebo condition with only three out of 19 patients completing the study [32]. In contrast, 63% of participants of the fluoxetine arm remained in the study. This was a significant difference compared to the placebo condition, which was interpreted as reduced relapse rates in patients receiving fluoxetine. The second, larger trial reported that 20% of eligible patients had no interest in trial participation and that 57% of trial participants terminated the trial prematurely [31], with similar dropout rates in both arms. There was no significant group difference in time to relapse in this trial, indicating that fluoxetine had no benefit as a post-inpatient aftercare treatment for patients with AN [31].

RCTs reporting on guided self-help interventions

Three trials investigated the efficacy of digital guided self-help interventions versus TAU following inpatient treatment for AN to prevent relapse [25, 26, 35]. The rationale for using digital treatment approaches in the aftercare for AN was to exploit the potential of these low-threshold interventions for patients living in a large catchment area and to make evidence-based treatments more available [35].

In one of these trials, patients were offered to participate in an internet-based program which involved nine modules of online self-help content together with monthly therapist-guided chats with other participants as well as email contact with therapists over nine months [35]. The self-help modules were based on principles of CBT and covered topics such as motivation and goal-setting, body acceptance, coping with ED symptoms and depression, emotion regulation,

Table 1 Overview on main characteristics and findings of RCTs investigating the efficacy of post-inpatient aftercare interventions for anorexia nervosa

Study	Aftercare intervention	Comparator	Adjunctive treatment	Duration	N	BMI at inclusion	Primary outcome	Definition of relapse	Main findings
Fichter et al. [28]	Internet-based guided self-help intervention (IGSH)	TAU	Outpatient or inpatient treatment and medication possible	9 months	258	IGSH: 17.8 ± 1.4 TAU: 17.7 ± 1.2	BMI	None provided	*Primary outcome* No significant group difference in weight gain after controlling for dosage of adjunctive inpatient treatment as the GSH group received more inpatient treatment as the TAU group *Secondary outcomes* Patients of the GSH had improved scores on some self-report dimensions related to ED cognitions and behaviors
Kaye et al. [25]	20 mg Fluoxetine/day (adjustment possible by a blinded physician)	Placebo	Optional adjunctive outpatient CBT	One year	35	89% average body weight	Prevention of relapse	Dropout from trial due to deteriorating clinical course (e.g. severe weight loss or severe ED symptoms), initiated by the patient, carer or physician	*Primary outcome* Significantly more patients receiving placebo had a relapse (dropped out) as compared to those receiving fluoxetine *Secondary outcomes* Patients who completed fluoxetine treatment over one year had higher weight, less ED symptoms, less obsessive thoughts, less depression and anxiety than the remaining group
Neumayr et al. [23]	Smartphone-based guided self-help intervention (SGSH)	TAU	SGSH is additional to TAU	8 weeks	40	SGSH: 19.1 ± 1.9 TAU: 18.6 ± 1.0	BMI self-reported ED symptoms	None provided	*Primary outcome* No significant group difference in weight gain or self-reported ED symptoms *Secondary outcomes* High levels of adherence and acceptance of SGSH

Table 1 (continued)

Study	Aftercare intervention	Comparator	Adjunctive treatment	Duration	N	BMI at inclusion	Primary outcome	Definition of relapse	Main findings
Parling et al. [29]	Acceptance and commitment therapy (ACT)	TAU	Optional additional daycare and other treatments; no additional psychotherapy for ACT patients	19 sessions	42	ACT: 17.5 ± 2.3 TAU: 18.1 ± 2.6	Good outcome defined as BMI ≥ 19 and EDE-Q global score ≤ 2.83	None provided	*Primary outcome* No significant group difference in good outcome *Secondary outcomes* Significant improvements in BMI and ED symptoms across time in both groups
Pike et al. [30]	Cognitive-behavior therapy (CBT)	Nutritional Counselling (NC)	Adjunctive pharmacotherapy possible	50 sessions over one year	33	Not reported BMI at admission: CBT: 16.0 ± 2.1 NC: 15.2 ± 1.5	Time to relapse	(a) BMI below 17.5 for more than 10 days (b) severe ED-related medical complications requiring inpatient care (c) exacerbation of non-ED psychopathology requiring other care	*Primary outcome* Patients in the CBT group had a significant longer relapse-free interval than patients receiving NC *Secondary outcomes* Patients in the CBT group showed a lower relapse rate and were more likely to meet criteria for good outcome
Sternheim et al. [26]	Internet-based guided self-help intervention based on MANTRA (iMANTRA) added to TAU	TAU	iMANTRA is additional to TAU	12 months	41	iMANTRA: 18.1 ± 2.2 TAU: 17.9 ± 1.4	Not defined due to feasibility focus	None provided	iMANTRA feasible and acceptable Effect sizes for BMI, ED pathology and general psychopathology at 6 months were small and tended to favor iMANTRA at 12 months assessment
Walsh et al. [24]	60 mg Fluoxetine/day (adjustment possible)	Placebo	Adjunctive outpatient CBT with specific focus on relapse prevention	One year	93	Fluoxetine: 20.2 ± 0.5 Placebo: 20.5 ± 0.5	Time to relapse	(a) BMI below 16.5 for 2 consecutive weeks (b) severe ED-related medical complications (c) imminent suicide risk (d) development of other severe psychiatric disorder	*Primary outcome* No difference in time to relapse between the fluoxetine and placebo group *Secondary outcomes* No difference in any secondary outcome between the fluoxetine and placebo group

ACT, Acceptance and Commitment Therapy; BMI, Body Mass Index; CBT, Cognitive Behavior Therapy; ED, eating disorder; EDE-Q, Eating Disorder Examination Questionnaire; IGSH, Internet-based Guided Self-help; iMANTRA, internet-based Maudsley Model of Anorexia Nervosa Treatment for Adults; NC, Nutritional Counselling; SGSH, Smartphone-based Guided Self-help; TAU, Treatment as usual

Table 2 Risk of bias assessment for included RCTs

Study	Randomization process	Deviations from intended intervention	Missing outcome data	Measurement of the outcome	Selection of reported results	Overall
Fichter et al. [28]	Some concerns	Some concerns	Low risk	Low risk	Low risk	Some concerns
Kaye et al. [25]	Low risk	Low risk	Low risk	Low risk	Some concerns	Some concerns
Neumayr et al. [23]	Some concerns	Some concerns	Low risk	Low risk	Some concerns	Some concerns
Parling et al. [29]	Low risk	Some concerns	High risk	High risk	Some concerns	High risk
Pike et al. [30]	Low risk	Some concerns	Low risk	Low risk	Low risk	Some concerns
Sternheim et al. [26]	Low risk	Low risk	Low risk	Some concerns	Low risk	Some concerns
Walsh et al. [24]	Low risk	Low risk	Low risk	Some concerns	Low risk	Some concerns

Table 3 Calculated effect sizes for the included RCTs

Study	n	P value main outcome	CI	Effect size
Fichter et al. [28][a]	258	.076		.22
Kaye et al. [25][a]	35	.006		.93
Neumayr et al. [23][b]	40		− 0.90, 0.41	− .24
Parling et al. [29][a]	42	.15	0.3–16.1	.64
Pike et al. [30][a,c]	33	p < 0.004		1.00
Sternheim et al. [26][b]	35		−0.28 to 1.09	0.40
Walsh et al. [24][a]	39	.64		.20

[a] Calculation of effect size from p-value via t-value and sample size

[b] Calculation of effect size from CI via standard error and sample size

[c] p-value was set to 0.004

problem solving, social relationships and self-esteem [35]. In this trial, a minimum BMI increase during inpatient treatment was necessary for inclusion as well as "sufficient motivation" to take part in the study [35] which was defined by several criteria related to treatment history and compliance, including a prognostic assessment by the therapist. A later feasibility trial also offered a guided internet-based program, however, this was based on the MANTRA treatment concept, which is the Maudsley Model of Anorexia Nervosa Treatment for Adults [7, 26, 36, 37] and also involved regular email therapist contact. This intervention was offered over one year and in order to be included into this study, patients had to have a minimum weight gain of one BMI point during inpatient treatment [26]. Core aspects of the intervention which were specifically added to MANTRA for the aftercare intervention comprised a traffic light system of relapse risk, a nutritional plan designed for weight maintenance as well as module on anxiety-related processes [26]. In the other, more recent pilot RCT, patients were offered the use of an eight weeks long smartphone app *Recovery Record* as post-inpatient aftercare intervention [25]. This app

includes interventions which are based on principles of CBT, dialectic-behavioral therapy (DBT) and motivational enhancement therapy (MET) [25], covering topics such as self-monitoring strategies, goal-setting, meal planning, coping strategies and guided meditations. Regular therapist contacts and feedback via the app were also included in this study [25].

One of these trials defined BMI as primary outcome [35], a further feasibility trial did not specify a primary outcome [26] and the second feasibility study primarily looked at BMI and self-reported ED symptoms as assessed by the Eating Disorder Examination Questionnaire (EDE-Q) [25]. None of these trials provided an explicit definition of relapse [25, 26, 35].

In the earlier larger study [35], 61% of eligible patients enrolled into the trial on internet-guided self-help, of those, 24.2% did not use the self-help program and 39.8% participants completed the full program. After controlling for adjunctive inpatient treatment, there was no significant group difference in weight gain between patients of the guided self-help group and those receiving TAU [35]. In the iMANTRA feasibility trial [26], 19.5% of inpatients screened for the study were found eligible and agreed to participate and 87.5% of those took up the iMANTRA intervention. Effect sizes for BMI, ED pathology and general psychopathology tended to favor iMANTRA at end of treatment, however, no significant differences were found [26]. In the later pilot study, 71.9% of eligible patients enrolled in the trial on smartphone-based guided self-help [25]. One patient terminated the intervention prematurely, all other participants showed regular daily use of the intervention [25]. At end of the aftercare intervention, there was no significant group difference in BMI or self-reported ED symptoms between those using the smartphone-based guided self-help adjunctive to TAU and those receiving TAU only [25]. The effect sizes in the feasibility trial at post-intervention were nonsignificant small to moderate favoring the intervention group regarding BMI (d = − 0.24; 95% confidence interval [CI] [− 0.90, 0.41]) and ED symptoms (Eating Disorder Examination-Questionnaire global: d = 0.56; 95% CI [− 0.10, 1.22]) [25]. Effects between the groups were absent at 6-months follow-up [25].

RCTs reporting on psychotherapy interventions

Two trials investigated the efficacy of psychotherapy interventions versus either TAU or nutritional counselling following inpatient treatment for AN to prevent relapse [27, 38]. One of the studies investigated a CBT intervention [38], while a second trial tested Acceptance and Commitment Therapy (ACT) as aftercare approach [27]. Differences in study design makes direct comparisons of the two trials difficult and each study is therefore reviewed separately.

Cognitive-behavior therapy (CBT)

In one trial, patients were randomly assigned to receive fifty sessions of either CBT or nutritional counselling as a control condition [38]. The CBT approach comprised topics including ED pathology, self-esteem and interpersonal functioning. Patients had to achieve a minimum weight gain up to 90% of ideal body weight maintained for at least two weeks during inpatient care in order to be eligible for the study [38]. *Time to relapse* was chosen as primary outcome [38], and relapse was defined similarly as in one of the later fluoxetine trials [31] based on several criteria reflecting severe deterioration of AN symptoms or comorbidities (see Table 1). In case of a relapse, trial participation was terminated [38]. Of those meeting inclusion criteria 76.7% took part in the study [38]. There was a high rate of treatment failure of 73% for the control group (a relapse rate of 53% plus a dropout rate of 20%), while the significantly lower rate of treatment failure in the CBT group was 22% (22% relapse, no dropout). There was a significant group difference in time to relapse, favoring CBT over the control condition [38].

Acceptance and commitment therapy (ACT)

Another trial investigated the efficacy of Acceptance and Commitment Therapy (ACT) as compared to TAU [27] for patients after intensive day-hospital treatment. Weight gain was not a primary focus of the day program, except for an optional final three weeks of the admission. Consequently, there was no eligibility criterion regarding minimum weight gain or BMI at randomization. The ACT therapy was a modified version of a treatment protocol developed for substance misuse (shortened from 48 to 19 sessions) and covered topics such as costs and benefits of the ED, emotional control and acceptance, experiential willingness, values and goals [27]. In both arms of the study patients were able to access additional clinical

care if this was required. Primary focus of the analyses was change in BMI and in self-reported ED symptoms as assessed by the Eating Disorder Examination Questionnaire (EDE-Q) [25]; additionally, this trial compared proportions in both groups reaching a *good outcome*, defined as a BMI ≥ 19 and an EDE-Q global score ≤ 2.83. Roughly 84% of eligible patients consented to be enrolled into the trial, 41.7% of the ACT group completed less than 16/19 treatment sessions and significantly more (15.8%) dropped out of the TAU condition [27]. There was no significant group difference regarding good outcome at the end of the aftercare intervention [27].

Ongoing trials

Our search for registered ongoing RCTs investigating the efficacy of aftercare interventions for AN [28–30] identified three studies which are currently in progress: The TRIANGLE study aims to strengthen self-management skills in a combined patient-carer approach [28]. A second study is based on the above outlined pilot RCT [25] testing the efficacy of a guided app-based self-help intervention as add-on to TAU in a larger sample [29]. The SUSTAIN trial conducted by our group investigates the efficacy of a novel post-inpatient psychotherapy which is predominantly delivered via videoconference [30].

Operationalization of recovery processes

Most studies operationalized recovery/relapse through BMI, focusing either on time until the BMI fell below a cutoff, or on BMI at the end of the observation period. Further, all studies reported dropout rates as a marker of treatment adherence, although definitions of dropout varied considerably between studies.

Discussion

The aim of this systematic review is to synthesize evidence from RCTs on the efficacy of treatments which aim to help patients with AN to maintaining benefits after inpatient or day-hospital treatment. We identified seven RCTs, two of them with a pilot and feasibility focus. The interventions they tested can be classified into pharmacotherapy, guided self-help and psychotherapy approaches.

Synthesis and discussion of results

The evidence from pharmacological efficacy trials is mixed, with one trial reporting superiority of fluoxetine vs. placebo in terms of reduced relapse rates [32] and a further, larger trial reporting no benefit of fluoxetine [31]. This heterogeneity could be due to methodological differences between the trials, concerning sample size, sample characteristics as well as definition and specificity of the primary outcome [31, 32]. It should also be considered that in both trials, adjunctive psychotherapy was included as part of the study protocol which also has an effect on the main outcome [31, 32]. Moreover, these studies suggest that post-inpatient pharmacotherapy is less acceptable to patients, as evidenced by low uptake and high dropout rates [31, 32]. Additionally, efficacy trials in this field of interventions are especially affected by ethical concerns about offering placebo treatments to severely ill patients [31, 32]. Pharmacotherapy plays a minor role in the treatment of AN as there is no evidence for its efficacy e.g. with respect to weight gain as a primary treatment goal [8, 13, 33]. In light of this, it is not surprising that there is no clear evidence for the efficacy of pharmacological agents in preventing relapse.

Guided self-help interventions have the potential to improve aftercare as they are more readily accessible and can be used more easily by patients who are ambivalent towards treatment. Moreover, they have the ability to bridge discontinuity of care, if disseminated via digital tools [39]. However, the efficacy of such digital guided self-help approaches as post-inpatient intervention for AN in terms of weight gain has not been demonstrated [25, 26, 35]. In one study, the self-help program was predominantly offered via homepage content, and the lack of superiority in this case might be partly due to a large proportion of patients not regularly engaging in the self-help program [35]. Those patients who fully completed the program did benefit [35], but the limited uptake might indicate reduced acceptability of this intervention, suggesting that this approach might not be intensive enough for a majority of patients. A later feasibility trial probing a guided internet-based self-help intervention in addition to TAU showed that this approach was well accepted and feasible, however, the trial was not powered to test efficacy [26]. A recent pilot study showed that contemporary mobile approaches like a smartphone application seem to meet many patients' needs, in terms of ease of uptake, acceptance and satisfaction which was high [25]. However, the intervention had also a comparably short duration which tends to foster acceptability. The study did not demonstrate additional beneficial effects of using the app in comparison to the control group, but this needs to be seen in the context of a pilot RCT with the main focus on feasibility and acceptability [25]. The pilot data are encouraging regarding feasibility and acceptability and therefore, a larger appropriately powered confirmatory RCT probing the efficacy of the app is currently in progress [29]. Overall, the studies on internet-based guided self-help for patients with AN are adding important information to the literature in an emerging field, as a recent review outlines that studies investigating self-help have so far mainly focused on other ED diagnoses like bulimia nervosa (BN) and binge eating disorder

(BED) [40]. For BN and BED, guided self-help interventions are superior to waitlist or delayed treatment regarding ED symptoms and abstinence rates [40], however, evidence is mixed and hard to interpret for comparisons with other (more intensive) treatments, partly also due to heterogeneous study designs [40]. Therefore, it will be important to investigate whether any form of self-help is a useful addition to current treatment options for AN, for instance, in terms of tailoring to patient needs with respect to content, speed and amount of guidance and feedback [41], but also regarding different levels of care and care pathways [12, 40–42].

The evidence on psychotherapy as aftercare strategy is mixed, too, with findings that a CBT intervention compared to nutritional counselling has the potential to delay relapse, while an ACT intervention did not result in better outcomes than TAU. Both trials had small sample sizes and variable dropout and treatment discontinuation [27, 38]. In the CBT study there was considerable drop out in the control condition, indicating that nutritional counselling was less accepted by patients [38], while in the ACT trial, engagement was actually higher in the TAU condition, although no difference was found in treatment outcome. In this latter trial, both study arms were able to access a range of additional treatment support [27], making it less likely to find differences.

To summarize, there is no clear evidence favoring a specific approach for post-inpatient aftercare in adult patients with AN. The effects of RCTs in this field are so far rather limited, partly due to various methodological challenges. Pharmacotherapy and low-threshold guided self-help suffer from limited uptake and high dropout [31, 32, 35]. Novel mobile guided self-help approaches seem more promising due to high patient satisfaction, but their efficacy has yet to be fully investigated [25, 29]. CBT might be beneficial in delaying relapse, but this is based on a single study with small sample size and high dropout in the control condition [38]. The CBT findings warrant replication in a larger well-powered trial. Recent reviews have emphasized that although considerable progress has been made in advancing evidence-based therapies for this patient group, there still is a long way to go [10, 21], and the present review shows that this also holds true for the more specific treatment stage of post-inpatient aftercare.

Methodological aspects

As defined by the scope of the present review, all of the included studies had implemented a RCT design, which is a methodological strength, constituting the gold standard for efficacy research. With one exception [35], studies were conducted in small or modest samples, i.e. most have been insufficiently powered. This is also indicated by the calculated effect sizes which also underline the large heterogeneity of existing trials. Regarding sample size it should be taken into account that it is especially challenging to conduct large-scale RCTs in AN research, due to a lack of funding opportunities, low prevalence rates and ambivalence of patients [43]. Partly also related to patients' ambivalence, most trials report comparably high dropout rates, especially from control conditions. Two major sources of heterogeneity between trials were choice of outcome as well as the sample characteristics. Some studies did not provide a definition of relapse, others did define relapse based on several outcome criteria and some studies primarily relied on BMI as primary outcome and indicator for relapse or recovery (see Table 1). This heterogeneity makes it difficult to compare trials, however, as outlined earlier, there is a general need for the field of ED to work towards a more unified definitions of relapse and recovery [20, 44]. Regarding sample characteristics, the BMI at inclusion into the aftercare intervention substantially varied between trials, and some studies defined a minimum weight gain, sufficient motivation or weight restoration as eligibility criteria [31, 35, 38]. This point again relates to the question how recovery or relapse are defined, and it is also tied to the situation that many adult patients with AN are not (weight) recovered or remitted when leaving inpatient or day-hospital treatment, posing the question to whom aftercare should be offered and tailored. A higher BMI at discharge from inpatient treatment is a positive prognostic predictor [45] and therefore is also likely to influence outcome of the aftercare intervention. At the same time, it could be argued that especially those patients who have not reached weight restoration are in need of ongoing support after discharge, as they have a higher relapse risk [6]. However, it might also be that this group of patients needs a specific form of aftercare. Finally, most trials allowed for or implemented adjunctive treatments as part of the trial (see Table 1). This was done for good reasons, especially regarding ethical and safety aspects in severely ill patients, nevertheless, it makes it hard to interpret the efficacy of a single novel aftercare intervention. For instance, pharmacotherapy was often combined with CBT, and therefore, the effects of psychotherapy might be to some extent responsible for a lack of group differences [31].

Strengths and limitations of the present review

To the best of our knowledge, this is the first systematic review to summarize evidence on the efficacy of aftercare interventions specifically tailored at the treatment of patients with AN after inpatient or day-hospital treatment. We performed this work according to the PRISMA guideline for systematic reviews [23]. We have only included trials with an RCT design as this is the gold standard for efficacy research. We have used broad search terms, searched several large databases, performed an additional hand search and also included ongoing trials. Nevertheless, the number of included trials is small. Overall, the studies reviewed in this work are heterogeneous and disparate, and it is therefore important to take into account that this puts limitations on summarizing findings. Due to the heterogeneous sample characteristics and outcomes chosen, it was not possible to conduct a meta-analysis, however, we did calculate effect sizes and report the range. Further limitations comprise that the review was not pre-registered and that the quality rating was performed by one researcher.

Future directions for research and treatment

Previous efficacy research demonstrates that there are several challenges in the development and implementation of effective aftercare for patients with AN: Patients with AN often experience ambivalence towards treatment [1], and also 'treatment fatigue'. Especially after completion of intensive inpatient therapy, many patients might feel ambivalent towards continuing with another treatment. In this critical stage of transition, it is important to offer a treatment which meets patients' needs, is not too low-threshold, and at the same time also fosters patients' autonomy and supports them on their way to recovery. In light of this, the development and advancement of efficient aftercare interventions would benefit from stronger integration of the perspective of people affected by the disorder, either as a patient or carer. Their lived experience is invaluable for the development of tailored intervention modules, supporting those who are about to overcome the disorder. Two recent reviews synthesize findings from predominantly qualitative insights into personal views on the recovery process from an ED [20, 46], identifying fundamental aspects contributing to long-term recovery based on patient perspectives, and these contain surprisingly few domains which are directly tied to core ED symptoms or behaviors. Themes include social-emotional dimensions such as positive interpersonal relationships and personality-related aspects such as autonomy, developing an identity beyond the ED and self-acceptance [20, 46]. The ongoing trial by Cardi et al. [28] consequently implements this approach by investigating a novel combined patient-carer approach which partly relies on interventions which were developed by patients and carers. Integrating patients' perspectives is also important towards the development of a consensus concept of recovery and relapse, as the use of heterogeneous outcomes in treatment trials is a further challenge in the field which makes comparability between interventions difficult.

Another issue which has yet to be investigated is that of interventions targeted to specific patient subgroups, for instance patients with the restrictive versus binge/purging subtype or those with comorbidities or longstanding illness. Overall, the variability between studies reviewed here could suggest that different people may benefit from different types of aftercare depending on the nature of previous treatment(s), stage of recovery, other support they have etc.

Beyond this, more research on mechanisms underlying the maintenance and progression of AN, but also recovery from this ED, will be important to inform novel treatment strategies, both for acute treatment as well as aftercare interventions [47]. Recently, novel innovative treatments which widely rely on insights from mechanism research have been probed for the treatment of AN, predominantly including non-invasive brain stimulation [21], and they might also unfold their effects in the stage of aftercare.

In order to extend current treatment options for adult patients with AN directly after inpatient or day-hospital treatment, our work group is currently conducting the SUSTAIN trial which is a multi-centre, randomized controlled confirmatory superiority trial investigating the efficacy of a novel post-inpatient psychotherapy as compared to optimized TAU [30]. The SUSTAIN aftercare intervention is based on the cognitive-interpersonal maintenance model of AN [7, 36, 37] and specifically tailored to achieve sustained recovery in AN following inpatient treatment. Patients randomized to the SUSTAIN aftercare intervention receive 20 treatment sessions over eight months. In order to ensure continuity of care for patients from a large catchment area, most treatment sessions take place via videoconference. Patients randomized to TAU-O receive routine outpatient psychotherapy. We will include 190 patients into this RCT who have reached a minimum BMI of 15 kg/m^2 during acute treatment. Change in BMI between baseline and end of aftercare treatment (T2) adjusted for baseline BMI is the primary outcome. As part of the SUSTAIN trial, we have established a lived experience council whose members are patients with AN and carers. The council members contribute their perspectives throughout the whole trial period and have, for instance, also contributed to a revision of the treatment manual.

Conclusion

Evidence on aftercare interventions for patients with AN is very limited, with a small number of randomized controlled intervention studies published. The field faces many challenges which generally affect intervention research in AN. Previous trials suggest that there lies potential in psychotherapy in terms of CBT-oriented aftercare interventions. Moreover, guided self-help approaches and the dissemination via digital dissemination strategies potentially have high acceptance and increase intervention uptake, however, their efficacy has yet to be demonstrated. A specific challenge is to increase uptake of aftercare interventions and to reduce dropout rates, calling for a better tailoring of interventions to patient needs and the integration of patient perspectives. Intensified research and care efforts are needed to address the problem of recurrent relapse after intensive inpatient treatment for AN and to eventually improve prognosis for this ED.

Acknowledgements
Not applicable.

Authors' contributions
KEG, SCB, KS, US, FJ and SZ conceived the review topic and research question. KEG and SCB developed the search term and eligibility criteria, performed the independent literature search and screening as well as the inclusion of trials. SCB performed the quality rating. KEG, SCB and KS analyzed the included studies. PM provided statistical expertise. SH, TH, EMS, UV, JvW, BW and AZ are trial site investigators of the SUSTAIN trial. KEG drafted the manuscript and all co-authors critically revised it and approved the final manuscript.

Funding
Open Access funding enabled and organized by Projekt DEAL. This work is funded by a grant from the German Federal Ministry of Science and Education (grant number 01KG2009). KS is receiving a grant from the Margarete von Wrangell Program funded by the Ministry of Science and Education Baden-Württemberg. US is supported by a National Institute of Health Research (NIHR) Senior Investigator Award and receives salary support from the NIHR Mental Health Biomedical Research Centre at the South London and Maudsley NHS Foundation Trust and King's College London, UK.

Competing interests
The authors declare that they have no competing interests.

Author details
Department of Psychosomatic Medicine and Psychotherapy, Medical University Hospital Tübingen, Eberhard Karls University, Osianderstr. 5, 72076 Tübingen, Germany. ^{2}Center of Excellence in Eating Disorders, Tübingen, Germany. Institute for Clinical Epidemiology and Applied Biostatistics, Medical Faculty, Eberhard Karls University Tübingen, Tübingen, Germany. ^{4}Department of Psychosomatic Medicine and Psychotherapy, LWL-University Hospital Bochum, Ruhr University Bochum, Bochum, Germany. ^{5}Department of Psychosomatic Medicine, Center for Internal Medicine and Dermatology, Charité - Universitätsmedizin Berlin, Freie Universität Berlin and Humboldt-Universität Zu Berlin, Berlin, Germany. ^{6}Clinic for Psychosomatic Medicine and Psychotherapy, LVR University-Hospital Essen, University of Duisburg-Essen, Essen, Germany. Schoen Clinic Roseneck, Prien am Chiemsee, Germany. ^{8}Department Psychiatry and Psychotherapy, University Hospital LMU Munich, Munich, Germany. ^{9}Department Psychiatry and Psychotherapy, University Hospital Freiburg, Freiburg, Germany. ^{10}Department of Psychosomatic Medicine and Psychotherapy, Ulm University Medical Center, Ulm, Germany. ^{11}Department of General

Internal Medicine and Psychosomatics, University Hospital Heidelberg, Heidelberg, Germany. [12]Department of Psychosomatic Medicine und Psychotherapy, Center for Mental Health, Faculty of Medicine, University of Freiburg, Freiburg, Germany. [13]Section of Eating Disorders, Department of Psychological Medicine, Institute of Psychiatry, Psychology and Neuroscience, King's College London, London, UK. [14]Department of Psychosomatic Medicine and Psychotherapy, University Hospital Magdeburg, Otto von Guericke University, Magdeburg, Germany.

References

1. Zipfel S, et al. Anorexia nervosa: aetiology, assessment, and treatment. Lancet Psychiatry. 2015;2(12):1099–111.
2. Fichter MM, et al. Long-term outcome of anorexia nervosa: results from a large clinical longitudinal study. Int J Eat Disord. 2017;50(9):1018–30.
3. Arcelus J, et al. Mortality rates in patients with anorexia nervosa and other eating disorders. A meta-analysis of 36 studies. Arch Gen Psychiatry. 2011;68(7):724–31.
4. Fichter MM, Quadflieg N. Mortality in eating disorders-results of a large prospective clinical longitudinal study. Int J Eat Disord. 2016;49(4):391–401.
5. DeJong H, Broadbent H, Schmidt U. A systematic review of dropout from treatment in outpatients with anorexia nervosa. Int J Eat Disord. 2012;45(5):635–47.
6. Schlegl S, et al. Specialized inpatient treatment of adult anorexia nervosa: effectiveness and clinical significance of changes. BMC Psychiatry. 2014;14:258.
7. Schmidt U, Treasure J. Anorexia nervosa: valued and visible. A cognitive-interpersonal maintenance model and its implications for research and practice. Br J Clin Psychol. 2006;45(3):343–66.
8. Resmark G, et al. Treatment of anorexia nervosa-new evidence-based guidelines. J Clin Med. 2019;8(2):153.
9. Hilbert A, Hoek HW, Schmidt R. Evidence-based clinical guidelines for eating disorders: international comparison. Curr Opin Psychiatry. 2017;30(6):423–37.
10. Zeeck A, et al. Psychotherapeutic treatment for anorexia nervosa: a systematic review and network meta-analysis. Front Psychiatry. 2018;9:158.
11. Treasure J, Stein D, Maguire S. Has the time come for a staging model to map the course of eating disorders from high risk to severe enduring illness? An examination of the evidence. Early Interv Psychiatry. 2015;9(3):173–84.
12. Treasure J, et al. Optimising care pathways for adult anorexia nervosa. What is the evidence to guide the provision of high-quality, cost-effective services? Eur Eat Disord Rev. 2021;29:306–15.
13. National Institute for Health and Care Excellence (NICE). Eating disorders: recognition and treatment. 2017; Available from: https://www.nice.org.uk/guidance/ng69/chapter/Recommendations#treating-anorexia-nervosa.
14. Herpertz, S., et al. S3-Leitlinie Diagnostik und Behandlung der Essstörungen (Online). 05.02.2021]; Available from: https://www.awmf.org/leitlinien/detail/ll/051-026.html.
15. Cruz AM, et al. Eating disorders-related hospitalizations in Portugal: a nationwide study from 2000 to 2014. Int J Eat Disord. 2018;51(10):1201–6.
16. Berends T, Boonstra N, van Elburg A. Relapse in anorexia nervosa: a systematic review and meta-analysis. Curr Opin Psychiatry. 2018;31(6):445–55.
17. Khalsa SS, et al. What happens after treatment? A systematic review of relapse, remission, and recovery in anorexia nervosa. J Eat Disord. 2017;5:20.
18. van Hoeken D, Hoek HW. Review of the burden of eating disorders: mortality, disability, costs, quality of life, and family burden. Curr Opin Psychiatry. 2020;33(6):521–7.
19. Brandon TH, Vidrine JI, Litvin EB. Relapse and relapse prevention. Annu Rev Clin Psychol. 2007;3:257–84.
20. de Vos JA, et al. Identifying fundamental criteria for eating disorder recovery: a systematic review and qualitative meta-analysis. J Eat Disord. 2017;5:34.
21. Brockmeyer T, Friederich HC, Schmidt U. Advances in the treatment of anorexia nervosa: a review of established and emerging interventions. Psychol Med. 2018;48(8):1228–56.
22. Watson HJ, Bulik CM. Update on the treatment of anorexia nervosa: review of clinical trials, practice guidelines and emerging interventions. Psychol Med. 2013;43(12):2477–500.
23. Moher D, et al. Preferred reporting items for systematic reviews and meta-analyses: the PRISMA statement. PLoS Med. 2009;6(7):e1000097.
24. Higgins J, et al. Assessing risk of bias in a randomized trial, in cochrane handbook for systematic reviews of interventions version 6.2, J. Higgins, et al., Editors. 2021.
25. Neumayr C, et al. Improving aftercare with technology for anorexia nervosa after intensive inpatient treatment: a pilot randomized controlled trial with a therapist-guided smartphone app. Int J Eat Disord. 2019;52(10):1191–201.
26. Sternheim L, Schmidt U. Preventing deterioration and relapse in severe anorexia nervosa: randomised controlled feasibility trial of an e-mail-guided manual-based self-care programme based on the Maudsley Model of Anorexia Nervosa Treatment for Adults, in Treatment of anorexia nervosa: a multimethod investigation translating experimental neuroscience into clinical practice., U. Schmidt, et al., Editors. 2017, NIHR Journals Library: Southampton (UK).
27. Parling T, et al. A randomised trial of acceptance and commitment therapy for anorexia nervosa after daycare treatment, including five-year follow-up. BMC Psychiatry. 2016;16:272.
28. Cardi V, et al. Transition care in anorexia nervosa through guidance online from peer and carer expertise (TRIANGLE): study protocol for a randomised controlled trial. Eur Eat Disord Rev. 2017;25(6):512–23.
29. Schlegl S, Neumayr C, Voderholzer U. Therapist-guided smartphone-based aftercare for inpatients with severe anorexia nervosa (SMART-AN): study protocol of a randomized controlled trial. Int J Eat Disord. 2020;53(10):1739–45.
30. Giel KE, et al. Specialized post-inpatient psychotherapy for sustained recovery in anorexia nervosa via videoconference-study protocol of the randomized controlled SUSTAIN trial. J Eat Disord. 2021;9(1):61.
31. Walsh BT, et al. Fluoxetine after weight restoration in anorexia nervosa: a randomized controlled trial. JAMA. 2006;295(22):2605–12.
32. Kaye WH, et al. Double-blind placebo-controlled administration of fluoxetine in restricting- and restricting-purging-type anorexia nervosa. Biol Psychiatry. 2001;49(7):644–52.
33. Davis H, Attia E. Pharmacotherapy of eating disorders. Curr Opin Psychiatry. 2017;30(6):452–7.
34. Carter JC, et al. Maintenance treatment for anorexia nervosa: a comparison of cognitive behavior therapy and treatment as usual. Int J Eat Disord. 2009;42(3):202–7.
35. Fichter MM, et al. Does internet-based prevention reduce the risk of relapse for anorexia nervosa? Behav Res Ther. 2012;50(3):180–90.
36. Schmidt U, et al. The maudsley outpatient study of treatments for anorexia nervosa and related conditions (MOSAIC): comparison of the maudsley model of anorexia nervosa treatment for adults (MANTRA) with specialist supportive clinical management (SSCM) in outpatients with broadly defined anorexia nervosa: a randomized controlled trial. J Consult Clin Psychol. 2015;83(4):796–807.
37. Schmidt U, et al. Two-year follow-up of the MOSAIC trial: a multicenter randomized controlled trial comparing two psychological treatments in adult outpatients with broadly defined anorexia nervosa. Int J Eat Disord. 2016;49(8):793–800.
38. Pike KM, et al. Cognitive behavior therapy in the posthospitalization treatment of anorexia nervosa. Am J Psychiatry. 2003;160(11):2046–9.
39. Bauer S, Moessner M. Harnessing the power of technology for the treatment and prevention of eating disorders. Int J Eat Disord. 2013;46(5):508–15.
40. Yim SH, Schmidt U. Self-help treatment of eating disorders. Psychiatry Clin North Am. 2019;42(2):231–41.
41. Aardoom JJ, Dingemans AE, Van Furth EF. E-health interventions for eating disorders: emerging findings, issues, and opportunities. Curr Psychiatry Rep. 2016;18(4):42.
42. Wu A, et al. Smartphone apps for depression and anxiety: a systematic review and meta-analysis of techniques to increase engagement. NPJ Digit Med. 2021;4(1):20.

43. Brockmeyer T, et al. Sample size in clinical trials on anorexia nervosa: a rejoinder to Jenkins. Psychol Med. 2019;49(9):1581–2.

44. Bardone-Cone AM, Hunt RA, Watson HJ. An overview of conceptualizations of eating disorder recovery, recent findings, and future directions. Curr Psychiatry Rep. 2018;20(9):79.

45. Glasofer DR, et al. Predictors of illness course and health maintenance following inpatient treatment among patients with anorexia nervosa. J Eat Disord. 2020;8(1):69.

46. Wetzler S, et al. A framework to conceptualize personal recovery from eating disorders: a systematic review and qualitative meta-synthesis of perspectives from individuals with lived experience. Int J Eat Disord. 2020;53(8):1188–203.

47. Glashouwer KA, et al. Time to make a change: a call for more experimental research on key mechanisms in anorexia nervosa. Eur Eat Disord Rev. 2020;28(4):361–7.

Permissions

All chapters in this book were first published by BioMed Central; hereby published with permission under the Creative Commons Attribution License or equivalent. Every chapter published in this book has been scrutinized by our experts. Their significance has been extensively debated. The topics covered herein carry significant findings which will fuel the growth of the discipline. They may even be implemented as practical applications or may be referred to as a beginning point for another development.

The contributors of this book come from diverse backgrounds, making this book a truly international effort. This book will bring forth new frontiers with its revolutionizing research information and detailed analysis of the nascent developments around the world.

We would like to thank all the contributing authors for lending their expertise to make the book truly unique. They have played a crucial role in the development of this book. Without their invaluable contributions this book wouldn't have been possible. They have made vital efforts to compile up to date information on the varied aspects of this subject to make this book a valuable addition to the collection of many professionals and students.

This book was conceptualized with the vision of imparting up-to-date information and advanced data in this field. To ensure the same, a matchless editorial board was set up. Every individual on the board went through rigorous rounds of assessment to prove their worth. After which they invested a large part of their time researching and compiling the most relevant data for our readers.

The editorial board has been involved in producing this book since its inception. They have spent rigorous hours researching and exploring the diverse topics which have resulted in the successful publishing of this book. They have passed on their knowledge of decades through this book. To expedite this challenging task, the publisher supported the team at every step. A small team of assistant editors was also appointed to further simplify the editing procedure and attain best results for the readers.

Apart from the editorial board, the designing team has also invested a significant amount of their time in understanding the subject and creating the most relevant covers. They scrutinized every image to scout for the most suitable representation of the subject and create an appropriate cover for the book.

The publishing team has been an ardent support to the editorial, designing and production team. Their endless efforts to recruit the best for this project, has resulted in the accomplishment of this book. They are a veteran in the field of academics and their pool of knowledge is as vast as their experience in printing. Their expertise and guidance has proved useful at every step. Their uncompromising quality standards have made this book an exceptional effort. Their encouragement from time to time has been an inspiration for everyone.

The publisher and the editorial board hope that this book will prove to be a valuable piece of knowledge for researchers, students, practitioners and scholars across the globe.

List of Contributors

Johanna Keeler, Ellen Lambert, Judith Owen, Jingjing Xia, Hubertus Himmerich and Janet Treasure
Section of Eating Disorders, Institute of Psychiatry, Psychology and Neuroscience, King's College London, 103 Denmark Hill, London SE5 8AF, UK

Miriam Olivola
Section of Eating Disorders, Institute of Psychiatry, Psychology and Neuroscience, King's College London, 103 Denmark Hill, London SE5 8AF, UK
Department of Mental Health and Addictions, Azienda Socio-Sanitaria Territoriale di Pavia, Pavia, Italy

Sandrine Thuret
Department of Basic and Clinical Neuroscience, Institute of Psychiatry, Psychology and Neuroscience, King's College London, London, UK
Department of Neurology, University Hospital Carl Gustav Carus, Technische Universität Dresden, Dresden, Germany

Valentina Cardi
Section of Eating Disorders, Institute of Psychiatry, Psychology and Neuroscience, King's College London, 103 Denmark Hill, London SE5 8AF, UK
Department of General Psychology, University of Padova, Padova, Italy

Liv Nilsen
Division of Mental Health and Addiction, Oslo University Hospital, Nydalen, Oslo, Norway

Veronica Lockertsen and Jan Ivar Røssberg
Division of Mental Health and Addiction, Oslo University Hospital, Nydalen, Oslo, Norway
Institute of Clinical Medicine, Faculty of Medicine, University of Oslo, 0318 Oslo, Norway

Lill Ann Wellhaven Holm
Oslo, Norway

Øyvind Rø
Institute of Clinical Medicine, Faculty of Medicine, University of Oslo, 0318 Oslo, Norway
Regional Department for Eating Disorders, Division of Mental Health and Addiction, Oslo University Hospital, Ullevål HF, Postboks 4950 Nydalen, 0424 Oslo, Norway

Linn May Burger
Drammen, Norway

Alexandra Gaál Kovalčíková, Ľubica Tichá, Alžbeta Čagalová and Ľudmila Podracká
Department of Paediatrics, The National Institute of Children's Diseases and Faculty of Medicine, Comenius University, Limbová 1, 83340 Bratislava, Slovakia

Katarína Šebeková
Institute of Molecular Biomedicine, Faculty of Medicine, Comenius University, Bratislava, Slovakia

Peter Celec
Institute of Molecular Biomedicine, Faculty of Medicine, Comenius University, Bratislava, Slovakia
Institute of Pathophysiology, Faculty of Medicine, Comenius University, Bratislava, Slovakia
Department of Molecular Biology, Faculty of Natural Sciences, Comenius University, Bratislava, Slovakia

Fatma Sogutlu
Department of Medical Biology, Faculty of Medicine, Ege University, Bornova, Izmir, Turkey

Ann F. Haynos, Lisa M. Anderson, Autumn J. Askew and Carol B. Peterson
Department of Psychiatry and Behavioral Sciences, University of Minnesota, 2450 Riverside Ave., Minneapolis, MN 55454, USA

Michelle G. Craske
Department of Psychology and Department of Psychiatry and Biobehavioral Sciences, University of California, Los Angeles, Los Angeles, CA, USA

Helen Startup, William Barber and Nicola Gilbert
Sussex Partnership NHS Foundation Trust, Sussex Eating Disorders Service, Brighton, UK

Mary Franklin-Smith
Leeds Partnership NHS Foundation Trust, CONNECT: The West Yorkshire Adult Eating Disorder Service, Leeds, UK

Yael Brown, Danielle Glennon and Akira Fukutomi
South London and Maudsley NHS Foundation Trust, Eating Disorders Outpatient Service, London, UK

Catherine Broomfield and Paul Rhodes
School of Psychology, Griffith Taylor Building, The University of Sydney, Sydney, NSW 2006, Australia

Stephen Touyz
InsideOut Institute, Charles Perkins Centre, The University of Sydney, Sydney, NSW 2006, Australia

Brooks B. Brodrick
Department of Psychiatry, University of Texas Southwestern Medical Center, 5323 Harry Hines Blvd., Suite BL6.110, Dallas, TX 75390-9070, USA
Department of Internal Medicine, University of Texas Southwestern Medical Center, 5323 Harry Hines Blvd., Dallas, TX 75390-9070, USA

Adrienne L. Adler-Neal, Jayme M. Palka and Carrie J. McAdams
Department of Psychiatry, University of Texas Southwestern Medical Center, 5323 Harry Hines Blvd., Suite BL6.110, Dallas, TX 75390-9070, USA

Virendra Mishra
Advance MRI LLC, Frisco, TX 75034, USA

Sina Aslan
Department of Psychiatry, University of Texas Southwestern Medical Center, 5323 Harry Hines Blvd., Suite BL6.110, Dallas, TX 75390-9070, USA
Advance MRI LLC, Frisco, TX 75034, USA

Kari Eiring
Institute of Psychology, Faculty of Social Sciences, University of Oslo, Oslo, Norway

Trine Wiig Hage and Deborah Lynn Reas
Regional Department of Eating Disorders, Division of Mental Health and Addiction, Oslo University Hospital-Ullevål, 0424 Nydalen Oslo, Norway

Elizabeth Kumiko Parker
Department of Dietetics and Nutrition, Westmead Hospital, Wentworthville, NSW 2145, Australia
Sydney School of Health Sciences, Faculty of Medicine and Health, The University of Sydney, Sydney, NSW 2006, Australia

Victoria Flood
Sydney School of Health Sciences, Faculty of Medicine and Health, The University of Sydney, Sydney, NSW 2006, Australia
Western Sydney Local Health District, Westmead, NSW 2145, Australia

Mark Halaki
Sydney School of Health Sciences, Faculty of Medicine and Health, The University of Sydney, Sydney, NSW 2006, Australia

Christine Wearne
Department of Medical Psychology, Westmead Hospital, Westmead, NSW 2145, Australia

Gail Anderson and Linette Gomes
Department of Adolescent and Young Adult Medicine, Westmead Hospital, Westmead, NSW 2145, Australia

Simon Clarke and Michael Kohn
Department of Adolescent and Young Adult Medicine, Westmead Hospital, Westmead, NSW 2145, Australia
Centre for Research Into Adolescents' Health (CRASH), Westmead Hospital, Westmead, NSW 2145, Australia
Sydney School of Medicine, Faculty of Medicine and Health, The University of Sydney, Sydney, NSW 2006, Australia

Frances Wilson
Department of Psychiatry, Westmead Hospital, Westmead, NSW 2145, Australia

Janice Russell
Sydney School of Medicine, Faculty of Medicine and Health, The University of Sydney, Sydney, NSW 2006, Australia
NSW Statewide Eating Disorder Service, Peter Beumont Unit, Professor Marie Bashir Centre, Royal Prince Alfred Hospital, Camperdown, NSW 2050, Australia

Elizabeth Frig
Department of Nutrition and Dietetics, Royal Prince Alfred Hospital, Camperdown, NSW 2050, Australia

Lot C. Sternheim
Department of Clinical Psychology, Universiteit Utrecht, Heidelberglaan 1, 3508, TC, Utrecht, The Netherlands
Utrecht, The Netherlands

Miriam I. Wickham
Department of Social Health and Organisation Psychology, Universiteit Utrecht, Heidelberglaan 1, 3508, TC, Utrecht, The Netherlands

Unna N. Danner
Department of Clinical Psychology, Universiteit Utrecht, Heidelberglaan 1, 3508, TC, Utrecht, The Netherlands
Altrecht Eating Disorders Rintveld, Wenshoek 4, 3705, WE, Zeist, The Netherlands

Todd W. Maddox
Department of Psychology, University of Texas, Austin, USA

Vincent J. Filoteo
Department of Psychiatry, University of California San Diego, La Jolla, CA, USA

Megan E. Shott and Guido K. W. Frank
Department of Psychiatry, University of California San Diego, La Jolla, CA, USA
Eating Disorders Center for Treatment and Research, University of California San Diego, San Diego, CA, USA

A. Austin, M. Flynn and K. L. Richards
Department of Psychological Medicine, King's College London, Institute of Psychiatry, Psychology and Neuroscience, 16 De Crespigny Park, London, UK

H. Sharpe
School of Health in Social Sciences, University of Edinburgh, Edinburgh, UK

K. L. Allen and U. Schmidt
Department of Psychological Medicine, King's College London, Institute of Psychiatry, Psychology and Neuroscience, 16 De Crespigny Park, London, UK
South London and Maudsley NHS Foundation Trust, London, UK

V. A. Mountford
Department of Psychological Medicine, King's College London, Institute of Psychiatry, Psychology and Neuroscience, 16 De Crespigny Park, London, UK
South London and Maudsley NHS Foundation Trust, London, UK
Maudsley Health, Abu Dhabi, UAE

D. Glennon and N. Grant
South London and Maudsley NHS Foundation Trust, London, UK

A. Brown
Sussex Partnership NHS Foundation Trust, Brighton, UK

K. Mahoney
North East London NHS Foundation Trust, London, UK

L. Serpell
North East London NHS Foundation Trust, London, UK
Division of Psychology and Language Sciences, University College London, London, UK

G. Brady, N. Nunes and F. Connan
Central and North West London NHS Foundation Trust, London, UK

M. Franklin-Smith, M. Schelhase and W. R. Jones
Leeds and York Partnership NHS Foundation Trust, Leeds, UK

G. Breen
Department of Social, Genetic & Developmental Psychiatry, King's College London, London, UK

Bethan Dalton, Savani Bartholdy, Maria Kekic, Jessica McClelland and Iain C. Campbell
Section of Eating Disorders, Department of Psychological Medicine, Institute of Psychiatry, Psychology & Neuroscience, King's College London, London, UK

Erica Maloney, Samantha J. Rennalls and Owen G. O'Daly
Department of Neuroimaging, Institute of Psychiatry, Psychology & Neuroscience, King's College London, London, UK

Ulrike Schmidt
Section of Eating Disorders, Department of Psychological Medicine, Institute of Psychiatry, Psychology & Neuroscience, King's College London, London, UK
South London and Maudsley NHS Foundation Trust, Maudsley Hospital, London, UK

Janet Conti
School of Psychology and Translational Research Institute, Western Sydney University, Locked Bag 1797, Penrith 2751, Australia

Caroline Joyce, Simone Natoli and Kelsey Skeoch
School of Psychology, Western Sydney University, Penrith, Australia

Phillipa Hay
Chair of Mental Health, School of Medicine, Translational Health Research Institute, Western Sydney University, Penrith, Australia

Annaleise Robertson
The Children's Hospital at Westmead, Sydney, Australia

Chris Thornton
The Redleaf Practice, Sydney, Australia

Sarah Byford, Hristina Petkova, Barbara Barrett and Ruth Stuart
Institute of Psychiatry, Psychology & Neuroscience at King's College London, PO24 David Goldberg Centre, De Crespigny Park, London SE5 8AF, UK

Tamsin Ford
Department of Psychiatry, University of Cambridge, Level 5 Clifford Allbutt Building, Cambridge Biomedical Campus, Hills Road, Cambridge CB2 0AH, UK

Dasha Nicholls
Imperial College London, Division of Psychiatry, Department of Brain Sciences, Commonwealth Building, Du Cane Road, London W12 0NN, UK

Mima Simic
South London and Maudsley NHS Foundation Trust, Michael Rutter Centre for Children and Young People, De Crespigny Park, London SE5 8AZ, UK

Simon Gowers
University of Liverpool, Mount Pleasant, Liverpool L69 3BX, UK

Geraldine Macdonald
University of Bristol, School for Policy Studies, 8 Priory Road, Bristol BS8 1TZ, UK

Nuala Livingstone
Queen's University Belfast, School of Social Sciences, Education & Social Work, 6 College Park Ave, Belfast BT7 1PS, UK

Grace Kelly
Queen's University Belfast, University Road, Belfast BT7 1NN, UK

Jonathan Kelly
Beat, Unit 1 Chalk Hill House, 19 Rosary Road, Norwich, Norfolk NR1 1SZ, UK

Kandarp Joshi
NHS Grampian and University of Aberdeen, CAMHS, City Hospital, Park Road, Aberdeen AB24 5AU, UK

Helen Smith
NHS Ayrshire and Arran, South CAMHS/NSAIU, CAMHS, Arrol Park Resource Centre, House 1, Doonfoot Road, Ayr KA7 2DW, UK

Ivan Eisler
South London and Maudsley NHS Foundation Trust, Maudsley Centre for Child and Adolescent Eating Disorders, Michael Rutter Centre for Children and Young People, De Crespigny Park, London SE5 8AZ, UK

Laurence Reuter, Denise Kästner, Justine Schmidt, Angelika Weigel, Bernd Löwe and Antje Gumz
Department of Psychosomatic Medicine and Psychotherapy, University Medical Center Hamburg-Eppendorf, Martinistr. 52, W37, 20246 Hamburg, Germany

Ulrich Voderholzer
Department of Psychiatry and Psychotherapy, University Hospital, LMU Munich, Munich, Germany
Schön Clinic Roseneck, Prien am Chiemsee, Germany

Department of Psychiatry and Psychotherapy, University Hospital of Freiburg, Freiburg, Germany

Marion Seidel
Schön Clinic for Psychosomatic Medicine and Psychotherapy, Bad Arolsen, Germany

Bianca Schwennen
Medclin Seepark Clinic for Acute Psychosomatic Care, Bad Bodenteich, Germany

Helge Fehrs
Department of Psychosomatic Medicine and Psychotherapy, Asklepios Westklinikum Hamburg, Hamburg, Germany

D. Blake Woodside
Program for Eating Disorders, University Health Network, Toronto, Canada
Centre for Mental Health, University Health Network, Toronto, Canada
Department of Psychiatry, Faculty of Medicine, University of Toronto, Toronto, Canada
Institute of Medical Science, University of Toronto, Toronto, Canada

Katharine Dunlop
Feil Family Brain and Mind Research Institute, Weill Cornell Medicine, New York, USA

Charlene Sathi, Eileen Lam and Brigitte McDonald
MRI-Guided rTMS Clinic, University Health Network, Toronto, Canada

Jonathan Downar
Centre for Mental Health, University Health Network, Toronto, Canada
Department of Psychiatry, Faculty of Medicine, University of Toronto, Toronto, Canada
MRI-Guided rTMS Clinic, University Health Network, Toronto, Canada
Krembil Research Institute, University Health Network, Toronto, Canada

Karolina Rymarczyk
Institute of Psychology, Cardinal Stefan Wyszyński University in Warsaw, Warsaw, Poland

Katrin E. Giel, Simone C. Behrens, Stephan Zipfel and Kathrin Schag
Department of Psychosomatic Medicine and Psychotherapy, Medical University Hospital Tübingen, Eberhard Karls University, Osianderstr. 5, 72076 Tübingen, Germany
Center of Excellence in Eating Disorders, Tübingen, Germany

Peter Martus
Institute for Clinical Epidemiology and Applied Biostatistics, Medical Faculty, Eberhard Karls University Tübingen, Tübingen, Germany

Stephan Herpertz
Department of Psychosomatic Medicine and Psychotherapy, LWL-University Hospital Bochum, Ruhr University Bochum, Bochum, Germany

Tobias Hofmann
Department of Psychosomatic Medicine, Center for Internal Medicine and Dermatology, Charité – Universitätsmedizin Berlin, Freie Universität Berlin and Humboldt-Universität Zu Berlin, Berlin, Germany

Eva-Maria Skoda
Clinic for Psychosomatic Medicine and Psychotherapy, LVR University-Hospital Essen, University of Duisburg-Essen, Essen, Germany

Jörn von Wietersheim
Department of Psychosomatic Medicine and Psychotherapy, Ulm University Medical Center, Ulm, Germany

Beate Wild
Department of General Internal Medicine and Psychosomatics, University Hospital Heidelberg, Heidelberg, Germany

Almut Zeeck
Department of Psychosomatic Medicine und Psychotherapy, Center for Mental Health, Faculty of Medicine, University of Freiburg, Freiburg, Germany

Florian Junne
Department of Psychosomatic Medicine and Psychotherapy, Medical University Hospital Tübingen, Eberhard Karls University, Osianderstr. 5, 72076 Tübingen, Germany
Center of Excellence in Eating Disorders, Tübingen, Germany
Department of Psychosomatic Medicine and Psychotherapy, University Hospital Magdeburg, Otto von Guericke University, Magdeburg, Germany

Index